Drug Interactions
in Psychiatry

Third Edition

Drug Interactions
in Psychiatry

THIRD EDITION

Edited By

Domenic A. Ciraulo, MD
Psychiatrist-in-Chief
Boston Medical Center
Professor and Chairman
Division of Psychiatry
Boston University School of
  Medicine
Boston, Massachusetts

David J. Greenblatt, MD
Professor and Chairman
Department of Pharmacology
  and Experimental
  Therapeutics
Professor of Psychiatry,
  Medicine, and Anesthesia
Tufts University School of
  Medicine
Chief, Division of Clinical
  Pharmacology
Tufts-New England Medical
  Center Hospital
Boston, Massachusetts

Richard I. Shader, MD
Professor of Pharmacology and
  Experimental Therapeutics
  and Psychiatry
Tufts University School of
  Medicine
Division of Clinical
  Pharmacology
Tufts-New England Medical
  Center Hospital
Boston, Massachusetts

Wayne L. Creelman, MD
Clinical Professor
Department of Psychiatry
Michigan State University
East Lansing, Michigan
Executive Vice President/
  Medical Director
Pine Rest Christian Mental
  Health Services
Grand Rapids, Michigan

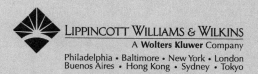

LIPPINCOTT WILLIAMS & WILKINS
A **Wolters Kluwer** Company
Philadelphia • Baltimore • New York • London
Buenos Aires • Hong Kong • Sydney • Tokyo

Acquisitions Editor: Charles W. Mitchell
Developmental Editor: Louise Bierig
Managing Editor: Nicole Dernoski
Project Manager: Alicia Jackson
Senior Manufacturing Manager: Benjamin Rivera
Senior Marketing Manager: Adam Glazer
Cover Designer: Terry Mallon
Production Service: TechBooks
Printer: RR Donnelley-Crawfordsville

© 2006 by LIPPINCOTT WILLIAMS & WILKINS
530 Walnut Street
Philadelphia, PA 19106 USA
LWW.com

2nd Edition, ©1995 by Williams & Wilkins

Library of Congress Cataloging-in-Publication Data
Drug interactions in psychiatry / edited by Domenic A. Ciraulo . . . [et al.].—3rd ed.
    p. ; cm.
  Includes bibliographical references and index.
  ISBN 0-7817-4817-8
  1. Psychotropic drugs—Side effects. 2. Drug interactions. I. Ciraulo, Domenic A.
  [DNLM: 1. Psychotropic Drugs—pharmacology. 2. Drug Interactions. QV 77.2 D789 2005]
RM315.D792 2005 615′ 788—dc22

                                                     2005016736

10 9 8 7 6 5 4 3 2 1

Contents

Editors

Domenic A. Ciraulo, M.D.
Psychiatrist-in-Chief
Boston Medical Center
Professor and Chairman
Division of Psychiatry
Boston University School of Medicine
Boston, Massachusetts

Wayne L. Creelman, M.D.
Clinical Professor
Department of Psychiatry
Michigan State University
East Lansing, Michigan
Executive Vice President/Medical Director
Pine Rest Christian Mental Health Services
Grand Rapids, Michigan

David J. Greenblatt, M.D.
Professor and Chairman
Department of Pharmacology and Experimental Therapeutics
Professor of Psychiatry, Medicine, and Anesthesia
Tufts University School of Medicine
Chief, Division of Clinical Pharmacology
Tufts-New England Medical Center Hospital
Boston, Massachusetts

Richard I. Shader, M.D.
Professor of Pharmacology and Experimental Therapeutics
    and Psychiatry
Tufts University School of Medicine
Division of Clinical Pharmacology
Tufts-New England Medical Center Hospital
Boston, Massachusetts

Contributors

Ann Marie Ciraulo, R.N.
Assistant Professor
Division of Psychiatry
Boston University School of Medicine
Boston, Massachusetts

Donna Jean Ecklesdafer, R.N.
Manager of Electroconvulsive Therapy Clinic
Electroconvulsive Therapy Clinic
Pine Rest Christian Mental Health Services
Grand Rapids, Michigan

Oliver Freudenreich, M.D.
Instructor in Psychiatry
Department of Psychiatry
Harvard Medical School
Director, MGH First Episode Schizophrenia Program
Department of Psychiatry
Massachusetts General Hospital
Boston, Massachusetts

Donald C. Goff, M.D.
Associate Professor of Psychiatry
Department of Psychiatry
Harvard Medical School
Director of Schizophrenia Program
Department of Psychiatry
Massachusetts General Hospital
Boston, Massachusetts

Clifford M. Knapp, Ph.D.
Assistant Professor
Division of Psychiatry
Boston University School of Medicine
Boston, Massachusetts

Manuel N. Pacheco, M.D.
Division of Psychiatry
Boston University School of Medicine
Boston, Massachusetts

Ofra Sarid-Segal, M.D.
Assistant Professor
Division of Psychiatry
Boston University School of Medicine
Boston, Massachusetts

Michael R. Slattery, M.D.
Medical Director
UMA Sleep Disorders Center
UMA Neurodiagnostic Center
Binghamton, New York

Karthik Venkatakrishnan, Ph.D.
Senior Research Scientist
Department of Pharmacokinetics, Dynamics and Metabolism
Pfizer Incorporated
Grotin, Connecticut

Charles A. Welch, M.D.
Instructor in Psychiatry
Harvard Medical School
Director of Somatic Therapies Consultation Service
Massachusetts General Hospital
Boston, Massachusetts

Preface

Twenty-five years have passed since the publication of the first edition of *Drug Interactions in Psychiatry*. We are grateful for our colleagues' kind comments about the previous editions and their helpful suggestions for the current edition. The goal of the third edition remains true to the original—to critically analyze drug interactions of importance to psychiatrists, nurses, pharmacists, and mental health professionals who prescribe and dispense psychotropic medication or practice psychotherapy with patients taking these medications. All chapters have been revised and updated. We have added appendices on herbals, medications used to treat substance abuse, and cytochromes, a table that has been expanded from the second edition.

The editors would like to thank Charley Mitchell, Nicole Dernoski, Louise Bierig, and the rest of the staff at Lippincott Williams & Wilkins for their help in editing the third edition. Special thanks are also due Meghan Zysik and Jeantel DeGazon for their assistance in research and manuscript preparation. Most of all, we would like to thank our families for their support and encouragement, and the sacrifices they made in support of this work.

The Editors

1

Concepts and Mechanisms of Drug Disposition and Drug Interactions

KARTHIK VENKATAKRISHNAN
RICHARD I. SHADER
DAVID J. GREENBLATT

Adverse drug reactions are a significant cause of deaths in the United States, with drug interactions being a key contributor. In today's regulatory, scientific, clinical, and marketing environments, drug interaction liabilities associated with medications are viewed as an important safety risk and have formed the basis of several recent safety-related market withdrawals by the Food and Drug Administration (FDA) in the last decade. Examples of these market withdrawals include the nonsedating antihistaminic drugs terfenadine (Seldane) and astemizole (Hismanal), the prokinetic agent cisapride (Propulsid), and the calcium channel blocker cardiovascular drug mibefradil (Posicor). Because several psychotherapeutic agents have a narrow therapeutic index (e.g., tricyclic antidepressants, lithium, monoamine oxidase inhibitors, and mood-stabilizing anticonvulsants), they are easy victims of pharmacokinetic and/or pharmacodynamic interactions. Further, the metabolism (and thus systemic exposure, pharmacodynamics, and toxic effects) of several of these drugs are subject to genetic variation and extensive interindividual variability due to a predominant contribution of polymorphic drug-metabolizing enzymes (e.g., nortriptyline and zuclopenthixol metabolism is primarily mediated by CYP2D6, which is absent in approximately 7% to 10% of whites). In addition, many psychopharmacologic agents are notable modulators of drug-metabolizing CYP enzymes (e.g., fluvoxamine inhibits the CYP1A2-mediated metabolism of theophylline, a drug with a narrow therapeutic index).

Of particular note is the increasing use of over-the-counter herbal remedies and natural products that provide an additional dimension of clinically significant risk beyond that associated with prescription agents. Unfortunately, such risks are often hidden and may not be readily apparent to the health care provider unless a patient's history is carefully obtained, with specific questions to capture the use of nonprescription products. For example, the seemingly innocuous over-the-counter herbal antidepressant St. John's wort is an established perpetrator of drug interactions with the immunosuppressant cyclosporin A that may cause a transplant rejection with a potentially fatal outcome.

Given the impact of drug interactions on patient safety and medical costs, the recognition of such interactions as a preventable cause of adverse drug reactions, and our ability to forecast and prevent (or manage) interactions without compromising pharmacologic efficacy in most cases, the obligate cannot be overemphasized that clinicians must be cognizant of the drug interaction liabilities associated with the medications they prescribe. The identification and strategic management of drug interaction risks and the appropriate education of the patient have thus become an integral component of successful and responsible psychiatric medical practice in the 21st century.

Approaching Drug Interactions in the 21st Century

The topic of drug interactions in today's scientific and clinical pharmacologic environments is heavily mechanistically driven and relies on an understanding of the processes of drug absorption, distribution, metabolism, and elimination; the molecular determinants of these processes; the genetic variability in these molecular determinants, and the diverse mechanisms of their modulation by co-administered agents, each having distinct clinical consequences. With the rapid introduction of new psychopharmacologic agents (as well as drugs in other therapeutic areas) having novel mechanisms of action and clearance mechanisms, not only do clinicians and their patients have more treatment options, but a concomitant rise has occurred in the incidence of polypharmacy and the associated risk of drug interactions. Despite their key role in modern pharmacy practice, the clinical management of drug interactions cannot rely solely on the use of computerized drug interaction databases to avoid contraindicated drug combinations. Clinicians must determine an individualized treatment regimen for their patients, based not only on accurate diagnosis but with due consideration to comorbid medical conditions and concomitant medications. Selected examples of clinical scenarios that highlight the importance of the individualized selection of psychotropic drug and/or patient education around drug interaction risks are summarized in Table 1.1.

It should be clear from these examples that the underlying bases of drug interactions can be diverse. This information further highlights the need for clinicians to have a basic understanding of the mechanisms of drug interactions, because it is almost impossible to remember every single contraindicated drug pair without some understanding of the biochemical basis of interaction risks associated with the perpetrator and/or victim drug. It must also be emphasized that it is incorrect to think in terms of "class effects" while assessing drug interaction risks. As will be apparent from discussions that follow in this chapter, the molecular mechanisms of pharmacokinetic interactions produced by a drug are unrelated to the pharmacologic mechanisms underlying its therapeutic effects. Thus, whereas fluoxetine, paroxetine, sertraline, fluvoxamine, and citalopram are all selective serotonin reuptake inhibitor (SSRI) antidepressants, their propensity to perpetrate pharmacokinetic drug interactions are distinctly different. Whereas fluoxetine and paroxetine are clinically significant inhibitors of CYP2D6 and produce extensive increases in the exposures of drugs requiring activity of this enzyme for their clearance, the same is not true for sertraline or citalopram, which do not perpetrate clinically significant interactions with CYP2D6 substrates. Similarly, fluoxetine impairs the clearance of CYP3A substrates, whereas paroxetine, sertraline, and citalopram are devoid of clinically significant effects. Of the aforementioned SSRI antidepressants, fluvoxamine is the only drug that inhibits CYP1A2 to a clinically significant extent. Thus, the terms "CYP inhibitor" and "mixed function oxidase inhibitor," which have been used historically to describe the effects of drugs on oxidative metabolism are meaningless in the 21st century. The CYP system is a heterogeneous collection of enzymes with distinct yet overlapping substrate/inhibitor selectivities. Unless the effects of each drug of interest are systematically evaluated on the activity of each enzyme isoform, clinical implications cannot be inferred.

In the last decade, in vitro approaches have been increasingly used to assess the risk of metabolic drug interactions. In many cases, these assessments have formed the basis for the conduct of controlled clinical drug interaction studies to determine clinical relevance. Thus, a basic understanding of the available in vitro models to assess metabolic inhibition, enzyme induction, transporter inhibition, and the like, together with an appreciation of key underlying assumptions and potential caveats can be useful for 21st-century clinicians. These models and the information they supply will enable the informed judgement

(text continues on page 6)

TABLE 1.1. CLINICAL SCENARIOS WITH PSYCHOTROPIC AGENT AS EITHER VICTIM OR PERPETRATOR OF DRUG INTERACTION AND STRATEGIC SELECTION OF CO-ADMINISTERED AGENT TO MINIMIZE DRUG INTERACTION RISK

Clinical Scenario	Selection of Therapeutic	Mechanistic Basis
Patient on **paroxetine** requiring antihypertensive treatment.	Choose **atenolol** rather than **metoprolol** as antihypertensive.	Paroxetine is a mechanism-based inactivator of CYP2D6 and clearance of metoprolol will be substantially impaired in a patient receiving this SSRI, resulting in increased plasma levels and augmented effects of metoprolol when administered at usual therapeutic doses. Atenolol's major clearance mechanism is renal excretion of unmetabolized drug; as a result, its pharmacokinetics and pharmacodynamic effects will not be affected by paroxetine.
Patient on self-medication with **St. John's wort**.	Advise against use of **oral contraceptive agents** as the sole mode of contraception.	St. John's wort contains hyperforin, a potent agonist of pregnane X receptor; it produces CYP3A induction. Clearance of ethinyl estradiol can thus be accelerated, resulting in decreased exposure and compromise of contraceptive efficacy.
Patient titrated to a stable dose of **desipramine** for treatment of depression, requiring systemic antifungal treatment for onychomycosis.	Choose **itraconazole** rather than **terbinafine** as antimycotic.	Desipramine's clearance is largely mediated by CYP2D6, and terbinafine is a potent CYP2D6 inhibitor. Co-administration can result in elevated desipramine levels (unless a compensatory dosage reduction of desipramine is made prior to initiation of terbinafine treatment) and TCA toxicity. Itraconazole is not a clinically meaningful CYP2D6 inhibitor and thus can be safely co-administered with desipramine without risk of a drug interaction.
Patient on a stable dose of **metoprolol** for control of hypertension, requiring antidepressant therapy.	Choose **citalopram** rather than **paroxetine** or **fluoxetine** as SSRI antidepressant.	Metoprolol's clearance is largely mediated by CYP2D6, and both paroxetine and fluoxetine are potent inhibitors of this enzyme. In contrast, citalopram does not inhibit CYP-mediated metabolism.

(continued)

TABLE 1.1. CLINICAL SCENARIOS WITH PSYCHOTROPIC AGENT AS EITHER VICTIM OR PERPETRATOR OF DRUG INTERACTION AND STRATEGIC SELECTION OF CO-ADMINISTERED AGENT TO MINIMIZE DRUG INTERACTION RISK (CONTINUED)

Clinical Scenario	Selection of Therapeutic	Mechanistic Basis
Patient with bipolar disorder receiving a stable dose of **lithium**, requiring an antihypertensive agent.	Choose a β-blocker rather than an **ACE inhibitor** as the antihypertensive agent.	ACE inhibitors impair the renal clearance of lithium and can elevate lithium levels, leading to lithium toxicity. β-Blockers do not impair lithium clearance and are thus preferred for treatment of hypertension in patients receiving lithium.
Transplant recipient on immunosuppression with **cyclosporin A** or **tacrolimus,** presenting with symptoms suggestive of depression.	Advise against self-medication with **St. John's wort** and initiate antidepressant treatment, if needed, with an **SSRI** but not **nefazodone.**	CYP3A and P-glycoprotein induction by St. John's wort can decrease cyclosporin A or tacrolimus exposure below therapeutic levels and potentially result in transplant rejection. SSRI antidepressants can be safely used, because they do not induce CYP3A or P-glycoprotein. On the other hand, nefazodone is a potent CYP3A inhibitor and is preferably avoided in patients receiving cyclosporin A or tacrolimus due to the potential for increased immunosuppressant levels and toxicity.
Patient receiving **itraconazole** for onychomycosis, requiring sedative-hypnotic for insomnia.	Choose **lorazepam, temazepam,** or **zolpidem** rather than **triazolam** as sedative-hypnotic.	Itraconazole is a potent inhibitor of CYP3A, the enzyme that solely mediates the clearance of triazolam. Co-administration can result in increased triazolam exposure and exaggerated pharmacodynamic effects. In contrast, lorazepam and temazepam are directly glucuronidated and thus are not victims of itraconazole-mediated CYP3A inhibition; zolpidem undergoes oxidative metabolism, but via multiple CYP isoforms, minimizing the contribution of CYP3A and the magnitude of interactions with CYP3A-selective inhibitors like itraconazole.

(continued)

TABLE 1.1. CLINICAL SCENARIOS WITH PSYCHOTROPIC AGENT AS EITHER VICTIM OR PERPETRATOR OF DRUG INTERACTION AND STRATEGIC SELECTION OF CO-ADMINISTERED AGENT TO MINIMIZE DRUG INTERACTION RISK (CONTINUED)

Clinical Scenario	Selection of Therapeutic	Mechanistic Basis
Patient receiving **buspirone** for anxiety disorder, requiring antibacterial treatment with a macrolide antibiotic.	Choose **azithromycin** rather than **erythromycin** or **clarithromycin** as antibiotic.	Buspirone's pharmacokinetics are characterized by extensive first-pass metabolism largely mediated by CYP3A. Both erythromycin and clarithromycin are mechanism-based inactivators of CYP3A and can impair buspirone clearance, whereas azithromycin does not impair clearance of CYP3A substrates and thus can be safely co-administered with buspirone.

of, and appropriate reaction to emerging experimental (in vitro) data that are routinely featured in the peer-reviewed clinical psychopharmacology literature (e.g., *Journal of Clinical Psychopharmacology* and *British Journal of Clinical Pharmacology*). The available experimental approaches to study drug interactions in vitro are briefly discussed later in this chapter, with emphasis on the principles and challenges associated with in vivo extrapolation.

SOME DEFINITIONS, AND A MECHANISTIC CLASSIFICATION OF DRUG INTERACTIONS

A clinically significant interaction between two drugs is said to have occurred when the therapeutic and/or toxic effects of one drug are altered as a consequence of co-administration of another drug. The drug whose effects are altered (diminished, with therapeutic efficacy lost; or enhanced, with resulting toxicity) is generally referred to as the *victim* of the interaction, and the co-administered agent responsible for the interaction is referred to as the *perpetrator* drug.

The pharmacologic or toxic effects of a drug following its administration are generally related to its exposure (concentration) at the site of activity (brain, for psychopharmacologic agents) or toxicity (e.g., heart muscle for cardiotoxic effects of thioridazine). This, in turn, is generally related to the exposure in systemic circulation (blood or plasma concentrations as described by the drug's pharmacokinetic profile). The pharmacokinetics of a drug, in turn, are a function of several factors, including but not limited to the rate and extent of absorption in the intestine following an oral dose, passive and/or active processes of distribution to various tissues, enzymatic catabolism (metabolism) by the liver, and the rate of elimination in the urine by the kidneys via glomerular filtration and active tubular secretion. When a drug alters the performance of any of these processes governing the absorption, distribution, metabolism, or excretion of another drug, the pharmacokinetics of the second drug will be altered when the two agents are co-administered; this results in a *pharmacokinetic drug interaction*. It must be emphasized that a pharmacokinetic interaction does not always imply a clinically significant drug interaction; the clinical consequence of a pharmacokinetic interaction depends not only on the magnitude of the interaction (alteration of systemic exposure) but also on the therapeutic window (or index) of the drug whose pharmacokinetics have been altered. When a drug has a narrow therapeutic window (low therapeutic index), the clinical consequences of the impairment of its clearance by another drug and increase in systemic concentrations are generally significant; in these cases, the drug interaction can result in toxicity unless a dosage adjustment of the victim drug is made. For example, lithium has a narrow therapeutic window, and even a 50% reduction in lithium clearance produced by thiazide diuretics is clinically meaningful, necessitating a corresponding reduction in lithium dosage when co-administered, for example, with hydrochlorothiazide. On the other hand, SSRI antidepressants (citalopram, sertraline, paroxetine, and fluvoxamine) have a relatively high therapeutic index and, as a class, generally are not victimized by drug interactions that result in the impairment of their clearance and an increase in their plasma levels.

When the co-administration of two drugs results in a modulation of the therapeutic and/or toxic effects of either drug, without a readily apparent alteration of the pharmacokinetics of either agent, a *pharmacodynamic drug interaction* is said to have occurred. The simplest kinds of pharmacodynamic interactions are those of *additivity* and *antagonism*, which generally are readily predictable from the mechanisms of action of each agent at the level of the target receptor or enzyme. For example, co-administration of two drugs with sedative-hypnotic effects (say, a benzodiazepine and a sedating antihistamine) would obviously lead to increased sedation and central nervous system (CNS) depression than would be expected from either agent alone, simply because of the additive effect of receptor occupation and downstream pharmacodynamics. In some cases, such enhanced pharmacodynamic effects are even more pronounced when the mechanisms of action of the two agents are distinct; this results in a net effect that exceeds the sum of each individual effect—a phenomenon referred to as *synergism*. Synergistic interactions can provide therapeutic benefit in some cases, although the risks for adverse events using the combination also may be higher, when compared to those associated with each agent alone. This increased risk may necessitate a gradual dose escalation of the second, added agent and titration to effect. For example, although generally regarded as a contraindicated combination due to the risks of serotonin syndrome, the careful addition of a monoamine oxidase inhibitor (MAOI) to ongoing tricyclic antidepressant (TCA) therapy may have significant benefits for some patients with treatment-resistant depression.

Pharmacodynamic antagonism is said to have occurred when the pharmacologic effects of one drug are diminished or abrogated upon the co-administration of another drug, without a decrease in the systemic exposure of the victim drug (i.e., with the underlying mechanism not being pharmacokinetic in nature). The simplest mechanism of pharmacodynamic antagonism is that involving the administration of a receptor antagonist. (A receptor antagonist is a drug that binds to a receptor but fails to elicit downstream pharmacodynamics; it prevents either an endogenous agonist or co-administered agonist drug from eliciting its maximal pharmacodynamic effect, thereby interfering with that agent's activity and therapeutic outcome.) Antagonism can be useful in the treatment of overdosage. Examples illustrating the application of antagonism in psychiatry include the use of flumazenil in the treatment of benzodiazepine overdose, the use of naloxone in the reversal of respiratory depression secondary to acute opioid overdosage, the use of the α-adrenergic antagonist phentolamine in the emergency management of a cheese reaction in patients receiving MAOIs, and the use of the $5HT_{1A}$ receptor antagonist cyproheptadine in the treatment of drug-induced serotonin syndrome. A more complex example of antagonism is the interaction between TCAs and the antihypertensive agent guanethidine, which results in diminished therapeutic efficacy. The mechanism of action of TCAs partly involves the inhibition of neurotransmitter reuptake at the noradrenergic synapse. The site of action of guanethidine is at the presynaptic adrenergic neuron, where it acts as a "substitute" or false neurotransmitter and depletes catecholamine-containing vesicles of their native neurotransmitter, thereby producing an antihypertensive effect. Interestingly, guanethidine reaches its site of action within the neuron by active uptake via the same transporter that mediates norepinephrine reuptake, which is inhibited by TCAs. As a result, in patients receiving TCAs, guanethidine cannot reach its site of action, thus making it ineffective as an antihypertensive agent. As another example, atenolol (a β1-subtype selective adrenergic antagonist) rather than propranolol (a nonselective β-blocker) should be chosen to reduce the autonomic symptoms (tachycardia, tremor, etc.) of anxiety disorders or to manage performance anxiety in patients with asthma. The use of propranolol will worsen the bronchospasm and interfere with the bronchodilatory effects of β2-adrenergic agonists such as albuterol, thus compromising their efficacy in the management of an acute asthmatic episode. This example illustrates the importance of understanding the receptor sub-type selectivity of therapeutic agents and the risks of pharmacodynamic interactions to ensure appropriate drug selection when considering comorbid conditions and co-administered medications.

Due to the mechanism-specific nature of pharmacodynamic drug interactions, they are discussed in detail in the remaining chapters of this book, as an integral part of the discussion of each class of neuropsychopharmacologic agents. The remainder of this chapter focuses on the common underlying mechanisms of pharmacokinetic drug interactions, selected examples, and implications for psychiatric therapeutics.

Processes of Drug Absorption, Disposition, and Modulation

DRUG INTERACTIONS RESULTING FROM MODULATION OF ORAL ABSORPTION

Unless administered via the intravenous route, drugs reach circulation via an absorptive process of some kind. With the widely used oral route of administration, absorption is generally viewed as a physicochemical process that is determined by drug dissolution in the stomach, followed by absorption of dissolved drug in the small intestine through passive diffusion across the lipid bilayer of the enterocyte membrane. Absorption is thus influenced by several factors, including aqueous solubility, lipophilicity, gastric pH level (which can influence dissolution in the stomach), gastric emptying rate, intestinal pH level (which determines the net charge on the drug during absorption depending on pK_a of the molecule), bile secretion (a common mechanism that explains the increased absorption of poorly soluble lipophilic drugs in the postprandial state), and gastrointestinal motility. Because co-administered drugs can potentially alter one or more of these factors, drug interactions can result from a modulation (increase or decrease) of the rate and/or extent of oral absorption. When a drug interaction decreases the rate of oral absorption, the pharmacokinetic consequence is an alteration of the temporal course of drug concentrations in circulation, with a prolongation (increase) of the time at which maximal plasma concentrations are reached (T_{max}) and blunting (decrease) in the maximal concentration (C_{max}). If absorption rate is the only parameter that is altered, the net exposure (area under the plasma concentration–time curve, AUC) will not be altered, and steady-state average plasma concentrations will be unaffected by the interaction. If however, the interaction results in a decrease in the extent of oral absorption, the AUC will be decreased, resulting in a decrease in steady-state average concentrations and potentially compromising pharmacologic efficacy and therapeutic outcome. Increases in the rate and/or extent of oral absorption will result in pharmacokinetic effects opposite in direction to those described.

Direct physicochemical interactions represent the simplest kind of absorptive drug interactions. For example, divalent cations such as Ca^{2+} (e.g., nutritional calcium supplements, milk) inhibit the absorption of tetracycline due to chemical complexation. Charcoal, aluminum hydroxide (a common ingredient in OTC antacids), cholestyramine, and kaolin-pectin can adsorb or bind some drugs, thereby reducing the extent of their absorption.

Alternatively, an alteration of the pH level of the stomach by one drug can influence the dissolution and hence absorption of another drug. For example, the antifungal agent ketoconazole requires an acidic pH level in the stomach for dissolution. Thus, the absorption of ketoconazole is impaired by antacids, including H_2-receptor antagonists (e.g., cimetidine) and gastric proton pump inhibitors (e.g., omeprazole), and its antifungal efficacy is compromised. Antacids have been shown to decrease the rate of absorption of certain benzodiazepines (e.g., chlordiazepoxide), due to their elevation of gastric pH levels above the benzodiazepine's pK_a (4.8 for chlordiazepoxide), thereby affecting dissolution in the stomach.

For the antianxiety effects of chlordiazepoxide, a decrease in absorption rate alone without an alteration of the extent of absorption, is not of clinical significance in the context of multiple-dose administration, because pharmacologic effects and therapeutic outcome are driven by steady-state average concentrations. Exceptions include sedative-hypnotic agents for which the rate of increase of plasma concentrations is an important determinant of rapid onset of sleep. When the possibility of an antacid effect on the pharmacokinetics of a drug exists, it is recommended that the drug be dosed at least 2 hours before antacid administration to minimize interaction risk. The value of this approach, however, is generally limited to direct-acting (neutralizing) antacids and not generalizable to systemically acting antisecretory agents (H_2-receptor antagonists and proton pump inhibitors). Another valuable piece of advice to patients is to always take their prescription medications with a full glass of water, to minimize the effects of absorptive interactions and ensure consistent oral absorption.

Absorptive drug interactions can also result from effects on gastrointestinal motility. For example, lithium levels may be increased dramatically by concurrent marijuana use, and this may result in toxicity. This effect may be due to the anticholinergic activity of marijuana, which slows gut motility and allows an increased duration of contact of the lithium ion with the absorptive surface of the intestine. In contrast, the antiemetic agent metoclopramide enhances gastrointestinal motility and has been shown to decrease the extent of absorption of digoxin due to decreased residence of digoxin in the small intestine. Although the decrease in digoxin exposure is relatively small (~20%), the interaction may be clinically significant, given the narrow therapeutic range for digoxin. Interestingly, metoclopramide's effect on the gastrointestinal tract is also characterized by an increase in gastric emptying rate, which can actually increase the rate of absorption of certain drugs, especially in conditions of decreased gastric emptying rate (such as gastroparesis, which often is encountered in migraine patients). This effect forms the basis of its co-administration with agents used in the abortive treatment of migraine.

Although traditionally viewed as a passive process, active drug transporters are being increasingly recognized as determinants of oral absorption. Some drugs (e.g., cephalosporin antibiotics) are substrates for active influx transporters, such as the pepT1 peptide transporter, and their intestinal absorption is therefore dependent on the activity of this transporter. More commonly, several drugs are substrates of active efflux transporters, such as MDR1 P-glycoprotein (P-gp) and breast cancer resistance protein (BCRP). These transporters are expressed in the apical membrane of enterocytes lining the small intestinal lumen; because these transporters pump drugs out of the enterocyte and back into the lumen, they effectively act as a barrier and decrease the extent of oral absorption. The incomplete oral bioavailability of several therapeutically important drugs, such as cyclosporin A and saquinavir, is explained at least in part by P-gp–mediated efflux at the level of the small intestine. Thus, the inhibition of the activity of this transporter by co-administered agents (e.g., itraconazole, ritonavir) represents a mechanism of drug interactions at the level of absorption. It is important to recognize that the contribution of P-gp as a factor that limits drug absorption is determined not only by whether the drug is a substrate, but also by its intrinsic transmembrane permeability and its concentration in the intestinal lumen (determined by the clinical dose) in relation to the K_m (substrate concentration at which half the maximal active transport flux is achieved) for transport activity.

Because efflux transport by P-gp is a saturable process, the potentially high local drug concentrations in intestinal lumen, if in excess of the K_m for the transport process, can saturate the transporter, making its impact on the oral absorption of the drug negligible. No examples exist of psychopharmacologics whose absorption is limited by P-gp to a clinically significant extent. In addition, no examples exist of interactions explained by P-gp modulation in which a prescription psychopharmacologic agent has been identified and proved to be the perpetrator. Thus, drug interactions via this mechanism are relatively uncommon in psychopharmacology. As an exception, the over-the-counter antidepressant St. John's wort, is a well described inhibitor and inducer of this transporter, thereby perpetrating drug interactions of clinical importance.

The intestine is only one of several anatomical sites that express P-gp. Other sites of expression include the blood–brain barrier (BBB), kidney, and liver. As a result, P-glycoprotein is a determinant, not only of oral absorption, but also of drug distribution (BBB penetration, for example) and clearance (renal and biliary clearance, for example), all of which are potential targets for drug interactions. These topics are discussed in the following sections on distribution and clearance.

DRUG INTERACTIONS RESULTING FROM MODULATION OF DRUG DISTRIBUTION

Drugs are distributed to the tissues by the systemic circulation. Entrance into the CNS requires the penetration of the BBB. Highly perfused tissues (brain, heart, liver, and kidney) show a rapid blood–tissue equilibration of drugs. Following this initial transfer, the drug is redistributed to tissues with lower blood flow but higher drug affinity, such as adipose tissue. An example of this process is the rapid onset of anesthesia after the intravenous injection of thiopental. Thiopental is a lipophilic drug with high permeability across cellular lipid bilayer membranes. Therefore, thiopental displays perfusion rate–limited distribution and is rapidly distributed into the brain, a richly perfused tissue. The duration of action of thiopental is short, however, because it is rapidly and extensively redistributed into the muscle and fat. The single-dose effects of benzodiazepines are more influenced by distribution factors than by the terminal (elimination) half-life. In fact, the effect of a single dose of lorazepam may last longer than that of diazepam despite the latter drug's longer elimination half-life. This is due to the greater lipid solubility and more extensive distribution of diazepam. The extent of drug distribution is determined by its relative extent of binding to plasma proteins and to tissue macromolecules; this is quantitatively described by pharmaco-kineticists as the volume of distribution (V_d). Together with clearance, the V_d of a drug determines its half-life, which in turn is a clinically useful pharmacokinetic parameter that determines the frequency of dosing and the time to reach steady-state following multiple-dose administration. The smaller the V_d, shorter the half-life, provided clearance is constant. Drugs that are extensively bound to plasma proteins relative to tissue macromolecules tend to be "held" in systemic circulation (the *central compartment* in pharmacokinetic terms), exhibit lower distribution to tissues (the *peripheral compartment* in pharmacokinetic terms), and as a net result, have a low V_d. The reverse is true for drugs that are extensively bound to tissue macromolecules relative to plasma proteins. Two major drug binding proteins are present in plasma: serum albumin and α1-acid glycoprotein. Acidic drugs (e.g., valproic acid, warfarin) bind primarily to serum albumin, and basic drugs (e.g., chlorpromazine, propranolol) bind primarily to α1-acid glycoprotein. Tissue binding is largely determined by physicochemical factors, including lipophilicity and charge, although active uptake and/or efflux processes may be operational for certain drugs in certain tissues. The most common mechanism of altered distribution in a drug interaction is thus the displacement of one drug from its binding sites on plasma proteins by another drug, thereby resulting in an increase in the plasma unbound fraction of the victim drug, and consequently, altered distribution. Because changes in plasma protein binding not only result in changes in V_d but also influence clearance, displacement interactions are discussed separately following the discussion of clearance.

One potential mechanism of a drug interaction for psychoactive agents is an alteration in the rate and/or extent of distribution into the CNS at the level of the BBB. The BBB is comprised of a single layer of endothelial cells lining the capillary network of the brain. In addition to the physical tightness of the junctions between adjacent endothelial cells, which contributes to the high resistance for transport of drugs into the brain, the BBB also expresses a variety of active drug transporters that contribute to its ability to keep foreign chemicals out of the brain. These include P-gp, multidrug resistance related proteins (MRPs), BCRP, organic anion transporters (OATs), and organic anion transporting polypeptides (OATPs) among others. P-gp is the best studied transporter at the BBB, however, having a demonstrated ability to restrict CNS distribution of its substrates. It is thus not surprising that the majority of CNS-active drugs are generally not efficiently transported by this efflux transporter, because they would be excluded from their target organ, if they were. Thus, whereas P-gp in the BBB is not an important determinant of drug interactions in psychopharmacology, in principle it is possible that a potent P-gp inhibitory drug could increase the brain exposure of those substrates of this transporter that are typically excluded from the CNS. This may produce neurotoxicity that may resemble signs of an overdose of the victim drug and present as a neurologic and/or psychiatric emergency. An experimental clinical drug interaction study demonstrated that treatment with high-dose quinidine (a P-gp inhibitor) allowed the P-gp substrate antidiarrheal agent loperamide (administered at a suprapharmacologic dose) to elicit respiratory depressant effects via its activity at central opioid receptors. Interestingly, the central effects of loperamide upon quinidine co-administration were observed early, even when no readily observable changes occurred in the systemic pharmacokinetics of loperamide, thus suggesting that the primary mechanism of the interaction was at the level of drug distribution to the brain. Although the above example provides a "proof-of-concept" that P-gp inhibition at the BBB can result in CNS distributional drug interactions, the clinical relevance of such interactions remains to be established. Not many drugs at the systemic levels achieved in circulation are potent enough P-gp inhibitors at typical clinical doses to cause a complete transporter inhibition at the BBB. Further, the therapeutic index of the victim drug must be small enough to elicit an interaction of clinical significance. A candidate victim of such an interaction at the level of the BBB is the antiemetic, prokinetic agent domperidone, which is used for its peripheral activity in the gastrointestinal tract and is kept out of the brain by P-gp–mediated efflux. Domperidone possesses dopamine D2 receptor antagonistic properties. Potent P-gp inhibitors have been shown to increase the brain distribution of high-dose domperidone in mice and induce a catalepsy resembling that produced by typical antipsychotic agents.

Whether a similar interaction can occur in humans is not known, but if it does, the clinical sequelae of the interaction can be expected to be characterized by extrapyramidal symptoms of excess D2 receptor blockade that are no different from that observed with conventional antipsychotic agents.

CONCEPTS OF CLEARANCE AND MECHANISMS OF MODULATION

Clearance is the most important pharmacokinetic parameter. An understanding of the factors that determine this parameter and the consequences of its modulation is central to the understanding of the majority of drug interactions that are encountered both in psychiatry and in the medical practice at large. Clearance is a proportionality factor relating the rate of drug elimination (mass of drug removed per unit time) to the plasma concentration (mass of drug per unit volume of blood or plasma) (Equation 1). Clearance is expressed as units of volume divided by time (e.g., mL/min, L/hr). Clearance can thus be viewed as the volume of blood or plasma from which drug is completely removed in unit time.

$$\text{Elimination Rate} = CL \cdot C \tag{1}$$

Rearranging terms in the above equation and integrating from the time of drug dosing to infinity (i.e., until elimination of the entire dose [amount of drug A] is complete), an operational equation for clearance can be derived (Equation 2). This is generally used to calculate this parameter in clinical pharmacokinetic studies in which an intravenous dose of the drug is administered and the area under the plasma concentration–time curve is measured and extrapolated to time infinity ($AUC_{0-\infty}$).

$$CL = \frac{\text{Elimination Rate}}{C} = \frac{\left(\dfrac{dA}{dt}\right)}{C} = \frac{\displaystyle\int_0^\infty dA}{\displaystyle\int_0^\infty C \cdot dt} = \frac{\text{Dose}}{AUC_{0-\infty}} \tag{2}$$

Equation 2 is extremely useful, because it states that the drug exposure (concentration integrated over time, or AUC) following an intravenous dose is determined only by two factors: dose and clearance. It therefore highlights the importance of clearance as the single most important determinant of drug exposure and the pharmacologic response resulting from drug delivery to the systemic circulation. Together with V_d, clearance determines the elimination half-life of a drug:

$$t_{1/2} = \frac{0.693 \cdot V_d}{CL} \tag{3}$$

Clearance can be defined for the whole body, or specifically for an eliminating organ (e.g., hepatic clearance, renal clearance). When defined for an organ, a physiological approach to its definition is useful and allows an appreciation of the factors influencing its value and the effects of their modulation. The elimination (extraction) of drug by an organ upon presentation in perfusing blood (flow rate Q) is often described by an extraction ratio (E), which is defined as the ratio of the rate of drug extraction to the rate of drug delivery (Equation 4).

$$\text{Extraction Ratio (E)} = \frac{\text{Rate of Extraction}}{\text{Rate of Delivery}} = \frac{Q \cdot (C_{in} - C_{out})}{Q \cdot C_{in}} \quad (4)$$

$$= \frac{C_{in} - C_{out}}{C_{in}}$$

In this equation, C_{in} and C_{out} are the drug concentrations in the blood entering the organ and the blood leaving the organ, respectively. C_{in} is greater than C_{out} if the drug is extracted by the organ. Because clearance is the ratio of the rate of extraction to concentration (Equation 1), it follows that clearance is simply the product of blood flow rate to the organ and the organ extraction ratio (Equation 5).

$$CL = \frac{\text{Rate of Extraction}}{\text{Concentration}} = \frac{Q \cdot (C_{in} - C_{out})}{C_{in}} = Q \cdot E \quad (5)$$

It thus follows, intuitively, that the maximum value for organ clearance is simply the blood flow rate to the organ (e.g., hepatic blood flow for the liver) and that organ clearance is achieved when the drug is extracted completely by the organ (E = 1). The organ clearance of a drug is described in its simplest form by Equation 6, known as the *well-stirred model*:

$$CL = \frac{Q \cdot (f_u \cdot CL_{int})}{Q + (f_u \cdot CL_{int})} \quad (6)$$

Organ clearance is a function of two independent variables: blood flow to the organ (Q) and the intrinsic maximal efficiency of drug removal by the organ in the absence of flow limitations (intrinsic clearance). The latter is determined by the unbound intrinsic clearance (CL_{int}) and the unbound fraction of the drug in circulation (f_u). From equations 5 and 6, the extraction ratio is described in Equation 7:

$$E = \frac{CL}{Q} = \frac{(f_u \cdot CL_{int})}{Q + (f_u \cdot CL_{int})} \quad (7)$$

A closer examination of Equations 6 and 7 indicates that drugs having intrinsic clearances much greater than blood flow to the clearing organ ($f_u \cdot CL_{int} \gg Q$) will have a high extraction ratio, and their clearance will approximate blood flow to the clearing organ (Q). The situation is referred to as *flow-limited clearance*, and changes in intrinsic clearance (such as metabolic inhibition or induction) will not appreciably alter clearance. Hence, half-life (Equation 3) and intravenous exposure (Equation 2) will not be altered appreciably either. For example, the opioid analgesic fentanyl is extensively metabolized by CYP3A4. However, the potent CYP3A inhibitor itraconazole has no effect on the pharmacokinetics of intravenously administered fentanyl, an observation that is explained by the high extraction ratio of fentanyl in humans. On the other hand, for drugs that are poorly extracted ($f_u \cdot CL_{int} \ll Q$), clearance is approximately equal to their intrinsic clearance ($f_u \cdot CL_{int}$), and changes in this parameter will directly translate to changes in clearance and, therefore, elimination half-life and intravenous exposure.

When a drug is administered orally, it is important to recognize that only a fraction of the administered dose reaches the systemic circulation, due to various factors including incomplete oral absorption, presystemic extraction during first-pass through the liver, and in some cases, metabolism in the small intestine as well. Thus, for an extravascular dose, Equation 2 is modified (Equation 8), with the term F (oral bioavailability) representing the fraction of the dose that reaches the systemic circulation intact. F is simply the product of the fraction absorbed (f_a), the fraction escaping the gut intact (F_G), and the fraction that survives first-pass extraction by the liver (F_H, which equals 1 minus the hepatic extraction ratio E_H):

$$CL = \frac{F \cdot Dose}{AUC_{0-\infty}} = \frac{f_a \cdot F_G \cdot F_H \cdot Dose}{AUC_{0-\infty}} \tag{8}$$

For a drug that undergoes approximately complete oral absorption and is not subject to significant intestinal metabolism or other extrahepatic clearance mechanisms (i.e., $f_a \approx 1$ and $F_G \approx 1$), oral bioavailability (F) can be approximated by F_H, and is described in Equation 9:

$$F \approx F_H = 1 - E_H = \frac{Q_H}{Q_H + (f_u \cdot CL_{int})} \tag{9}$$

Although the determination of clearance is not possible without intravenous administration, it is possible to determine the CL/F ratio in a fashion analogous to the determination of clearance following intravenous administration. The CL/F ratio, calculated as dose divided by AUC following oral administration (Equation 8), is otherwise referred to as the *apparent oral clearance* (CL_{po}). Apparent oral clearance is a very useful parameter in clinical pharmacokinetics, because it is numerically equal to the intrinsic clearance ($f_u \cdot CL_{int}$) of the drug when the assumption of complete absorption and lack of extrahepatic clearance mechanisms is reasonably valid (verifiable by dividing Equation 6 by Equation 9). Thus, a change in intrinsic clearance (as would occur in a metabolic drug interaction) results in a corresponding change in apparent oral clearance; this is reflected as a change in AUC following oral dosing, independent of the drug's extraction ratio (unlike the situation with intravenous dosing, where exposure is not appreciably altered for highly extracted drugs). Although the effects of a change in intrinsic clearance on the apparent oral clearance (and thus, systemic AUC) of a drug are independent of extraction ratio, the effects on oral bioavailability and elimination half-life are not. An inspection of Equation 9 suggests that for poorly extracted drugs ($f_u \cdot CL_{int} \ll Q$), oral bioavailability is approximately complete ($F \approx 1$), and an alteration of intrinsic clearance due to a drug interaction should not be expected to appreciably change F. On the other hand, F will be sensitive to changes in intrinsic clearance for those drugs whose baseline pharmacokinetics are characterized by a high extraction ratio. As with intravenous dosing, following oral dosing, the elimination half-life of high-extraction drugs will not be altered when intrinsic clearance is modulated (because clearance is flow dependent), whereas the half-life of poorly extracted drugs will be inversely sensitive to intrinsic clearance changes (because clearance is approximately equal to intrinsic clearance for such drugs).

The following general conclusions can thus be made: For high-extraction ratio drugs, the alteration of intrinsic clearance does not appreciably affect intravenous pharmacokinetics. For low-extraction ratio drugs, a decrease (increase) in intrinsic clearance due to metabolic enzyme inhibition (induction) will result in an increase (decrease) in systemic exposure and a longer (shorter) elimination half-life. Irrespective of the baseline extraction ratio, systemic exposure (AUC) following oral dosing will increase (decrease) as a result of a decrease (increase) in intrinsic clearance. For high-extraction ratio drugs, these changes in oral AUC are, however, largely due to an increase (decrease) in C_{max} and F without an alteration of half-life; the reverse is true for low-extraction ratio drugs, whose half-life is increased (decreased) without a change in C_{max} or F, to produce a change in AUC of similar magnitude. Simulated pharmacokinetic profiles illustrating these concepts are shown in Figure 1.1.

Although not discussed here, alterations in liver blood flow (Q_H) represent yet another mechanism of clearance modulation. Drug interactions resulting from such a mechanism are relatively rare.

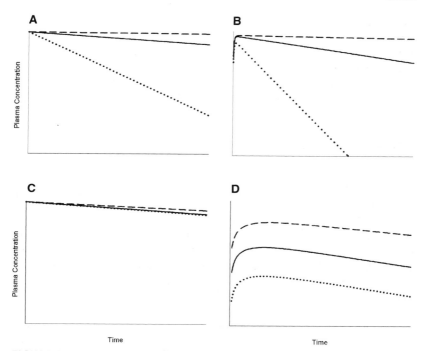

FIGURE 1.1. ■ Contrasting effects of inhibition or induction of hepatic clearance on the intravenous (panels **A** and **C**) and oral dose (panels **B** and **D**) pharmacokinetics of a drug with a low hepatic extraction ratio (panels **A** and **B**) and a drug with a high hepatic extraction ratio (panels **C** and **D**). Solid lines represent the control state profiles, with the induced and inhibited profiles represented as dotted and dashed lines, respectively. Simulations assume complete absorption and hepatic extraction ratios of 0.05 for the low-extraction drug and 0.95 for the high-extraction drug.

Thus far, we have repeatedly made reference to the term *intrinsic clearance* and alluded to the fact that this parameter is modulated in drug interactions that result from metabolic inhibition or induction. It is thus important to better appreciate the kinetic, biochemical, and molecular determinants of intrinsic clearance, and the mechanisms underlying its modulation. From a biochemical standpoint, drug extraction processes are simply metabolic reactions involving drug metabolizing enzymes (metabolic clearance) or active transport processes involving transporters in the liver (active biliary clearance) or kidney (renal clearance via active tubular secretion), for example. All these processes have a common feature: The rate of the process depends on substrate (drug) concentration and is saturable, with a maximal capacity. In their simplest form, the kinetics of drug metabolism and active transport are described using the Michaelis-Menten equation (Equation 10), as follows:

$$\text{Rate} = v = \frac{V_{max} \cdot S}{K_m + S} \tag{10}$$

In this equation, V_{max} is the maximum velocity of the metabolic or transport process (an indicator of the capacity of the process); S is the unbound concentration of the substrate at the level of the enzyme or transporter; and K_m, the Michaelis constant, is an inverse function of the affinity between the drug and enzyme (smaller the K_m, higher the affinity) and is empirically defined as the substrate concentration at which half the maximal velocity is attained. Applying the previous definition of clearance (Equation 1), intrinsic clearance can be described as illustrated in Equation 11, and is simply equal to the $V_{max} : K_m$ ratio when the unbound drug concentration at the metabolic site is well below the K_m (an assumption that is generally true for most drugs):

$$CL_{int} = \frac{\text{Rate}}{\text{Concentration}} = \frac{v}{S} = \frac{V_{max}}{K_m + S} \tag{11}$$

$$\approx \frac{V_{max}}{K_m} \quad \text{when } S \ll K_m$$

When a metabolic enzyme is induced (i.e., its intracellular content is increased due to an increase in gene expression or via a stabilization of the protein by protection from degradation), the result is an increase in V_{max}, and a corresponding increase in CL_{int}. For example, carbamazepine is an inducer of CYP3A. In patients taking carbamazepine, the concentration of this metabolic enzyme is increased, resulting in an increase in the V_{max} of the metabolism of its substrates, a corresponding increase in intrinsic clearance of such metabolic processes, and therefore a decrease in systemic exposure of co-administered CYP3A substrate drugs like triazolam or ethinyl estradiol. Several mechanisms of enzyme induction are possible, as will be discussed later for individual drug-metabolizing enzymes, in the section on molecular determinants of drug clearance.

Enzyme inhibition, on the other hand, decreases CL_{int}, and this can result in one of several ways: either due to a decrease in V_{max} alone, an increase in K_m alone, or a combination of both, depending on the exact mechanism of inhibition. Enzyme inhibition can be broadly classified into two categories: reversible inhibition and irreversible or pseudo-irreversible inhibition. Reversible inhibition can be further classified as competitive, noncompetitive, and uncompetitive, although mixed mechanisms displaying features of both competitive and noncompetitive interactions are often encountered. From the standpoint of drug-metabolizing enzymes and drug interactions, competitive inhibition is the most commonly encountered mechanism of reversible inhibition, with noncompetitive inhibition being less common, and uncompetitive inhibition being extremely rare. Whereas a competitive inhibitor decreases CL_{int} via an increase in K_m, a noncompetitive inhibitor does so by decreasing V_{max}. The kinetic parameter that is central to describing quantitatively the potency of an inhibitor (and therefore, the magnitude of interaction risk associated with the drug as a perpetrator) is the inhibition constant K_i. For reversible inhibition that is competitive or noncompetitive, with $S \ll K_m$, Equation 12 describes the effect of the inhibitor (concentration I) on intrinsic clearance:

$$CL_{int}\,(+\text{Inhibitor}) = \frac{CL_{int}\,(\text{Control})}{1 + \dfrac{I}{K_i}} \tag{12}$$

Because intrinsic clearance is numerically equal to apparent oral clearance if absorption is complete and if the liver is the sole organ of clearance for the victim drug, systemic exposure of the victim drug in the presence of the inhibitor can be described by Equation 13:

$$AUC_{po}\,(+\text{Inhibitor}) = \left(1 + \frac{I}{K_i}\right) \cdot AUC_{po}\,(\text{Control}) \tag{13}$$

An inspection of Equation 13 suggests that the $I:K_i$ ratio is the single most important determinant of the magnitude of increase of victim drug exposure following metabolic inhibition. Thus, the potency of the inhibitor and exposure collectively determine drug interaction magnitude, with the fold-increase in victim drug exposure being directly related to the $I:K_i$ ratio, as illustrated in Figure 1.2.

Unlike reversible inhibition, the mechanism-based inactivation of an enzyme (e.g., the inactivation of CYP2D6 by paroxetine, or the inactivation of CYP3A by erythromycin) results from a metabolism-dependent suicide inactivation of an enzyme and a decrease in the pool of active enzyme. This leads to a reduction in intrinsic clearance via a reduction of V_{max} (the opposite of enzyme induction, from the standpoint of pharmacokinetic consequence). Because enzyme inactivation is practically irreversible, the return of victim drug clearance to baseline will only occur following synthesis of active enzyme, resulting in complex time-dependent drug interactions. Thus, the time course of a

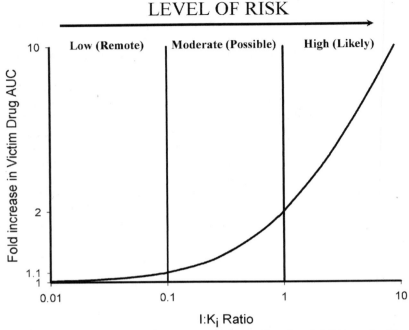

FIGURE 1.2. ▪ Relationship between the $I:K_i$ ratio of an inhibitor of metabolic clearance, the fold-increase in exposure to the victim drug, and a resulting classification of drug interaction risk.

drug interaction reversal resulting from mechanism-based inactivation is not only a function of the half-life of the perpetrator drug but is determined by biochemical physiologic factors, including the biosynthesis and degradation rates of the specific enzyme. For example, following the cessation of multiple-dose paroxetine administration, CYP2D6 activity returns back to baseline much more slowly (half-life of ~70 hours) than would be predicted based on the steady-state half-life of paroxetine (~18 hours). This is consistent with the practically irreversible inhibition of CYP2D6 by paroxetine via mechanism-based inactivation.

DISPLACEMENT INTERACTIONS RESULTING FROM MODULATION OF PLASMA PROTEIN BINDING

As discussed earlier, plasma protein binding is a determinant of V_d as well as clearance; therefore, changes in protein binding (either due to a disease state or a drug interaction) can influence pharmacokinetics. However, the clinical significance of such displacement interactions in most cases is remote and depends on the pharmacokinetic properties of the drug—most important, on its extraction ratio. In a recent commentary in *Clinical Pharmacology and Therapeutics*, Benet and Hoener provide a systematic analysis of the impact of a displacement interaction on the exposure of unbound drug (which drives pharmacologic effect), from first pharmacokinetic principles. Based on their analysis, the authors of this commentary elegantly demonstrate that a displacement interaction is of clinical relevance only if the victim drug (whose unbound fraction is increased) has a high extraction ratio and is administered intravenously, or if it is orally administered and subject to clearance via extrahepatic mechanisms having a high extraction ratio. Transiently exaggerated pharmacodynamics or toxicity may result if the displaced drug has a low therapeutic index and a very rapid pharmacokinetic-pharmacodynamic equilibration time (i.e., the effects are driven directly by plasma concentrations without a time delay for biophase distribution to the effect compartment containing the target receptor). Very few drugs (e.g., intravenous lidocaine) satisfy the above criteria to qualify as victims of displacement interactions of clinical relevance. Low therapeutic index drugs like warfarin, tolbutamide, phenytoin, carbamazepine, and valproic acid have been traditionally considered as likely victims of displacement interactions. This is in part due to the observation of clinically significant interactions in which the extent of their plasma protein binding was decreased. We now understand, in retrospect, that the mechanisms underlying many such interactions (e.g., warfarin–phenylbutazone, tolbutamide–sulfaphenazole) is in fact, metabolic inhibition by the perpetrator agent. Interestingly, all of the drugs mentioned have low extraction ratios that are less than 0.1, making an alteration of plasma protein binding inconsequential from a clinical standpoint.

RENAL CLEARANCE AND ITS MODULATION

The excretion of unmetabolized drug in the urine can be a significantly important clearance mechanism for some drugs. Examples include lithium, digoxin, and penicillins. Equation 14 for renal clearance (CL_r) follows from Equation 1:

$$CL_r = \frac{\text{Excretion Rate}}{\text{Concentration}} = \frac{\frac{dA_e}{dt}}{C} = \frac{\int_0^\infty dA_e}{\int_0^\infty C \cdot dt} = \frac{A_{e,0-\infty}}{AUC_{0-\infty}} \quad (14)$$

Thus, renal clearance can be determined from the total amount of unchanged drug excreted in the urine (A_e) following a single dose of the drug (via any route of administration) and the corresponding area under the plasma concentration-time curve ($AUC_{0-\infty}$). The processes at the level of the nephron that govern the extent of drug excretion in the urine are no different from those applicable for endogenous substances. Net excretion of a drug in urine is determined by glomerular filtration of unbound drug in plasma, active secretion in the proximal tubule, and reabsorption (passive and/or active) in the distal and proximal tubules. Filtration is determined by the glomerular filtration rate (GFR, 120 mL/min in healthy 70-kg 20-year old man) and the unbound fraction of the drug in plasma. When the unbound renal clearance of a drug exceeds GFR, it can be inferred that a net secretion of drug into the urine is present, a process that largely occurs in the proximal tubule of the nephron. On the other hand, if the unbound renal clearance of a drug is lower than GFR, the observation is consistent with net reabsorption that usually occurs in the distal as well as proximal tubules of the nephron. In reality, both secretion and reabsorption occur, and depending on which process quantitatively predominates to influence the extent of urinary excretion of a drug, either net secretion or net reabsorption occurs. Proximal renal tubular epithelial cells express a variety of drug transporters (e.g., P-gp, organic cation transporters, organic anion transporters, and organic anion transporting polypeptides) that can mediate active secretion as well as active reabsorption. For example, the cardiac glycoside digoxin is a substrate for P-gp, and efflux by this transporter at the level of the kidney's proximal tubular epithelial cells is a quantitatively important mechanism of digoxin clearance. The renal clearance of lithium is characterized by net reabsorption, occurring largely in the proximal tubule via mechanisms that are similar to those that apply for the related endogenous sodium ion. Thus, renal clearance of lithium is well below GFR and is influenced by physiological conditions that modulate sodium homeostasis, as well as by drugs that modulate renal sodium reabsorption. For example, thiazide diuretics increase lithium blood levels, due to enhanced lithium retention by the nephron, secondary to enhanced sodium excretion. Passive reabsorption in the distal tubule is generally a function of the physicochemical properties of the drug, including lipophilicity and charge at urinary pH levels, with reabsorption being significant only for those drugs that are nonpolar and uncharged at urinary pH levels. Thus, the reabsorption of drugs can be sensitive to changes in urinary pH level, depending on the drug's pKa. This has important implications in clinical toxicology settings, in which drug interactions at the level of reabsorption can be utilized favorably to aid detoxication. For weak acids (e.g., phenobarbital, having a pKa level of ~7.3), urinary alkalinization via the intravenous administration of sodium bicarbonate to achieve a urinary pH level of 7.5 results in a "trapping" of the acidic drug in its ionized form in the renal tubules, thereby minimizing reabsorption and enhancing renal excretion. The reverse is true for weakly basic drugs like methamphetamine, whose renal excretion is enhanced by urinary acidification, although the approach is no longer recommended due to its unfavorable risk–benefit ratio. Antidepressants and antipsychotics are eliminated mainly by hepatic metabolism, rendering excretion interactions clinically insignificant.

Biochemical and Molecular Determinants of Drug Disposition

CONCEPTS OF BIOTRANSFORMATION

Biotransformation (or metabolism) is an integral component of the four-step absorption-distribution-metabolism-elimination (ADME) process that determines pharmacokinetics. Biotransformation generally converts nonpolar, lipophilic, pharmacologically active drug molecules into polar inactive or nontoxic metabolites that are readily eliminated by the kidneys. The liver is the major site of drug metabolism, with intestinal drug extraction playing a secondary, yet important role in the presystemic extraction of several orally administered agents. Traditionally, biotransformation pathways are classified into two groups: Phase I reactions that involve functionalization of drug substrates to yield more polar derivatives such as alcohols, phenols, or carboxylic acids; and Phase II reactions that involve bimolecular conjugation with hydrophilic moieties to yield products such as glucuronides and sulfates that are readily excreted by the kidneys. Although the products of Phase I oxidative reactions are generally substrates for subsequent Phase II conjugation, prior to excretion in urine or bile, the direct conjugation of a drug via glucuronide or sulfate formation can also occur, although less commonly. Examples of oxidative Phase I biotransformations include the hydroxylations of aliphatic or aromatic carbon centers, O-dealkylations, N-dealkylations, N-oxygenations (N-oxide and hydroxylamine formation), S-oxygenations (sulfoxide and sulfone formation), epoxidations, and the like. Although less common, reductive Phase I biotransformations also are observed for some drugs. A notable example in psychopharmacology is the nitro reduction of the nitrated benzodiazepine clonazepam. The majority of Phase I metabolic reactions are catalyzed by an enzyme superfamily known as the cytochromes P450 (CYP), although other enzyme systems, including flavin containing monooxygenases (FMO), aldehyde oxidase (AO), aldehyde dehydrogenases, monoamine oxidases (MAO), carbonyl reductases and esterases, also are important for the metabolism of certain drugs. The major drug-metabolizing enzymes of relevance to psychopharmacology are reviewed in the following sections.

CYTOCHROMES P450

Cytochromes P450 (CYPs) constitute a superfamily of hemoproteins that catalyze the Phase I biotransformation of numerous therapeutic agents. These enzymes are estimated to account for the biotransformation of approximately 60% of the commonly prescribed drugs in the United States.

Although expressed in several tissues, the human drug-metabolizing CYPs are concentrated in the smooth endoplasmic reticulum of the Zone III hepatocytes in the liver, with lower levels of expression in the intestine, lungs, kidneys, and brain. The multiple CYP enzymes are classified into families, subfamilies, and isoforms based on a systematic nomenclature. The first number designates the family (>40% sequence identity within family members); the letter that follows designates the subfamily (>59% sequence identity), which is followed by a number indicating a particular CYP isoform. The major human drug-metabolizing CYPs belong to families 1, 2, and 3, the specific isoforms being 1A1, 1A2, 2A6, 2B6, 2C8, 2C9, 2C19, 2D6, 2E1, 2J2, 3A4, 3A5, and 3A7.

The following is a brief overview of the human drug-metabolizing CYP isoforms and clinically relevant substrates, inhibitors, inducers, and genetic polymorphisms.

CYP1A Subfamily

CYP1A1 is predominantly extrahepatic in humans and is not expressed in uninduced human liver. High CYP1A1 expression and inducibility have been associated with an enhanced risk of bronchogenic lung carcinoma in smokers, probably related to the increased activation of carcinogens in cigarette smoke. The induction of CYP1A1 gene expression by polycyclic aromatic hydrocarbons occurs via the activation of the aromatic hydrocarbon receptor. Higher levels of CYP1A expression and of associated enzymatic activities can result from increased cigarette smoking, physical exercise, and the ingestion of charbroiled meats. CYP1A1 is polymorphically expressed in human intestine. In vitro, CYP1A1 activity in the human small intestine is inhibited by the azole antifungal agent ketoconazole, but is resistant to inhibition by the SSRI antidepressant fluvoxamine, which strongly inhibits CYP1A2. However, a meaningful quantitative contribution of CYP1A1 to the oral clearance of any drug substrate in humans remains to be demonstrated.

CYP1A2 is universally expressed in human liver and is reported to account, on average, for ~13% of total immunoquantified levels of human hepatic CYP. CYP1A2 is the primary enzyme responsible for the human hepatic metabolism of phenacetin, tacrine, caffeine, and theophylline, and also plays a role in the metabolism of clozapine, olanzapine, and imipramine. Due to a major role of CYP1A2 in the metabolism of clozapine, enzyme induction via the activation of the Ah receptor (as with cigarette smoking or chronic therapy with the proton pump inhibitory antiulcer drug omeprazole) are factors that contribute to a reduction in steady-state clozapine exposures. Clinically significant CYP1A2 inhibitors include the SSRI antidepressant fluvoxamine and the fluoroquinolone antibiotics ciprofloxacin and enoxacin.

CYP2A6

CYP2A6 has a relatively minor role in the biotransformation of drugs and accounts for only ~4% of total immunoquantified levels of human hepatic CYP. This enzyme has been characterized as a coumarin 7-hydroxylase; it is an important molecular determinant of nicotine metabolism in humans, and it plays a role in the reductive metabolism of the anesthetic halothane. Genetic polymorphisms in CYP2A6 have been identified with the discovery of several inactive and/or expression-deficient variants (*2, *3, *4, *5, and *10 alleles). These polymorphisms result in a poor metabolizer phenotype, as do variants that encode an enzyme with lower activity (*6, *7, and *12 alleles), when compared with the wild-type enzyme. Pharmacogenetic studies suggest that individuals bearing these defective alleles have a reduced ability to metabolize nicotine and therefore a decreased risk of tobacco dependence. This finding led to the design of a pharmacological approach to the treatment of smoking dependence in humans by the co-administration of the CYP2A6 inhibitory drug methoxsalen, the therapeutic utility of which requires further investigation.

CYP2B6

CYP2B6 is usually considered as a low abundance isoform in human liver, and it was initially reported to account for an average of only 0.2% of total immunoquantified levels of human hepatic CYP. However, recent studies suggest that large interindividual variations may exist in the level of expression of this isoform, with the protein accounting for as much as 24% of total human liver microsomal CYP in some livers. CYP2B6 is the sole mediator of the hydroxylation of the antidepressant bupropion, and it contributes significantly to the metabolism of the antiretroviral agent efavirenz, the anticonvulsant S-mephenytoin, the barbiturate S-mephobarbital, the MAO-B inhibitor selegiline, the anticancer agent cyclophosphamide, and the anesthetics propofol and ketamine. Hormone replacement therapy and ethinyl estradiol-containing contraceptive treatments have been shown to impair bupropion clearance via inhibition of CYP2B6-mediated hydroxylation. In vitro data indicate that CYP2B6 activity is potently inhibited by the thrombolytic agents ticlopidine and clopidogrel (via irreversible mechanism-based inactivation), the SSRI antidepressant paroxetine, and the antiretroviral agent ritonavir, although controlled pharmacokinetic studies investigating the magnitude and clinical implications of these interactions remain to be done. The implications of the inhibition of CYP2B6 activity on the safety profile of bupropion deserves clinical investigation.

CYP2C Subfamily

The human CYP2C subfamily consists of four isoforms: 2C8, 2C9, 2C18, and 2C19. CYP2C9 and 2C19 catalyze the biotransformation of several therapeutically important drugs, including nonsteroidal anti-inflammatory drugs (NSAIDs), oral hypoglycemic agents, S-warfarin, anticonvulsants, sulfonamide antibiotics, and antidepressants. CYP2C isoforms are highly abundant in human liver (average of ~18% of total immunoquantified levels of human hepatic CYP), second only to CYP3A. CYP2C9 is the most abundant human hepatic CYP2C isoform, followed by CYP2C8 and CYP2C19. CYP2C18 is a minor isoform without any demonstrated role of clinical significance in drug metabolism. CYP2C9 and 2C19 show a 91% identity in amino acid sequence. Thus, most substrates of CYP2C9 are metabolized by CYP2C19 as well, albeit with lower values of intrinsic clearance, attributable to a lower affinity and lower level of expression of the latter isoform in human liver.

CYP2C8 plays an important role in the metabolism of the antidiabetic agents repaglinide and rosiglitazone and the anticancer agent paclitaxel (Taxol), and contributes to the epoxidation of the anticonvulsant carbamazepine. CYP2C8 activity is inhibited by gemfibrozil and the flavone quercetin.

CYP2C9 is the primary enzyme responsible for the metabolism of the oral hypoglycemic agent tolbutamide, the anticoagulant S-warfarin, the anticonvulsant phenytoin, the angiotensin receptor antagonist antihypertensive agent losartan, and NSAIDs such as ibuprofen, flurbiprofen, diclofenac, indomethacin, and the selective COX-2 inhibitor celecoxib. Clinically significant CYP2C9 inhibitors include the sulfon-amide antimicrobials sulfamethoxazole and sulfinpyrazone, and the azole antifungal agents miconazole and fluconazole. Clinically significant inducers of CYP2C9 include barbiturates, carbamazepine, and rifampin. CYP2C9 displays multiallelism, with the two major variant proteins of clinical importance differing from the wild type enzyme by point substitutions at positions 144 (cysteine in place of wild-type arginine resulting from the CYP2C9*2 allele) and 259 (leucine in place of wild-type isoleucine resulting from the CYP2C9*3 allele). Although these polymorphisms can affect enzymatic activity in a sub-strate-dependent manner, in the majority of cases, the *2 variant exhibits decreased activity, whereas the *3 variant results in an almost complete loss or dramatic reduction in enzyme activity. Thus, individuals homozygous for the *3 allele are classified as CYP2C9 poor metabolizers (PMs) and have significantly lower clearance of CYP2C9 substrate drugs. In the cases of drugs with narrow therapeutic windows, such as warfarin or phenytoin, such individuals have significantly lower dosage requirements to produce the desired level of anticoagulation or antiepileptic effects without bleeding or CNS toxicity, respectively. The population frequency of the *3 allele displays interethnic variation, with a frequency of ~8 % on average in whites (resulting in the homozygous PM phenotype at a very low frequency of approximately 0.5% or lower) and lower frequencies of ~1% in blacks and ~2% in Asians (and correspondingly negligible frequencies of the homozygous PM phenotype in these subpopulations). Other allelic variants such as the *4, *5, and *6 alleles have been described, but the body of information available on their clinical pharmacologic relevance is limited.

CYP2C19 is polymorphically expressed, is solely responsible for the 4-hydroxylation of the anticonvulsant S-mephenytoin, and contributes significantly to the clearance of the benzodiazepine diazepam, the proton pump inhibitor antiulcer drug omeprazole, the antimalarial agent proguanil, the SSRI antidepressant citalopram, and the tricyclic antidepressant amitriptyline. Clinically significant CYP2C19 inhibitors include fluvoxamine, omeprazole, and the antithrombotic agent ticlopidine, and inducers of clinical importance include the antituberculosis drug and PXR ligand rifampin and the antimalarial agent artemisinin. Several CYP2C19 PM alleles have been identified (*2, *3, *4, *5, *6, *7, *8) and interethnic differences in their distribution have been reported. The major alleles that account for the majority of CYP2C19 PMs are the *2 and *3 variants, both of which result in a truncated enzymatically inactive protein. These genetic polymorphisms result in a poor metabolizer phenotype at a frequency of 1% to

6% in whites and at a greater frequency of 12% to 23% in Asian populations.

CYP2D6

CYP2D6 represents an average of ~1.5% of total immunoquantified levels of human hepatic CYP and is partially or entirely responsible for the metabolism of a variety of psychopharmacologic and cardio-vascular drugs including atomoxetine, risperidone, thioridazine, zuclopenthixol, perphenazine, desipramine, nortriptyline, paroxetine, venlafaxine, codeine, metoprolol, encainide, flecainide, propafenone, and mexiletine. Clinically significant CYP2D6 inhibitors include the SSRI antidepressants fluoxetine and paroxetine, the allylamine anti-fungal agent terbinafine, the antithrombotic drug ticlopidine, and the antiarrhythmic agent quinidine. CYP2D6 is polymorphically expressed. The molecular bases of the CYP2D6 polymorphism are diverse: At least 70 distinct alleles of CYP2D6 have been identified, with a wide spectrum of phenotypic consequences. In whites, the major mutant alleles that account for the PM phenotype (~7% fre-quency) are *3, *4, and *5 (all of which result in a complete loss of CYP2D6 activity), of which *4 is fairly white subpopulation–specific. The frequency of the PM phenotype in Asians is much lower (~1%). Alleles such as *2, *10, and *17 encode an enzyme with decreased functional activity, accounting in large part for the intermediate metabolizer (IM) phenotype in whites, Asians, and blacks, respec-tively. Approximately 10% to 15% of whites and 40% of Asians are CYP2D6 IMs. CYP2D6 activity can be increased dramatically by gene duplication, multiplication, and amplification, resulting in the ultrara-pid metabolizer (URM) phenotype. The incidence of CYP2D6 gene duplication/multiplication (URM phenotype) displays a European-African north-south gradient. The frequency of this phenotype is rela-tively low in Northern Europeans (e.g. ~1–2% in Swedes) with a higher frequency in Southern regions of the continent (~4% in Ger-mans and up to 10% in Spanish and Italians). Going east, the fre-quency increases to as high as 20% in Saudi Arabians and 29% in black Ethiopians. The pharmacokinetic consequences of the pharma-cogenetic diversity of CYP2D6 have been clearly demonstrated using nortriptyline as the substrate, in studies that show a gene–dosage effect of CYP2D6 upon systemic exposure to this tricyclic antidepressant.

CYP2E1

CYP2E1 accounts for an average of ~7% of total immunoquantified levels of human hepatic CYP and is of greater importance to toxicant metabolism than drug metabolism. The skeletal muscle relaxant chlorzoxazone is metabolized primarily by CYP2E1. In addition, this isoform plays a role in the metabolism of acetaminophen, dapsone, aniline, and ethanol. CYP2E1 is inhibited by the acute administration of ethanol and by diethyldithiocarbamate (the principal metabolite of disulfiram), and is induced by chronic ethanol consumption and by isoniazid. Examples illustrating the importance of this enzyme in clinical psychopharmacology are limited.

CYP3A Subfamily

The human CYP3A subfamily consists of four isoforms: 3A4, 3A5, 3A7, and 3A43. Only CYPs 3A4 and 3A5 are of relevance to drug metabolism in adult humans (CYP3A7 is a fetal liver enzyme and CYP3A43 is a minor isoform of no established clinical importance). CYPs 3A4 and 3A5 are expressed abundantly in both human liver and small intestine, and they account for an average of ~29% of total immunoquantified levels of human hepatic CYP. Although CYP3A4 is expressed in everyone, CYP3A5 is polymorphically expressed in approximately 30% of whites and in >50% of African Americans. Almost all CYP3A substrates are metabolized by both isoforms. However, the catalytic activity for most substrates is higher with CYP3A4 (although exceptions to this general trend exist), making it a dominant contributor to net CYP3A activity in most individuals.

Examples of drugs that are metabolized primarily by CYP3A span all therapeutic classes and include immunosuppressants such as cyclosporin A and tacrolimus; sedative-hypnotic agents such as midazolam and triazolam; antidepressants such as nefazodone and trazodone; anxiolytic agents such as alprazolam and buspirone; calcium channel blockers such as nifedipine, felodipine, and diltiazem; antiarrhythmic agents such as amiodarone, quinidine, and lidocaine; antiinfectives such as erythromycin, quinine, ritonavir, saquinavir, and amprenavir; antineoplastic agents such as etoposide, ifosfamide, tamoxifen, and vinblastine; synthetic opioids such as fentanyl, alfentanil, and sufentanil; and the nonsedating antihistaminic drugs terfenadine, loratadine, and astemizole. Examples of clinically significant CYP3A inhibitors include the macrolide antibiotics erythromycin and clarithromycin, the calcium channel blocker diltiazem, the azole antifungal agents ketoconazole and itraconazole, the human immunodeficiency viral protease inhibitor ritonavir, the antidepressants nefazodone and fluoxetine (due to the potent inhibitory effect of its active metabolite norfluoxetine), and grapefruit juice (due to the potent inhibitory effect of its constituent furanocoumarins, particularly, 6′,7′-dihydroxybergamottin). Inhibition of CYP3A by grapefruit juice is only at the level of the small intestine (i.e., E_G), without any effects on hepatic extraction. Inducers of CYP3A4 primarily act by enhancing gene transcription via the activation of the nuclear pregnane X receptor (PXR), and include rifampin, St. John's wort (by the constituent hyperforin), dexamethasone, phenytoin, carbamazepine, phenobarbital, ritonavir, and nevirapine. As an added complexity, some of these agents are both inhibitors and inducers (e.g., ritonavir, St. John's wort), thus leading to complex time- and dose-dependent interactions that are difficult to predict without controlled clinical studies evaluating various dosing regimes of the perpetrator drug. CYP3A induction by St. John's wort has important implications for patient education by physicians, because self-medication with this seemingly innocuous over-the-counter antidepressant can result in deleterious effects for patients receiving narrow therapeutic index CYP3A substrates like ethinyl estradiol-containing oral contraceptives or immunosuppression with cyclosporin A or tacrolimus.

The CYP3A5 polymorphism is explained by the existence of the variant alleles *3 and *6, which are associated with the lack of enzyme expression due to alternative splicing and enzyme truncation. Although several studies have investigated the impact of the CYP3A5 polymorphism to drug disposition, its significance still remains unclear. Whereas in vitro data have suggested higher CYP3A enzyme activity in livers and intestines expressing CYP3A5, compared with those lacking the enzyme, in vivo studies have failed to demonstrate consistent effects. It thus appears from the collective data that the constitutive activity of CYP3A in humans is not influenced by CYP3A5 expression to an important extent. However, isoform-specific differences in the potency of CYP3A inhibitors have been described in vitro, with the general trend suggestive of more potent inhibition of CYP3A4 compared with CYP3A5. The clinical significance of these in vitro observations for interindividual variability in drug interaction risk remains to be elucidated.

FLAVIN-CONTAINING MONOOXYGENASES

Like the CYP enzymes, flavin-containing monooxygenases (FMO) catalyze the oxidative biotransformation of drugs, although their scope is generally limited to the oxygenation of the soft nucleophilic heteroatoms in drugs. The most common FMO-mediated metabolic reactions include N- and S- oxygenations to produce N-oxide and S-oxide metabolites. Multiple isoforms of FMO exist, with FMO3 being the major human liver microsomal isoform. FMO1 in humans is primarily expressed in the kidneys, where it can contribute to the renal metabolism of its substrates. Although psychopharmacologic agents such as imipramine have been shown to be metabolized by human FMO1, a meaningful contribution of this enzyme to the overall clearance of the tricyclic antidepressant has not been established, due to the greater capacity and contribution of hepatic CYP enzymes to its total metabolic clearance. FMO2, a lung enzyme across species, is truncated and not expressed in active form in most human beings, with the exception of a small subset of blacks who express full-length FMO2. FMO4 and FMO5 are minor human enzymes without any established clinical significance for drug metabolism. Although FMO3, the major adult human isoform, has been shown to metabolize several therapeutic agents (examples in psychiatry include clozapine and olanzapine, which undergo N-oxidation by this enzyme), no examples exist of therapeutic agents whose clearance is entirely dependent on this enzyme. Most oxidations catalyzed by FMOs are either catalyzed by CYPs as well (as in the case of clozapine and olanzapine), or other, parallel CYP-mediated metabolic pathways exist. As a result, no examples exist of clinically significant drug interactions involving the inhibition of FMO3. However, metabolism by FMO3 does have important physiological consequences. This enzyme is the sole catalyst of the N-oxidation of the diet-derived substance trimethyl amine. Thus, loss-of-function mutations in the FMO3 gene form the molecular basis of the "fish-odor syndrome" trimethylaminuria.

Aldehyde Oxidase

Aldehyde oxidase (AO) is an enzyme that is mainly localized in hepatic cytosol (as well as extrahepatic sites). It contributes to the metabolism of the antiviral agent famciclovir; the hypnotic zaleplon; the atypical antipsychotic ziprasidone; a downstream aldehyde metabolite of the SSRI citalopram; and the anticonvulsant zonisamide. The role of AO in famciclovir metabolism is critical to its pharmacology, because it is responsible for its conversion to the active metabolite penciclovir. Cimetidine is a weak AO inhibitor in vitro and produces a small impairment of zaleplon clearance, an effect that is thought to be explained at least in part by AO inhibition. However, cimetidine does not significantly alter famciclovir or ziprasidone pharmacokinetics, suggesting that the effects of this drug on AO activity in vivo are modest, at best. Although recent in vitro studies have identified several potent AO inhibitors, the clinical significance of AO inhibition on the pharmacokinetics of its substrates in humans remains to be established. For psychopharmacologics, ziprasidone is probably one of the best examples where AO contribution to clearance is significant. Because only one-third of the overall clearance of ziprasidone is

CYP3A mediated, and two-thirds is mediated by AO, the pharmacokinetic consequences of CYP3A inhibition are small for this atypical antipsychotic agent.

Carbonyl Reductases

Carbonyl reductases comprise of a group of enzymes with ketone and aldehyde reduction properties. They are localized both in the microsomal and cytosolic compartments of cells, distributed not only in the liver but at other extrahepatic sites, including red blood cells and brain and heart tissue. Carbonyl reduction contributes importantly to the reductive metabolism of endogenous prostaglandins and steroids, the antiemetic dolasetron, the antidepressant bupropion, the antipsychotic agent haloperidol, the anticancer drugs doxorubicin and daunorubicin, and the methylxanthine derivative pentoxifylline. It has been suggested that carbonyl reductase-mediated metabolism of doxorubicin in the heart may play a role in modulating the cardiotoxic effects of this anticancer agent. The relative contribution of carbonyl reduction and CYP2B6-mediated hydroxylation to the overall clearance of bupropion is unknown and deserves investigation.

Monoamine Oxidases

Two isoforms of monoamine oxidase (MAO) exist: MAO-A and MAO-B. Whereas human MAO-A shows substrate selectivity for serotonin, MAO-B is the primary catalyst of dopamine and β-phenethylamine oxidation. MAO enzymes are expressed in several tissues, including liver, intestine, brain, blood platelets (MAO-B only), and placenta (MAO-A only), with their localization primarily restricted to mitochondria. Several isoform-selective and nonselective inhibitors of MAO (MAOIs) are clinically used in psychiatry for their beneficial effects as antidepressants (e.g., phenelzine, tranylcypromine, isocarboxazid, moclobemide) or in Parkinson's disease (MAO-B-selective inhibitor selegiline). When combined with SSRI antidepressants, bupropion, or meperidine, MAOIs can produce clinically significant pharmacodynamic drug interactions, generally contraindicating such combinations. These dynamic interactions are not discussed here, but are detailed in the chapter on the drug interactions of antidepressants. MAO-A significantly contributes to the primary metabolism of the "triptan" antimigraine drugs sumatriptan and rizatriptan, as well as the secondary metabolism of the desmethyl metabolite of zolmitriptan. Moclobemide is a clinically significant inhibitor of MAO-A and produces a twofold increase in rizatriptan exposure and a fivefold increase in exposure of its desmethyl metabolite, thus augmenting its hypertensive effects. Whereas moclobemide is a reversible inhibitor of the enzyme, many other clinically used MAOIs, such as phenelzine and isocarboxazid, are irreversible mechanism-based inactivators. Therefore, it may take up to 2 weeks following discontinuation of therapy with irreversible MAOIs for the regeneration of enzyme activity via biosynthesis of the enzyme and elimination of drug interaction risk with a MAO substrate.

Uridine Diphosphate Glucuronosyltranferases

Traditionally classified as "Phase II" enzymes, the uridine diphosphate glucuronosyltransferases mainly catalyze the bimolecular conjugation of polar (e.g., hydroxylated, hydrolyzed, etc.) metabolites of drugs with the hydrophilic sugar glucuronic acid (from uridine diphosphate-glucuronic acid), to enable their excretion in urine and bile. Although somewhat less common, several examples of drugs undergo direct conjugation by UGTs to form primary metabolites. The clearance of such drugs is thus governed by the activity of these enzymes, and factors (inhibition, induction, genetic polymorphisms) influencing UGT activity will impact drug clearance. At least 15 different UGT isoforms occur in humans, belonging to two distinct families: UGT1 and UGT2. Enzymes of the UGT1 family include UGT1A1, UGT1A3, UGT1A4, UGT1A6, UGT1A7, UGT1A8, UGT1A9, and UGT1A10. Enzymes of the UGT2 family include UGT2A1, UGT2B4, UGT2B7, UGT2B15, and UGT2B17. Several of the UGTs are expressed extrahepatically in tissues such as the esophagus (1A7, 1A8, 1A10, 2B7, 2B10, 2B15), intestine (1A8, 1A10, 2B7) and brain (1A6, 2A1, 2B7). In fact, some isoforms are expressed exclusively extrahepatically (e.g., UGTs 1A7, 1A8, and 1A10 are expressed primarily in the gastrointestinal tract, including the esophagus; UGT2A1 is expressed primarily in olfactory epithelium and the brain; and UGT2B17 appears to be a prostate-specific enzyme). Although UGTs have been shown to metabolize therapeutic agents, their significance to drug clearance remains to be systematically evaluated. In addition to their ability to metabolize drugs, UGTs play an important role in the metabolism of endobiotics, such as bilirubin, and steroids. UGT1A1 is the principal bilirubin conjugating enzyme, with genetic deficiency in the enzyme (as in Crigler-Najjar syndromes and Gilbert syndrome) resulting in inheritable unconjugated bilirubinemia.

Examples of drugs for which direct conjugation by UGTs is an important clearance mechanism include lorazepam, temazepam, valproic acid, lamotrigine, morphine, codeine, propofol, ketoprofen, zidovudine, acetaminophen, chloramphenicol, mycophenolic acid, clofibric acid, and ezetimibe. For many other drugs, such as imipramine, amitriptyline, olanzapine, and furosemide, direct glucuronidation represents a minor clearance mechanism, with CYP-mediated oxidation and/or renal clearance playing a major role. Information on the identity and relative contributions of the various UGT isoforms to the overall glucuronidation rate of drugs is limited. However, it is growing because of the increasing availability of tools to study glucuronidation in vitro. For example, we now know that (S)-oxazepam is glucuronidated primarily by UGT2B15, whereas the R isomer is glucuronidated primarily by UGTs 2B7 and 1A9. Valproic acid glucuronidation appears to be mediated by at least three UGT isoforms: 1A6, 1A9, and 2B7. The clinical implications of these emerging findings, from the standpoint of drug interaction risks, remain to be elucidated. Probenecid increases exposures of lorazepam, acetaminophen, zidovudine, and clofibric acid. Although these interactions are explained, at least in part by the inhibition of glucuronidation by probenecid, its effects on the renal clearance of the glucuronide metabolites via transporter inhibition and the possible deconjugation of glucuronides may also contribute to the decrease in metabolite excretion and increase in parent drug exposure observed in these studies. Valproic acid impairs the glucuronidation of zidovudine and lorazepam, and the immunosuppressant tacrolimus is a clinically significant inhibitor of the glucuronidation of mycophenolic acid. It is hoped that scientific progress in this area will allow a better understanding of the molecular determinants (at the level of specific enzyme isoforms) of inhibitory drug interactions at the level of glucuronidation. The induction of glucuronidation has been observed in cigarette smokers and following the administration of enzyme-inducing agents like rifampin, phenytoin, and barbiturates. Cigarette smoking (which produces enzyme induction via the activation of the aromatic hydrocarbon receptor) has been shown to modestly induce the glucuronidation of acetaminophen, codeine, and propranolol. Phenytoin and pentobarbital, ligands of the constitutive androstane receptor (CAR), have been shown to induce the glucuronidation of acetaminophen and oxazepam, respectively. Rifampin treatment increases the clearance of lamotrigine, zidovudine, acetaminophen, codeine, and morphine, suggesting that the UGTs mediating these biotransformations are inducible via PXR activation. Taken together, these observations suggest that UGTs in both subfamilies 1A and 2B may be inducible via all three mechanisms: Ah receptor activation, CAR activation, and PXR activation. Despite its inducibility by a variety of mechanisms, the magnitudes of pharmacokinetic interactions at the level of glucuronidation are smaller than that observed with CYP induction. For example, whereas the magnitude of rifampin effects on clearance via glucuronidation is generally small (approximately twofold or lower on average, with the exception of codeine glucuronidation that is induced at three- to fivefold), corresponding effects of this antitubercular agent on the clearance of CYP3A substrates are an order of magnitude or greater.

In Vitro Approaches and Challenges Associated with Extrapolation to In Vivo Drug Interaction Magnitude

The increasing application of reductionism in the biomedical sciences over the last two decades has significantly influenced our approach to studying drug interactions. Experimental, as well as mathematical, methods have been developed and reasonably validated to enable the prediction of drug interaction risk associated with the inhibition of CYP-mediated metabolism—without having to perform time-consuming and expensive clinical pharmacokinetic studies. Although the exact character of the drug interaction (relative magnitude of increase in C_{max}, AUC, or half-life; extent of change in pharmacodynamics; impact on patient safety; change in dosing regimen; etc.) cannot always be predicted solely using such methods, these in vitro approaches allow us to categorize, at least qualitatively, the risk as low (remote), moderate (possible), or high (likely), thereby helping prioritize the conduct of clinical drug interaction studies to confirm and characterize the clinical consequences (kinetic and/or dynamic).

Because of their localization in hepatocellular endoplasmic reticulum, metabolism by CYP enzymes is routinely studied in vitro using human liver microsomes (preparations of endoplasmic reticular membranes from tissue homogenates of autopsied or surgically biopsied human liver samples). With these preparations as the source of enzyme, in a physiological buffer containing the necessary cofactors to support CYP activity, the formation of drug metabolites (or depletion of the substrate) can be quantitatively characterized in vitro, and the potency of a perpetrator drug as an inhibitor of the biotransformation determined. Typical estimates of potency include the inhibition constant (K_i) and the half-maximal inhibitory concentration (IC_{50}). The determination of K_i requires the measurement of the biotransformation rate of interest as a function of both substrate and inhibitor concentration, followed by a formal enzyme kinetic analysis of the data. On the other hand, determination of IC_{50} is generally less cumbersome and only requires measurement of the biotransformation rate of interest as a function of inhibitor concentration, with the substrate concentration generally fixed at or below the K_m for metabolism. For the forms of reversible enzyme inhibition commonly encountered for drug metabolic reactions (competitive and noncompetitive), the IC_{50} value is generally reasonably close to the K_i or equal to the K_i value, provided the metabolic reaction was conducted at a substrate concentration below the K_m for the biotransformation. Inhibitor potency then is used in conjunction with the estimated in vivo concentration of the perpetrator drug (I) to estimate the magnitude of a drug interaction using Equation 13, as described earlier. As a general guide, $I:K_i$ ratios of <0.1, 0.1-1.0, and >1.0 are interpreted as low (remote), moderate (possible), and high (likely) levels of drug interaction risk, based on translations to <1.1-fold, 1.1-2-fold, and >2-fold increases in victim drug exposure, respectively (Figure 1.2). A significant challenge to the quantitative prediction of drug interaction magnitude is the uncertainty in estimates of enzyme-available concentrations of the inhibitor (I) in vivo. This is especially true when active hepatic uptake of the inhibitor drug occurs, leading to an underestimation of liver enzyme-available concentrations from systemic pharmacokinetic data. Despite these challenges and limitations, this in vitro–in vivo scaling approach has clearly demonstrated predictive utility for the qualitative prediction and rank ordering of drug interaction risks associated with several clinically used, potent CYP inhibitors, such as the azole antifungal agents, SSRI antidepressants, and the antiretroviral HIV protease inhibitors. For example, clinically significant drug interactions, such as the terfenadine–ketoconazole or midazolam–itraconazole interactions, can be readily predicted using in vitro models.

An additional challenge is the uncertainty in knowing what fraction of total clearance of the victim drug is mediated by the inhibited enzyme (f_m). When f_m is <1, Equation 13 requires the following modification (Equation 15).

$$AUC_{po}\,(+\text{Inhibitor}) = \frac{1}{\left(\left(\dfrac{f_m}{1 + \dfrac{I}{K_i}}\right) + (1 - f_m)\right)} \cdot AUC_{po}\,(\text{Control}) \quad (15)$$

This equation essentially describes in mathematical terms that those victim drugs that are more dependent on a given enzyme for their clearance experience interactions of larger magnitude when that enzyme is inhibited, compared to those that are less dependent on the enzyme. For example, consider the interaction of the antidepressant venlafaxine with the CYP2D6-selective inhibitor quinidine. Venlafaxine is a racemic drug. Based on differences in the pharmacokinetics of venlafaxine in CYP2D6 EM and PM subjects, it can be inferred that the f_m for CYP2D6 for (R)-venlafaxine is 0.9, whereas that for (S)-venlafaxine is 0.5. Consistent with these observations, treatment with quinidine results in a 12-fold increase in exposure of the R isomer but only a four-fold increase in exposure of the S-isomer. As another example, the potent CYP3A4 inhibitor ketoconazole produces an 11-fold increase in the exposure of the hypnosedative triazolam (CYP3A4 $f_m \sim 1.0$), but only a 1.7-fold increase in the exposure of another hypnosedative, zolpidem (estimated CYP3A4 $f_m \sim 0.5$). Similarly, ketoconazole produces a sixfold increase in exposure of the antipsychotic quetiapine (cleared almost entirely by CYP3A), but only a 1.3-fold increase in the exposure of ziprasidone (cleared by both aldehyde oxidase and CYP3A). Because aldehyde oxidase is a cytosolic enzyme, metabolism and inhibition studies in human liver microsomes alone would suggest a greater contribution of CYP3A to ziprasidone metabolism (and predict a larger magnitude of interaction with ketoconazole than actually occurs), leading to erroneous forecasting of interaction risk. Thus, this example highlights the importance of considering the role of a victim drug's alternative metabolic pathways and clearance mechanisms when assessing the risk of a drug interaction from in vitro inhibitor potency estimated in human liver microsomes. The relationships between f_m, $I:K_i$ ratio, and magnitude of a drug interaction are illustrated in Figure 1.3.

It is important to recognize that in vitro models only predict the victim drug's magnitude of increase in AUC and not the exact nature of the pharmacokinetic interaction that can determine its clinical consequences (i.e., whether the effect on AUC is primarily due to an increase in C_{max}, a prolongation of elimination half-life, or a combination of both). As discussed earlier, the latter is dependent on the baseline pharmacokinetic properties of the victim drug (i.e., high- vs. low-extraction drug). For example, caffeine and tacrine are both metabolized almost entirely by CYP1A2. The SSRI antidepressant fluvoxamine (a potent CYP1A2 inhibitor) produces qualitatively similar effects on the oral clearance of both these drugs (80% to 90% impairment). However, the increase in caffeine exposure ($E_H \sim 0.07$) manifests itself as a prolongation of elimination half-life (sixfold) without a significant effect on C_{max}. Conversely, an increase in C_{max} (sixfold) is noted for the victim drug tacrine ($E_H \sim 0.95$), without a significant effect on elimination half-life. In vitro experiments per se, would not predict these differences, unless the resulting data are interpreted within the context of the pharmacokinetic properties of the victim drug.

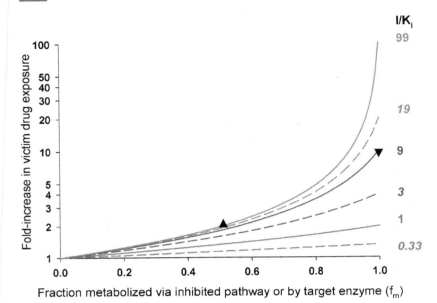

FIGURE 1.3. ■ Relationship between the fraction of a drug metabolized by the target enzyme that is inhibited in a drug interaction and the fold-increase in victim drug exposure, for inhibitors with a range of potencies relative to their exposure ($I:K_i$ ratio). Note that interaction magnitude increases with f_m as well as the $I:K_i$ ratio. If a drug is metabolized by multiple enzymes or clearance mechanisms so that f_m for the inhibited enzyme is only 0.5, even a very potent inhibitor ($I:K_i$ ratio of 99) will produce only a twofold increase in exposure due to the existence of compensatory clearance mechanisms (▲). Conversely, if a drug is metabolized entirely by a single enzyme, even inhibition by an 11-fold less potent inhibitor ($I:K_i$ ratio of 9) would result in a 10-fold increase in victim drug exposure (▼).

Several CYP3A substrates are also substrates for the ATP-dependent efflux transporter P-gp. Examples include cyclosporin A, indinavir, lovastatin, terfenadine, and erythromycin, among others. The same is true for inhibitors (e.g., itraconazole, ketoconazole, ritonavir). Fortunately, most commonly used prescription psychotropic agents are not clinically important P-gp substrates. In fact, avid P-gp substrates are generally excluded from the CNS due to the barrier function of this transporter in the BBB. Because the gene expression of P-gp is regulated by PXR as well, this transporter shares inducers with CYP3A as well. Thus, clinical interactions of St. John's wort with cyclosporin and indinavir, for example, are mediated by a combination of CYP3A induction as well as increased expression of P-gp in the intestine and liver. For drugs like digoxin, which are almost exclusively cleared renally (via active transport by P-gp), decreases in exposure following chronic dosing with St. John's wort are explained primarily by P-gp induction at the levels of the small intestine and the kidney. Thus, it is especially important to consider the role of P-gp in the disposition of a given drug (and its inhibition by the perpetrator drug) when predicting drug interactions involving CYP3A substrates.

CYP3A substrates pose yet another challenge to in vivo extrapolation from in vitro data. Given the abundant expression of the enzyme subfamily in the small intestine (in addition to the liver) and the victim-drug–specific relative contribution of the liver and intestine to overall oral clearance, it is difficult to quantitatively predict the exact magnitude of a drug interaction from in vitro human liver microsomal inhibition data alone. For example, alprazolam and triazolam are both exclusively metabolized by CYP3A. The potent and selective CYP3A inhibitor produces an 11-fold increase in triazolam exposure but only a threefold increase in alprazolam exposure, most likely explained by the significantly lower contribution of gut extraction to alprazolam's oral clearance (<10% intestinal contribution), compared to that for triazolam (~50% intestinal contribution). This difference, in turn, is explained by alprazolam having a much smaller intrinsic clearance than triazolam for metabolism by CYP3A. It is important to recognize that Equations 13 and 15 assume that the liver is the sole organ of victim drug clearance. Thus, when intestinal metabolism is significant, this model may substantially underestimate the magnitude of a drug interaction.

When a perpetrator drug is a mechanism-based inactivator of a drug-metabolizing enzyme, in vitro inhibition studies may suggest apparent competitive inhibition, unless specific experiments are performed to rule out a mechanism-based process. An empirical approach to diagnose the mechanism-based inhibition of CYP enzymes is to compare the potency of the inhibitor without and with preincubation with human liver microsomes in the presence of necessary cofactors for CYP activity. If mechanism-based inhibition is operational, the apparent inhibitory potency will be increased (i.e., the IC_{50} value is decreased) in the presence of preincubation. Equations 13 and 15 are not applicable when mechanism-based inactivation is observed and alternative mathematical models must be applied to account for the concentration- as well as time-dependent nature of the inhibition process. A formal enzyme kinetic analysis of the inactivation process is necessary in vitro to determine not only the potency of the inactivator (K_I) but also the maximal rate of enzyme inactivation (k_{inact}). When the perpetrator drug is a mechanism-based inactivator, the $I : K_I$ ratio is not the sole determinant of interaction magnitude, and clinically significant inhibition of clearance will be seen even in cases where $I \ll K_I$, if the k_{inact} is large enough.

In vitro models are being used increasingly to study enzyme induction. Primary cultures of human hepatocytes are the most common and best characterized. Because induction involves an indirect response mechanism (drug binding to a nuclear receptor in the cell and activation of gene transcription, for example), it is not only concentration-dependent but also time-dependent. This makes the in vitro–in vivo extrapolation of enzyme induction challenging, because cultured hepatocytes as opposed to the liver in an intact human being may not necessarily be kinetically equivalent with respect to the processes governing enzyme induction. Nevertheless, a qualitative assessment of the risk for the induction of specific CYP isoforms can be made in reference to established positive controls whose in vivo effects are known (e.g., rifampin for CYP3A4, omeprazole for CYP1A2) and can provide useful information to help prioritize clinical drug interaction studies.

Active metabolites must be considered when assessing the clinical significance of a potential metabolic drug interaction from in vitro data or data from controlled drug interaction studies having endpoints that are solely pharmacokinetic in nature. This can be illustrated by the interactions of the antipsychotic agents perphenazine and risperidone with the SSRI antidepressant paroxetine. Both antipsychotics are metabolized almost exclusively by CYP2D6 (f_m values for CYP2D6 of $\sim$0.9 for both drugs). Paroxetine at usual clinical doses produces a six- to sevenfold increase in the exposure of both drugs. Despite similar pharmacokinetic consequences, the clinical consequences of these two interactions are strikingly different. Whereas impairment of perphenazine clearance by paroxetine is associated with a significant increase in psychomotor impairment, sedation, and extrapyramidal side effects of this antipsychotic agent, the risperidone–paroxetine combination is generally well tolerated by the majority of patients. Perphenazine undergoes metabolic inactivation by CYP2D6, so that inhibition of the enzyme by paroxetine results in a significant elevation of active drug concentrations above the thresholds for CNS toxicity. Risperidone's pharmacologic activity, in contrast, is determined both by the parent drug and an active 9-hydroxy metabolite, which is generated by CYP2D6. Thus, while inhibition of the enzyme results in significantly elevated parent drug levels, exposure to the active metabolite is correspondingly lower, relative to the control state. As a result, the total exposure of pharmacologically active drug-related material following risperidone administration without and with paroxetine are comparable, explaining the lack of a clinically significant interaction despite the alteration of parent drug pharmacokinetics. This example highlights the importance of integrating kinetic results with the dynamic endpoints of clinical significance in appropriately interpreting and reacting to drug interactions of pharmacokinetic origin.

Cell-based models are widely used to study the transport of drugs by membrane transporters, such as P-gp, and to estimate the potency for inhibition by a perpetrator drug. Common cell-based systems for studying P-gp–mediated transport include Caco-2 cells and the Madin Darby canine kidney (MDCK) cell line overexpressing transfected human P-gp. They can be grown in culture in special "transwell" systems to develop into a monolayer of polarized cells that have a distinct apical and basolateral membrane, with P-gp expression confined to the apical membrane. Drug transport then can be measured as the flux of drug in both directions (A-to-B and B-to-A). When the drug is a P-gp substrate, efflux by the transporter results in an asymmetric flux in the two directions, with the B-to-A flux exceeding the A-to-B flux. If a perpetrator drug is an inhibitor of P-gp, co-incubation with the substrate (e.g., digoxin, rhodamine 123, quinidine, etc.) will result in a concentration-dependent decrease in the asymmetry of flux in the two directions. The resulting data can then be mathematically analyzed to determine inhibitor potency. Inhibition potencies for transporters (K_I or IC_{50} values) are interpreted in a manner analogous to those for drug-metabolizing enzymes. However, it is important to account for the differences in inhibitor concentration "seen" by the transporter, depending on the site of transporter expression. For example, whereas systemic concentrations of the inhibitor are most relevant when assessing the risk for P-gp inhibition in the liver, kidney, or BBB, luminal concentrations of the drug in the intestine (which would generally be orders of magnitude higher than systemic concentrations) are of relevance to assess the impact on drug absorption. The in vitro prediction of the in vivo magnitude of a drug interaction at the level of transporters is less straightforward, and validated quantitative models for scaling remain to be developed.

Conclusion

Pharmacokinetic drug interactions can stem from a variety of mechanisms. Although the molecular determinants of human drug metabolism and its modulation have been extensively studied and have helped explain the mechanisms of the majority of clinically significant interactions, occasional examples of puzzling interactions still remain to be rationalized mechanistically. For example, the antipsychotic agent quetiapine is primarily cleared by CYP3A-mediated metabolism.

Thioridazine, a CYP2D6 substrate, has not been reported to induce CYP3A in humans. Nevertheless, co-administration of the two drugs results in a clinically significant increase in quetiapine clearance. Despite our current fairly extensive knowledge of the clearance mechanisms of these two drugs and their effects on drug disposition mechanisms, this interaction unfortunately cannot be rationalized today. Of greater concern is that we cannot predict if thioridazine carries hidden risks as a potential perpetrator of similar interactions with other therapeutic agents via this unidentified "black box" mechanism. Examples like these highlight the importance of elucidating the clinical significance of new drug-metabolizing enzymes and transporters that are being discovered by molecular pharmacologists, and a continued refinement of our knowledge of clearance mechanisms of the drugs we prescribe. Thus, we are faced with an area of research that is highly interdisciplinary, relying on strong partnerships between scientists and physicians to strengthen the bridge between the biology of drug disposition and its implications for clinical therapeutics.

REFERENCES

Plasma Protein Binding

Benet LZ, Hoener BA: Changes in plasma protein binding have little clinical relevance: Clin Pharmacol Ther 71(3): 115–121, 2002.

Greenblatt DJ, Sellers EM, Koch-Weser J: Importance of protein binding for the interpretation of serum or plasma drug concentrations. J Clin Pharmacol. 22(5–6): 259–263, 1982.

Drug Transport and CNS Distribution

Ayrton A, Morgan P: Role of transport proteins in drug absorption, distribution and excretion. Xenobiotica 31(8–9): 469–497, 2001.

Sadeque AJ, Wandel C, He H, Shah S, Wood AJ: Increased drug delivery to the brain by P-glycoprotein inhibition. Clin Pharmacol Ther 68(3): 231–237, 2000.

von Moltke LL, Greenblatt DJ: Drug transporters in psychopharmacology—are they important? J Clin Psychopharmacol 20(3): 291–294, 2000.

Concepts of Clearance and Presystemic Extraction

Greenblatt DJ. Presystemic extraction: mechanisms and consequences. J Clin Pharmacol 33(7): 650–256, 1993.

Lin JH, Chiba M, Baillie TA: Is the role of the small intestine in first-pass metabolism overemphasized? Pharmacol Rev 51(2): 135–158, 1999.

Shen DD, Kunze KL, Thummel KE: Enzyme-catalyzed processes of first-pass hepatic and intestinal drug extraction. Adv Drug Deliv Rev 27(2–3): 99–127, 1997.

Wilkinson GR, Shand DG: Commentary: a physiological approach to hepatic drug clearance. Clin Pharmacol Ther 18(4): 377–390, 1975.

Cytochrome P450 Isoforms and Genetic Polymorphisms

Bertilsson L, Dahl ML, Dalen P, Al-Shurbaji A: Molecular genetics of CYP2D6: clinical relevance with focus on psychotropic drugs. Br J Clin Pharmacol 53(2): 111–122, 2002.

Daly AK: Pharmacogenetics of the major polymorphic metabolizing enzymes. Fundam Clin Pharmacol 17(1): 27–41, 2003.

Desta Z, Zhao X, Shin JG, Flockhart DA: Clinical significance of the cytochrome P450 2C19 genetic polymorphism. Clin Pharmacokinet 41(12): 913–958, 2002.

Dresser GK, Spence JD, Bailey DG: Pharmacokinetic-pharmacodynamic consequences and clinical relevance of cytochrome P450 3A4 inhibition. Clin Pharmacokinet 38(1): 41–57, 2000.

Ekins S, Wrighton SA: The role of CYP2B6 in human xenobiotic metabolism. Drug Metab Rev 31(3): 719–754, 1999.

Floyd MD et al.: Genotype-phenotype associations for common CYP3A4 and CYP3A5 variants in the basal and induced metabolism of midazolam in European- and African-American men and women. Pharmacogenetics 13(10): 595–606, 2003.

Hesse LM et al.: CYP2B6 mediates the in vitro hydroxylation of bupropion: potential drug interactions with other antidepressants. Drug Metab Dispos 28(10): 1176–1183, 2000.

Lamba JK, Thummel KE: Genetic contribution to variable human CYP3A-mediated metabolism. Adv Drug Deliv Rev 54(10): 1271–1294, 2002.

Lee CR, Goldstein JA, Pieper JA: Cytochrome P450 2C9 polymorphisms: a comprehensive review of the in-vitro and human data. Pharmacogenetics 12(3): 251–263, 2002.

Miners JO, Birkett DJ: Cytochrome P4502C9: an enzyme of major importance in human drug metabolism. Br J Clin Pharmacol 45(6): 525–538, 1998.

von Moltke LL et al.: Metabolism of drugs by cytochrome P450 3A isoforms. Implications for drug interactions in psychopharmacology. Clin Pharmacokinet 29 Suppl 1: 33–43, 1995.

Aldehyde Oxidase

Beedham C et al.: Ziprasidone metabolism, aldehyde oxidase, and clinical implications. J Clin Psychopharmacol 23(3): 229–232, 2003.

Lake BG et al.: Metabolism of zaleplon by human liver: evidence for involvement of aldehyde oxidase. Xenobiotica 32(10): 835–847, 2002.

Obach RS et al.: Human liver aldehyde oxidase: inhibition by 239 drugs. J Clin Pharmacol 44(1): 7–19, 2004.

Monoamine Oxidases

Dixon CM et al.: Characterization of the enzyme responsible for the metabolism of sumatriptan in human liver. Biochem Pharmacol 47(7): 1253–1257, 1994.

Van Haarst AD et al.: The effects of moclobemide on the pharmacokinetics of the 5-HT1B/1D agonist rizatriptan in healthy volunteers. Br J Clin Pharmacol 48(2): 190–196, 1999.

Glucuronidation

Court MH et al.: Stereoselective conjugation of oxazepam by human UDP-glucuronosyltransferases (UGTs): S-oxazepam is glucuronidated by

UGT2B15, while R-oxazepam is glucuronidated by UGT2B7 and UGT1A9. Drug Metab Dispos 30(11): 1257–1265, 2002.

Lin JH, Wong BK: Complexities of glucuronidation affecting in vitro in vivo extrapolation. Curr Drug Metab 3(6): 623–646, 2002.

Tukey RH, Strassburg CP: Human UDP-glucuronosyltransferases: metabolism, expression, and disease. Annu Rev Pharmacol Toxicol 40: 581–616, 2000.

Drug Interactions and In vitro Models

Bjornsson TD et al.: The conduct of in vitro and in vivo drug–drug interaction studies: a Pharmaceutical Research and Manufacturers of America (PhRMA) perspective. Drug Metab Dispos 31(7): 815–832, 2003.

Lin JH: Sense and nonsense in the prediction of drug–drug interactions. Curr Drug Metab 1(4): 305–331, 2000.

Obach RS: Drug–drug interactions: an important negative attribute in drugs. Drugs Today 39(5): 301–338, 2003.

Shader RI et al.: The clinician and drug interactions—an update. J Clin Psychopharmacol 16(3): 197–201, 1996.

Tucker GT et al.: Optimizing drug development: strategies to assess drug metabolism/transporter interaction potential—towards a consensus. Br J Clin Pharmacol 52(1): 107–117, 2001.

Venkatakrishnan K et al.: Human drug metabolism and the cytochromes P450: application and relevance of in vitro models. J Clin Pharmacol 41(11): 1149–1179, 2001.

Venkatakrishnan K et al.: Drug metabolism and drug interactions: application and clinical value of in vitro models. Curr Drug Metab 4(5): 423–459, 2003.

Von Moltke LL et al.: In vitro approaches to predicting drug interactions in vivo. Biochem Pharmacol 55(2): 113–122, 1998.

Antidepressants

DOMENIC A. CIRAULO   WAYNE L. CREELMAN
RICHARD I. SHADER   DAVID J. GREENBLATT

For the purposes of discussing drug interactions we have divided the antidepressants into three categories: (a) antidepressants, general; (b) selective serotonin reuptake inhibitors (SSRIs); and (c) monoamine oxidase inhibitors (MAOIs). The drugs comprising these three categories, their mechanisms of action, and their interactions are summarized in Tables 2.1, 2.2, and 2.3.

Section 2.1   General Antidepressants

Acetazolamide (Diamox)

EVIDENCE OF INTERACTION

Acetazolamide is a carbonic anhydrase inhibitor useful in the treatment of glaucoma, seizure disorders, and abnormal fluid retention (such as that seen with cardiac edema). It alkalizes urinary pH levels, thus potentially increasing the amount of an antidepressant that is not ionized, which promotes reabsorption of the drug by the kidney and increases serum levels.

MECHANISM

Pharmacokinetic alteration of renal reabsorption.

CLINICAL IMPLICATIONS

This type of interaction is important only when drugs are eliminated primarily through the kidney. Antidepressants are primarily eliminated through hepatic metabolism; thus it is unlikely that this interaction is of clinical importance (Gram et al. 1971, Sjoqvist et al. 1969).

Amantadine

EVIDENCE OF INTERACTION

After a cumulative dose of 450 mg bupropion over 72 hours, a 75-year-old man taking amantadine 300 mg daily for Parkinson's disease,

TABLE 2.1.   SELECTED NON-SSRI ANTIDEPRESSANTS AND THEIR METABOLITES

Tertiary Amines	Cytochrome Substrates
Amitriptyline	1A2, 2C19, 2C9, 2D6, 3A4
Imipramine	2C19, 2C9, 1A2, 3A4, 2D6
Clomipramine	3A4, 2D6 (also inhibits 2D6), 2C19
Trimipramine	2C19, 1A2, 3A4, 2D6
Doxepin	2C19, 3A4, 1A2, 2C9
Secondary Amines	
Nortriptyline	2D6
Desipramine	2D6
Protriptyline	2D6
Aminoketones	
Bupropion	2B6 (also inhibits 2B6), 2D6 (also inhibits 2D6)
Tetracyclics	
Mirtazapine	3A, 2D6, 1A2
Maprotiline	2D6, 1A2
Phenylethylamine	
Venlafaxine	2D6
Triazolopyridine	
Trazodone	3A4
Phenylpiperazine	
Nefazodone	3A4 (also inhibits 3A4), 2D6

(Reprinted with permission from Pharmacotherapy of Depression, DA Ciraulo and RI Shader (eds.) pg. 61, Humana Press, Totowa, New Jersey, 2004.)

haloperidol 2 mg daily, and benztropine 2 mg daily, became agitated and delirious, with visual and auditory hallucinations (Liberzon et al. 1990). After discontinuation of the bupropion, his symptoms cleared in 4 days.

MECHANISM
An interaction has not been established.

CLINICAL IMPLICATIONS
This single case report does not establish an interaction between amantadine and bupropion, because the symptoms may have been produced by bupropion alone.

Ammonium Chloride

Ammonium chloride acidifies the urine and could potentially reduce serum concentrations of antidepressants (Gram et al. 1971, Sjoqvist

TABLE 2.2. INHIBITION OF HUMAN CYTOCHROME P450 BY SELECTED ANTIDEPRESSANTS

Cytochrome P450 Inhibition

	1A2	2C9	2C19	2D6	2E1	3A	2B6
Fluoxetine	+	+ +	+ to + +	+ + +	—	+	+
Norfluoxetine	+	+ +	+ to + +	+ + +	—	+ +	0
Sertraline	+	+	+ to + +	+	—	+	+
Desmethyl-sertraline	+	+	+ to + +	+	—	+	0
Paroxetine	+	+	+	+ + +	—	+	+ + +
Fluvoxamine	+ + +	+ +	+ + +	+	—	+	+
Citalopram	+	0	0	0	0	0	0
Monodesmethyl-citalopram	0	0	0	+	0	0	0
Escitalopram	0	0	0	+	0	0	0
Nefazodone	0	0	0	0	—	+ + +	0
Triazole-dione	0	0	0	0	—	+	0
Hydroxy-nefazodone	0	0	0	0	—	+ + +	0
Venlafaxine	0	0	0	0/+	—	0	0
O-Desmethyl-venlafaxine	0	0	0	0	—	0	0
Mirtazapine	0	0	0	0	0	0	0
Bupropion	0	0	0	+ +	0	0	+

0 = Minimal or zero inhibition; +, + +, + + + = mild, moderate, or strong inhibition; Dash (—) indicates no data available
Metabolites are italicized
Adapted with permission from Greenblatt DJ et al.: Human cytochromes and some new antidepressants: kinetics, metabolism, and drug interactions. J Clin Psychopharmacol 19: 23S, 1999.

et al. 1969). Because hepatic metabolism is responsible for the elimination of cyclic antidepressants, this is not a clinically relevant effect.

Analgesics, Opioid (*See also* Methadone, this chapter)

EVIDENCE OF INTERACTION

Clomipramine, pargyline, and nialamide potentiate the analgesic effect of morphine and pentazocine in rodents (Lee et al. 1980). Morphine analgesia in rats was potentiated by amitriptyline, desipramine, and sertraline (Taiwo et al. 1985). This effect was blocked by the prior

(text continues on page 55)

TABLE 2.3.   CLINICALLY IMPORTANT ANTIDEPRESSANT DRUG INTERACTIONS: FOCUS ON THE NON-SSRI, NON-TCA AGENTS

BUPROPION

2B6, 2D6

2B6 is primary cytochrome responsible for metabolism. Bupropion slightly inhibits 2B6 and moderately inhibits 2D6. Pharmacokinetic interactions are probably underreported.

Amantadine

The combination produced agitation, ataxia, tremor in nursing home patients, which resolved within 72 hours of drug discontinuation.

Carbamazepine

Carbamazepine reduces bupropion levels.

MAOI

Bupropion poses as great a risk as other antidepressants when co-administered with MAOI. Hypertensive crises are possible. Allow 2 weeks washout if switching from MAOI to bupropion.

Ritonavir and related agents

These drugs impair bupropion metabolism and elevate levels. Toxicity is possible.

DULOXETINE

2D6, 1A2

Duloxetine is a 2D6 inhibitor and may impair the metabolism of drugs that use this cytochrome. Drugs that inhibit 1A2 such as quinolone antibiotics, increase duloxetine levels and can result in toxicity.

Protein binding

Duloxetine is highly protein bound; there is a potential for interactions with other highly bound drugs.

Limited experience

Experience with duloxetine is limited at the time of publication. Expect serious interactions with MAOI.

VENLAFAXINE

2D6, 3A4

Venlafaxine is a weak inhibitor of 2D6. 2D6 mediates the metabolism of venlafaxine to O-desmethylvenlafaxine, which is active. 3A4 is believed to be a minor pathway of venlafaxine metabolism. Venlafaxine does not inhibit 3A4 in vitro, and clinical studies show no effect on several drugs metabolized by 3A4 (e.g., alprazolam, diazepam, terfenadine).

Risperidone

150 mg venlafaxine at steady state inhibited risperidone metabolism and increased the risperidone AUC by 32%. There was a corresponding decrease in 9-hydroxyrisperidone levels so that the total concentration of parent and metabolite was not altered significantly.

(continued)

TABLE 2.3. CLINICALLY IMPORTANT ANTIDEPRESSANT DRUG INTERACTIONS: FOCUS ON THE NON-SSRI, NON-TCA AGENTS (CONTINUED)

Haloperidol	150 mg venlafaxine at steady state inhibited metabolism of an acute 2 mg oral dose of haloperidol and increased the haloperidol AUC by 70% and C_{max} by 88% without affecting elimination half-life.
Clozapine	There are clinical reports of seizures associated with elevated clozapine levels when venlafaxine has been administered concomitantly.
Imipramine and Desipramine	Although imipramine and 2-hydroxyimipramine pharmacokinetics are not altered by concurrent venlafaxine, the clearance of desipramine and 2-hydroxyimipramine is impaired resulting in higher levels. With venlafaxine 37.5 mg or 75 mg administered twice daily, the AUC of 2-hydroxydesipramine increased 2.5 and 4.5 times above that of monotherapy. Desipramine AUC increased by over one-third that of single drug therapy levels.
Indinavir	When indinavir (800 mg single oral dose) was administered with venlafaxine (150 mg daily, steady state condition), the antidepressant was associated with decreases in the AUC and C_{max} of indinavir (28% and 38%, respectively) compared to monotherapy.
Cimetidine	Although cimetidine can impair the metabolism of venlafaxine, it does not appear to affect O-desmethylvenlafaxine levels. Since the metabolite is present in greater concentrations than venlafaxine, in most patients the interaction should not have serious effects. In individuals at higher risk for venlafaxine adverse effects (e.g., elderly, medically ill) dosage reduction may be necessary. In such cases, alternatives to cimetidine should be considered.
Lithium	A pharmacokinetic study in healthy volunteers found that venlafaxine (150 mg daily, steady state condition) did not affect single dose lithium pharmacokinetics.
Warfarin	Case reports of increases in INR and prothrombin time when venlafaxine was added to warfarin therapy.
Serotonergic Agents	The serotonin syndrome can occur with venlafaxine and other agents that increase serotonin. Pharmacodynamic interactions with venlafaxine are essentially the same as SSRI. MAOIs are contraindicated.

(continued)

TABLE 2.3.   CLINICALLY IMPORTANT ANTIDEPRESSANT DRUG INTERACTIONS: FOCUS ON THE NON-SSRI, NON-TCA AGENTS (CONTINUED)

TRAZODONE

3A4 — Trazodone is a 3A4 substrate, and subject to interactions with drugs that inhibit or induce 3A4.

Ritonavir — Ritonavir inhibits 3A4 metabolism. Ritonavir reduced oral clearance of trazodone, prolonged elimination half-life, and increased C_{max}. Nausea, dizziness, hypotension, and syncope were reported with the combination. Other protease inhibitors such as indinavir also inhibit 3A4 and will probably interfere with metabolism.

Ketoconazole — Ketoconazole and itraconazole inhibit 3A4 and impair trazodone metabolism.

SSRIs — SSRIs that inhibit 3A4 will impair trazodone metabolism. A serotonin syndrome has been reported, but the combination is often used clinically without adverse effects.

Carbamazepine — Carbamazepine decreases levels of trazodone and its metabolite, m-chlorophenylpiperazine. Carbamazepine levels may be slightly increased.

Phenytoin — One case report found elevated phenytoin levels with trazodone, but the evidence is limited.

Thioridazine — Thioridazine increased trazodone levels by 36% and m-chlorophenylpiperazine levels by 54%.

Anticoagulants — A case report and retrospective chart review suggested that some patients could have a decrease in the anticoagulant effect of warfarin when trazodone was added to the regimen. There are many case reports of antidepressants interacting with warfarin, although the effect is not found consistently. It is probably advisable to monitor anticoagulation effects more closely when trazodone or other antidepressants are added or discontinued from a regimen that includes warfarin.

NEFAZODONE

2D6, 3A4 — Nefazodone is a substrate for 2D6 and 3A4, and inhibits 3A4. Doses of drugs metabolized by 3A4 should be reduced. If the co-administered drug is associated with toxicity (e.g., pimozide) co-administration should be avoided.

(continued)

TABLE 2.3.   CLINICALLY IMPORTANT ANTIDEPRESSANT DRUG INTERACTIONS: FOCUS ON THE NON-SSRI, NON-TCA AGENTS (CONTINUED)

Alprazolam Triazolam	Nefazodone impairs the metabolism of benzodiazepines metabolized by 3A4. Alprazolam dose should be reduced by 50%, triazolam by 75%. Lorazepam is not affected.
Carbamazepine	Very large reductions in nefazodone and hydroxynefazodone levels occur in the presence of carbamazepine. The combination should be avoided.
Buspirone	Some evidence suggests that buspirone levels are increased when administered with nefazodone. Some clinicians limit starting dose of buspirone to 5 mg daily if patients are taking nefazodone.
Cyclosporine	Nefazodone inhibits 3A4 metabolism of cyclosporine. Case reports suggest that cyclosporine levels may increase 2-fold at low nefazodone doses (25 mg twice daily) and even higher with therapeutic doses (100 mg twice daily). One case report describes an increase in cyclosporine levels from 78 ng/ml to 775 ng/ml thirteen days after starting nefazodone (150 mg twice daily).
Statins	There is a case report of a patient taking simvastatin 40 mg/day for 19 weeks who developed rhabdomyolysis and myositis 1 month after starting nefazodone 200 mg daily. Another patient developed symptoms 6 weeks after nefazodone was added. It is not possible to determine if rhabdomyolysis was caused by the combination because this is a known adverse effect of the statins.
Digoxin	Nefazodone (200 mg twice daily) increased digoxin levels in a study of healthy male volunteers (15% increase in AUC) but there was not an increase in adverse or cardiac effects.
Haloperidol	Nefazodone may moderately increase haloperidol levels but clinical importance is unlikely.
Propranolol	In a study of healthy male volunteers nefazodone (200 mg) decreased AUC of propranolol and extended the time to reach steady state by 1 day. There were no clinically important changes in propranolol's cardiovascular effects.

(continued)

TABLE 2.3. CLINICALLY IMPORTANT ANTIDEPRESSANT DRUG INTERACTIONS: FOCUS ON THE NON-SSRI, NON-TCA AGENTS (CONTINUED)

Tacrolimus	Tacrolimus toxicity has been reported in transplant patients when nefazodone was added to their regimen. Neurotoxicity characterized by headache, confusion, and delirium has been described.
Clozapine	Increased clozapine and norclozapine serum levels were reported in a 40-year old man taking nefazodone (300 mg/d). The interaction appears to be dose related with 200 mg causing 5% and 31%, and 300 mg 75% and 87% increases in parent and metabolite, respectively.
Nifedipine	Nefazodone inhibits metabolism (3A4).
Eplerenone (Inspra®)	Nefazodone inhibits metabolism (3A4). Since this may result in hyperkalemia, the combination should be avoided.
Methylprednisolone	Nefazodone inhibits metabolism (3A4) and may result in prolonged cortisol suppression.
Loratadine (Claritin®)	Nefazodone inhibits metabolism (3A4). Loratadine (20 mg/day) and nefazodone (300 mg twice daily) were studied in healthy men and women. There was an increase in the AUC of loratadine and its metabolite, which was correlated with an increase in the QTc interval (21.6 ms).
St. John's Wort	There is a report of a serotonin syndrome occurring in an elderly patient on nefazodone when St. John's Wort was added. The same report described the syndrome in patients taking SSRI and St. John's Wort.
MAOI	Serotonin syndrome possible. Since nefazodone also has norepinephrine reuptake inhibiting properties, adrenergic hyperstimulation may also occur.
MIRTAZAPINE 2D6, 1A2, 3A4	Mirtazapine is a substrate for 2D6, 1A2, 3A4, but does not inhibit them significantly. There is the potential for mirtazapine metabolism to be affected by inhibition or induction of these enzymes but studies are lacking.
CNS sedatives	The manufacturer reports additive impairment of cognitive and motor skills when venlafaxine is

(continued)

TABLE 2.3.   CLINICALLY IMPORTANT ANTIDEPRESSANT DRUG INTERACTIONS: FOCUS ON THE NON-SSRI, NON-TCA AGENTS (CONTINUED)

	administered with alcohol or diazepam. Mirtazapine probably poses as great a risk as other antidepressants when co-administered with MAOI.
MAPROTILINE	
2D6, 1A2	Maprotiline is a substrate for cytochromes 2D6, 1A2, but does not inhibit them significantly. There is the potential for maprotiline metabolism to be affected by inhibition or induction of these enzymes, but studies are lacking.
TCA-like interactions	Maprotiline's pharmacologic actions are similar to TCA and many interactions can be predicted. Blocking of guanethidine, and interactions with anticholinergic and sympathomimetic drugs are similar to TCA. Maprotiline poses as great a risk as other antidepressants when co-administered with MAOI.
Drugs that lower the seizure threshold	Maprotiline lowers the seizure threshold and should be avoided in patients taking other medications that do the same (TCA, antipsychotics).

administration of parachlorophenylalanine, which reduces brain serotonin to about 32% of normal levels (it may also reduce brain norepinephrine and dopamine to about 69% of normal levels; Koe 1966, Miller et al. 1970). The effect of parachlorophenylalanine was not reversed by serotonin, which suggests that other neurotransmitters may also be involved. Animal models of pain suggest that mixed-action and noradrenergic antidepressants may be more effective analgesics than SSRIs (Mochizucki 2004). The morphine-potentiating effects of the antidepressants were blocked by methysergide (a serotonin antagonist), yohimbine, and phentolamine (α-adrenergic antagonists), but not by propranolol (a β-adrenergic antagonist). Another study found that morphine analgesia in rats was potentiated by desipramine or clomipramine, but that by 8 to 15 days of treatment, this effect was no longer present and a reduction from baseline morphine analgesic activity occurred (Kellstein et al. 1984). Other studies have also demonstrated that desipramine potentiates morphine analgesia (Ossipov et al. 1982).

Nefazodone alone had an analgesic effect in one animal model of pain, and it potentiated the analgesic action of morphine fourfold, without affecting lethality in this mouse model (Pick et al. 1992). Naloxone did not block the analgesic effect of nefazodone alone, suggesting that the analgesic action of nefazodone is not mediated via the opiate system.

Propoxyphene may inhibit the metabolism of doxepin and perhaps other cyclic antidepressants (Abernethy et al. 1982). Elevated serum levels of doxepin developed in an 89-year-old man taking doxepin 150 mg daily, after propoxyphene 65 mg every 6 hours was administered. The patient became lethargic, and his symptoms did not clear completely until 5 days after propoxyphene was stopped.

MECHANISM

It is likely that the potentiation of serotonergic and noradrenergic systems are responsible for enhanced analgesic effects. This is supported by evidence that fluoxetine (a specific serotonin uptake inhibitor) and 5-methoxy-N,N-dimethyltryptamine (a specific serotonin agonist) potentiate the action of morphine, whereas serotonergic antagonists or depleting agents antagonize its action. Mixed action and noradrenergic antidepressants also have analgesic properties. Desipramine inhibits the metabolism of methadone and morphine and may increase plasma levels of these opioids (Goldstein et al. 1982, Liu et al. 1975, 1985). Methadone also inhibits the metabolism of desipramine (Maany et al. 1989).

Propoxyphene inhibits oxidative metabolism (CYP3A4, possibly 2D6 and 2C9), as evidenced by impaired antipyrine clearance in healthy volunteers who had taken eight doses of propoxyphene 65 mg every 4 hours (Abernethy et al. 1982).

CLINICAL IMPLICATIONS

Several anecdotal reports suggest that cyclic antidepressants relieve pain, and they are useful alone in the treatment of headache and neuropathic pain (Douglas et al. 2004, Namaka et al. 2004, Singleton et al. 2005, Vu 2004). Combinations of agents may allow lower doses of opioids to be used, although some evidence suggest that tolerance occurs with prolonged treatment. Further clinical studies are required (also see the section on Selective Serotonin Reuptake Inhibitors).

Anesthetics (General) (*See also* Sympathomimetics, this chapter)

EVIDENCE OF INTERACTION

Reports in the 1970s linked general anesthesia to an increased risk of cardiac arrhythmias (Edwards et al. 1979, Glisson et al. 1978). After the administration of halothane and pancuronium, tachyarrhythmias developed in two patients without cardiovascular disease who were receiving long-term imipramine treatment (Edwards et al. 1979). This same drug combination in dogs increased the risk of premature ventricular contractions, ventricular tachycardia, ventricular fibrillation, and cardiac arrest. Postoperative hypotension and delirium also have been reported in patients taking antidepressants (Berggren et al. 1987, Sprung et al. 1997). There is one prospective study of 80 patients with major depression treated with antidepressants (imipramine, clomipramine, maprotiline, mianserin), half of whom had antidepressants discontinued 72 hours prior to anesthesia (propofol and fentanyl induction; vecuronium for tracheal intubation; isoflurane in nitrous oxide for maintenance). Those whose antidepressants were discontinued were more likely to experience an increase in depressive symptoms and delirium postoperatively, compared with patients who continued antidepressant therapy. The incidence of hypotension and cardiac arrhythmias did not differ (Kudoh et al. 2002).

MECHANISM

Both imipramine and pancuronium have anticholinergic and adrenergic actions. When combined with halothane, which is known to predispose the myocardium to arrhythmias following administration of atropine or epinephrine, the likelihood of cardiac arrhythmias increases.

CLINICAL IMPLICATIONS

Although case reports have suggested an increased risk of hypotension, delirium, and cardiac arrhythmias in patients taking antidepressants undergoing general anesthesia, one prospective study (Kudoh et al. 2002) found no such relationship. In fact, this study found an increase in depressive symptoms and delirium in patients who had their antidepressants discontinued 72 hours prior to anesthesia.

Anticholinergic Agents

EVIDENCE OF INTERACTION

Tricyclic antidepressants and maprotiline have significant anticholinergic effects. When given with antiparkinsonian agents (benztropine, trihexyphenidyl, etc.), significant additive atropinic effects may occur in some antipsychotics (especially thioridazine, chlorpromazine), antihistamines, glutethimide, meperidine, and other medications.

Central nervous system (CNS) symptoms of the anticholinergic syndrome include anxiety, agitation, disorientation, dysarthria, impairment of memory, hallucinations, myoclonus, and seizures. Systemic signs include tachycardia, arrhythmias, mydriasis, elevated body temperature, hot dry flushed skin, decreased bowel motility, and urinary retention.

MECHANISM

Receptor site interaction.

CLINICAL IMPLICATIONS

Anticholinergic toxicity is an important syndrome, especially in geriatric patients. Cyclic antidepressants with strong anticholinergic effects include all tricyclics (amitriptyline, clomipramine, imipramine, protriptyline, trimipramine, nortriptyline, doxepin, and desipramine). Antidepressants with little or no anticholinergic effects include SSRIs, trazodone, nefazodone, bupropion, duloxetine, and venlafaxine (Richelson et al. 1984). Treatment for the anticholinergic syndrome includes a discontinuation of offending agents and slow intravenous or intramuscular administration of 1 to 2 mg of physostigmine, repeated as needed every 15 to 30 minutes. Peripheral anticholinergic symptoms can be treated with neostigmine, but this agent does not cross the blood–brain barrier (BBB).

Anticoagulants (*See also* SSRI)

EVIDENCE OF INTERACTION

A single case report describes a 40-year-old woman whose hypoprothrombinemic response to warfarin was reduced when trazodone was administered (Hardy et al. 1986). While receiving warfarin after mitral valve replacement, trazodone 300 mg/day was administered to treat depression. A 30% reduction in prothrombin times was observed after 5 weeks of trazodone therapy, which returned to pretreatment levels when the antidepressant was discontinued. A retrospective chart review of 75 patients found three cases in which changes in international normalized ratio (INR) of 1 or greater were associated with the administration of trazodone (Small et al. 2000). The addition of trazodone to warfarin therapy decreased INR and prothrombin time, whereas these values increased when trazodone was discontinued.

In a controlled study by Vesell et al. (1970), a single dose of dicumarol 4 mg/kg orally was given prior to the administration of nortriptyline 4 mg/kg orally. Following 8 days of nortriptyline administration, the serum half-life of dicumarol was significantly longer (105.7 ± 54.2 hours) than pretreatment half-life (35.3 ± 5.3 hours).

In a placebo-controlled study, Pond et al. (1975) found that warfarin elimination was not affected by concurrent nortriptyline or amitriptyline administration. The half-life of warfarin 25 mg, taken with a single dose of synthetic vitamin K 10 mg, was measured prior to the initiation of nortriptyline 40 mg/day (orally/divided dose) or amitriptyline 75 mg/day (orally/divided dose) and during the last 4 days of the 13-day course of nortriptyline or amitriptyline. No consistent effect on warfarin elimination was observed. A similar protocol was followed with dicumarol, 200 mg and 300 mg doses. Inconsistent effects were observed on dicumarol metabolism, with a suggestion that dicumarol absorption was increased in the presence of these highly anticholinergic antidepressants. An increase in elimination of the half-life of dicumarol was found in only 2 of 12 subjects.

In one report, it was suggested that concurrent treatment with amitriptyline contributed to hemorrhagic reactions in patients taking warfarin, although a causal relationship was not established (Koch-Weser 1973).

MECHANISM

No consistent evidence supports an interaction between warfarin or dicumarol and amitriptyline or nortriptyline. Some evidence suggests that nortriptyline may prolong dicumarol half-life, although a carefully controlled study found no interaction (Pond et al. 1975). These tricyclic antidepressants may increase dicumarol bioavailability by decreasing intestinal (gut) motility, thereby increasing absorption (Pond et al. 1975). Further complicating the matter is an animal study indicating that amitriptyline and nortriptyline impaired warfarin metabolism in the rat (Loomis et al. 1980). Antidepressant-induced displacement from protein binding sites and increases in unbound warfarin are possible when highly bound drugs are added to the anticoagulant.

CLINICAL IMPLICATIONS

Data on this interaction are limited. Due to genetic factors, dose, and route of administration, warfarin kinetics are complex and variable. If an interaction does occur, it is probably uncommon. Patients receiving this combination should be monitored for alterations in coagulation that would indicate that an adjustment in the warfarin dose is necessary. Anticoagulant response to warfarin, dicumarol, and related anticoagulants should be monitored closely when trazodone, nortriptyline, or other antidepressants are started or discontinued (also see the section on Selective Serotonin Reuptake Inhibitors).

Anticonvulsants (*See also* Chapter 5)

PHENYTOIN

Contradictory evidence has emerged concerning the possibility of interaction between tricyclic antidepressants and phenytoin. In one study, three subjects were given amitriptyline 25 mg twice daily with and without phenytoin (Pond et al. 1975). Phenytoin elimination half-lives did not differ during concurrent treatment. Another report, however, suggested that phenytoin levels increased in two patients after imipramine was discontinued (Perucca et al. 1977). These patients had been receiving imipramine 75 mg daily over a 3-month period, with increasing serum levels of phenytoin (1 patient increased from 30 to 60 mmol/L, 7.6 to 15.1 mg/L). When imipramine was discontinued, levels fell. This case was complicated by the co-administration of nitrazepam and clonazepam in one patient, and sodium valproate and carbamazepine in the other. Another study showed that nortriptyline 75 mg daily produced a small increase in phenytoin levels (Houghton et al. 1975). A case report described an elevation of phenytoin levels from therapeutic levels (10 to 20 μmg/mL) to 46 μmg/mL after 4 months of trazodone 500 mg/day. The patient complained of dizziness and weakness, which abated when trazodone was reduced to 400 mg/day and phenytoin from 300 mg to 200 mg/day (Dorn 1986).

VALPROATE

Conflicting data exist on the possible interaction of cyclic antidepressants and valproate. One study reported a rise in desipramine serum concentrations from 246 ng/mL to 324 ng/mL after valproate therapy was discontinued (Joseph et al. 1993). On the other hand, another report described increased levels of amitriptyline and nortriptyline when amitriptyline was prescribed with valproic acid (Vandel et al. 1988). Other studies also have reported increases in amitriptyline/nortriptyline levels in the presence of valproate (Bertschy et al. 1990). A similar interaction has been reported with clomipramine(Fehr et al. 2000).

CARBAMAZEPINE

In a study, 36 children with attention deficit disorder were treated either with imipramine alone or imipramine with carbamazepine (Brown 1992). Despite receiving higher doses of desipramine, children in the combined treatment group had lower serum antidepressant levels, suggesting that carbamazepine induced drug metabolism. Carbamazepine co-treatment also increased desipramine clearance (Spina et al. 1995) and lowered levels of desipramine in other studies (Baldessarini et al. 1988). Another study found lower total levels of imipramine and desipramine when the former drug was administered with carbamazepine, but free levels did not change (Szymura-Oleksiak et al. 2001). In a 10-year study of almost 3,000 patients, comparisons were made between the concentration-to-dose ratio of patients taking only an antidepressant and those taking an antidepressant plus carbamazepine (Jerling et al. 1994b). The mean ratio of amitriptyline and nortriptyline was 50% lower in patients taking both carbamazepine and an antidepressant, compared with those taking the antidepressant alone, suggesting significant enzyme induction by carbamazepine.

MECHANISM

The mechanism of interaction with phenytoin is unknown. Valproate may impair the metabolism of some cyclic antidepressants, but additional data are needed. Carbamazepine is a well-known enzyme inducer (CYP2C9, CYP3A4) and lowers the serum levels of many drugs that undergo oxidative hepatic metabolism.

CLINICAL IMPLICATIONS

The interaction with phenytoin is not well established, but clinicians should be aware that it is possible that phenytoin levels may increase with antidepressant co-administration. More frequent monitoring of phenytoin levels may be necessary. Frequent monitoring of antidepressant levels during concurrent therapy with valproate or carbamazepine is warranted.

Antihypertensives (*See also* Reserpine, this section)

EVIDENCE OF INTERACTION

The interaction between the tricyclic antidepressants and guanethidine is well established. Imipramine 75 mg/day antagonized the antihypertensive effects of guanethidine in three hypertensive patients (Leishman et al. 1963). In that study, the effective dose of guanethidine (or bethanidine, debrisoquin, or methyldopa) was determined clinically and given throughout the study period. After 5 days of antihypertensive treatment, desipramine (70 mg [$N = 9$], 125 mg [$N = 1$], 50 mg [$N = 3$], 150 mg [$N = 1$]), or protriptyline (20 mg daily [$N = 1$]) was added to the treatment regimen. Altogether, seven patients were taking guanethidine, three were taking bethanidine, two were taking debrisoquin, and three were taking methyldopa (two patients were studied twice). Desipramine and protriptyline reversed the antihypertensive effects of guanethidine in every patient. The reversal of the effect of guanethidine required 1 to 2 days for maximum antagonism, whereas reversal of bethanidine or debrisoquin occurred within a few hours. No patients had a rise in pressure greater than their pre-study level. After discontinuation of the antidepressant, 5 to 7 days were required for the antihypertensive action to reappear (for the two patients receiving 125 and 150 mg, 10 days were necessary for return of effect). The action of methyldopa was not antagonized by desipramine (*see below*).

Probably all cyclic antidepressants that inhibit the reuptake of norepinephrine block the antihypertensive effect of guanethidine. Amitriptyline 75 mg/day was administered to a patient receiving guanethidine 75 mg/day, methyldopa 750 mg/day, and trichlormethiazide 8 mg/day. Five days after the initiation of amitriptyline treatment, a reversal of antihypertensive effect was seen, requiring an increase in the guanethidine dose (to 300 mg/day). Amitriptyline was discontinued, and 18 days were required to overcome the antagonism (Meyer et al. 1970). Differences between the onset of, and recovery from, antagonism of amitriptyline and desipramine may be related to the relative abilities of the drugs and their metabolites to influence noradrenergic function. Desipramine is highly noradrenergic, whereas amitriptyline is less so (its demethylated metabolite, nortriptyline, has substantial noradrenergic effects).

Studies that have not found an antidepressant-induced reversal of the antihypertensive effects of guanethidine are misleading, because they observed patients for too short a period (8 and 12 hours), whereas the antagonism develops after 1 or 2 days (Gulati et al. 1966, Ober et al. 1973).

A single case report described cardiac standstill in a 37-year-old man taking both guanethidine 125 mg/day (after failure to control hypertension with methyldopa and intramuscular hydralazine) and imipramine 75 mg daily in divided doses. It is not possible to definitively attribute these cardiac complications to a drug interaction.

Other antihypertensives also have been investigated with respect to a possible interaction with antidepressants. Although animal data suggest that the hypotensive effect of methyldopa may be antagonized by antidepressants, human studies do not support an interaction. After the intravertebral artery infusion of tricyclic antidepressants to anesthetized cats, methyldopa 20 mg/kg was administered via the same route. The usual hypotensive effect of methyldopa was blocked by both imipramine and desipramine 300 μmg/kg (van Zwieten 1975). Similar findings have been reported after intraventricular injection in rats (Finch 1975). Studies of humans, on the other hand, have not confirmed the animal findings. Five male volunteers (one "mildly hypertensive") were given either desipramine 25 mg 3 times daily or placebo in a double-blind crossover design 2 weeks apart. After 4 days of antidepressant or placebo, methyldopa 750 mg was administered. Desipramine did not reduce the hypotensive effect. This study confirmed the findings of Mitchell et al. (1970), who found no interaction in three patients receiving that combination.

The hypotensive effect of clonidine may be antagonized during concurrent antidepressant therapy. Briant et al. (1973) studied five hypertensive patients maintained on clonidine plus a diuretic for

2 to 3 years. Desipramine 75 mg/day or placebo was added to the drug regimen, and the antidepressant caused a rise in blood pressure in four of five patients, averaging 22/15 mm Hg supine, 12/11 mm Hg standing. In one patient, the blood pressure increased within 24 hours of taking the active drug. Another report described a woman whose blood pressure was controlled with clonidine 0.4 mg daily until she was given 50 mg per day of imipramine for 2 days, after which her blood pressure rose to 230/130 mm Hg (Hui 1983). Trazodone also antagonized clonidine (Hansten 1984).

Animal data support these findings. Van Zwieten (1975) found that the hypotensive effect of intravenously administered clonidine 1 μmg/kg was antagonized in anesthetized cats pretreated with desipramine, imipramine, amitriptyline, protriptyline, and mianserin. Another study found that single doses of desipramine and amitriptyline attenuated clonidine-induced electroencephalogram synchronization in rats, whereas mianserin potentiated it (Kostowski et al. 1984). Chronic antidepressant administration (14 days) either completely (desipramine, amitriptyline) or partially (mianserin) reduced the effect of clonidine. Other evidence suggested that mianserin did not reverse the antihypertensive effects of clonidine or methyldopa (Elliott et al. 1981, Elliott et al. 1983). Although maprotiline reversed the antihypertensive effect of bethanidine, guanethidine, and debrisoquin, it did not alter the antihypertensive response to clonidine (Gundert-Remy et al. 1983).

Lower doses of cyclic antidepressants may be required when diltiazem, verapamil, or labetalol are prescribed concurrently. Twelve healthy male volunteers received a 7-day course of verapamil 120 mg every 8 hours, diltiazem 90 mg every 8 hours, labetalol 200 mg every 12 hours, or placebo (Hermann et al. 1992). On the 4th day of the study period, imipramine (a single 100-mg oral dose) was administered. Verapamil, diltiazem, and labetalol increased the imipramine plasma versus time area-under-the-curve (AUC) by 15%, 30%, and 53%, respectively. No consistent changes were found in the levels of the primary metabolites—desipramine, 2-hydroxyimipramine, or 2-hydroxydesipramine. Propranolol may impair the metabolism of maprotiline (Saiz-Ruiz et al. 1988, Tollefson et al. 1984). Nifedipine has been implicated in the reversal of antidepressant response (Fadden 1992, Hullett et al. 1988), but the effect of nifedipine in animal models of depression is not entirely consistent with the case reports (Kostowski et al. 1990).

MECHANISM

Guanethidine and related antihypertensives (bethanidine, debrisoquin) are taken up into noradrenergic neurons by the same pump that is responsible for the reuptake of norepinephrine. Tricyclic antidepressants block this pump, preventing guanethidine from reaching its site of action.

Clonidine is known to activate the presynaptic α-adrenoreceptors, which provide a negative feedback system in the peripheral and central nervous system. In vitro preparations of rat cerebral cortex slices were used to demonstrate that desipramine antagonized the inhibitory effect of clonidine on central adrenergic neurotransmission, perhaps by altering the sensitivity of the presynaptic receptor (Dubocovich et al. 1979). One study found no interaction between nortriptyline, imipramine, and desmethyldoxepin on platelet α_2-adrenoreceptors (Barnes et al. 1982).

Verapamil and diltiazem inhibit the metabolism of drugs oxidized by the cytochrome P450-3A4 isoenzyme.

Some β-blockers (e.g. propranolol, labetalol) may be susceptible to interactions involving CYP2D6.

CLINICAL IMPLICATIONS

Guanethidine (and the related antihypertensives bethanidine, debrisoquin) should not be used with antidepressants that block the neuronal noradrenergic reuptake pump (Table 2.4). Doses of doxepin less than 100 mg probably do not antagonize the hypotensive effect, but this may not produce an adequate antidepressant effect. Clonidine (and the related antihypertensives guanabenz and guanfacine) also should be avoided. Hypertensive crises have been reported when clonidine and tricyclics are co-administered (Briant et al. 1973, Hui 1983). Bupropion and maprotiline do not interact with clonidine. The withdrawal syndrome associated with clonidine, characterized by rebound hypertension and tachycardia, may be exacerbated by amitriptyline and possibly other antidepressants (Stiff et al. 1983).

Methyldopa and thiazide diuretics are safe to use, but caution must be observed to avoid hypotension, especially in the elderly. Potassium must be monitored when the thiazides are used, because hypokalemia may increase cardiac irritability and the chance of arrhythmia. Some evidence suggests that mianserin does not reverse the antihypertensive effects of clonidine or methyldopa (Elliott et al. 1981, Elliott et al. 1983). Although maprotiline reverses the antihypertensive effect of bethanidine, guanethidine, and debrisoquin, it does not alter the antihypertensive response to clonidine (Gundert-Remy et al. 1983).

Verapamil (Calan and others) and diltiazem (Cardizem) may impair the metabolism of imipramine and other psychotropic medications metabolized by the cytochrome P450-3A4 isoenzyme. Dosage reductions of the antidepressant may be required. Some β-blockers (e.g., propranolol, labetalol) may be susceptible to interactions involving CYP2D6. (Also see Reserpine, this section, and specific antihypertensive

(text continues on page 67)

TABLE 2.4. ANTIDEPRESSANT INTERACTIONS WITH COMMONLY USED ANTIHYPERTENSIVE AGENTS

THIAZIDE DIURETICS	Lithium levels are doubled with typical therapeutic doses of thiazides.
	Hypotensive response exaggerated with MAOI, but may be possible with any antidepressants that induce orthostatic hypotension (e.g., TCA).
β-BLOCKERS	
Cytochromes and β-Blockers	
Atenolol	Renal excretion
Bisoprolol	2D6, 3A4 substrate
Carteolol	2D6 substrate
Carvedilol	2D6, 2C9, 3A4 substrate
Esmolol	Esterases
Labelotol	2D6 substrate and inhibitor
Metoprolol	2D6 substrate
Nadolol	Renal
Penbutolol	2D6 substrate
Pindolol	2D6 substrate and inhibitor
Propranolol	2D6 substrate and inhibitor, 1A2, 2C19 substrate
Sotalol	Renal
Timolol	2D6 substrate
Antidepressants and β-Blockers	
Bupropion	Inhibits 2D6
MAOI	Bradycardia reported
SSRI (3A4 and 2D6 inhibitors may interact, use renally excreted β-blockers, such as atenolol)	
Fluoxetine	Metoprolol induced lethargy and bradycardia. Sotalol no interaction (not metabolized by 2D6)
Fluvoxamine	Large increases in propranolol concentration, but not in β-blockade or hypotensive effect. Also inhibits

(continued)

TABLE 2.4. ANTIDEPRESSANT INTERACTIONS WITH COMMONLY USED ANTIHYPERTENSIVE AGENTS (CONTINUED)

	metoprolol metabolism with adverse effects (hypotension, bradycardia).
Sertraline	No PK interaction
Paroxetine	In a PK study, paroxetine increased metoprolol C_{max}, elimination half-life, and produced prolonged β-blockade. There is also stereospecific inhibition of carvedilol metabolism. The AUC of the R(+) enantiomer increased 77% with the combination, but there was no increase in β-blockade or adverse effects.
Imipramine	Labetalol increases imipramine AUC and C_{max}. Propranolol leads to heartblock.
Maprotiline	Case report of increased propranolol levels, another of visual hallucinations.
ANGIOTENSIN CONVERTING ENZYME (ACE) INHIBITORS	
Quinapril (Accupril®), Captopril, Enalapril, Lisinopril	Renal excretion increases lithium levels and toxicity.
ANGIOTENSIN RECEPTOR BLOCKERS	
Candesartan	Not significantly metabolized by P450
Irbesartan	2C9 substrate
Olmesartan	Not significantly metabolized by P450
Losartan	2C9 (major) 3A4 (minor) substrate
Valsartan	Not identified, but not P450
Telmisartan	Eliminated unchanged, P450 not involved
Eprosartan	Eliminated unchanged, P450 not involved
CALCIUM CHANNEL BLOCKERS (3A4 inhibitors such as nefazodone interact)	
Verapamil	Verapamil is metabolized by 3A4, 1A2, and 2C. Important interactions reported with 3A4 inhibitors and inducers.
Diltiazem	Diltiazem is both a substrate and inhibitor of 3A4.
Nifedipine, Felodipine, Nisoldipine, Isradipine	3A4 substrate

agents under the sections on Selective Serotonin Reuptake Inhibitors and Monoamine Oxidase Inhibitors).

Antipsychotics (*See* Chapter 3)

Antimicrobials

EVIDENCE OF INTERACTION

Rifampin may induce the metabolism of tricyclic antidepressants. A patient treated with a combination of rifampin, isoniazid, pyrazinamide, and pyridoxine was given nortriptyline 175 mg daily, to achieve antidepressant serum levels of 193 mmol/L (Bebchuk et al. 1991). Following the discontinuation of rifampin and isoniazid, nortriptyline serum levels rose to 671 mmol/L, accompanied by adverse effects. The reduction of nortriptyline to 75 mg daily resulted in a return to therapeutic levels of the antidepressant. A 43-year-old woman who was taking nortriptyline (75 mg daily) did not have detectable serum nortriptyline levels while taking concomitant rifampin (Self et al. 1996). Nortriptyline levels of 76 ng/mL and 140 ng/mL were reported 2 and 4 weeks after rifampin was discontinued.

In another case report (Gannon et al. 1992), a 65-year-old woman was taking nortriptyline 75 mg daily for 1 year, prior to taking fluconazole (Diflucan). Twelve days after the addition of the antifungal agent, the serum nortriptyline level rose to 252 ng/mL from a baseline of 149 ng/mL. A similar interaction was reported in a 12-year-old boy taking amitriptyline and fluconazole (Robinson et al. 2000). In that case, amitriptyline 50 mg twice daily was prescribed for neuropathic pain. Four days after starting fluconazole (200 mg), the patient experienced syncopal episodes. Three other cases of a fluconazole–amitriptyline interaction have been reported in men, with two of them resulting in toxicity characterized by visual hallucinations, delirium, cardiac arrest, and death (Newberry et al. 1997). Elevated serum amitriptyline levels (724 ng/mL, 349 ng/mL, 1224 ng/mL) were reported despite doses of amitriptyline of only 50 to 150 mg daily. The combination has also been linked to torsades de pointes.

The interaction of ketoconazole (200 mg/day) for 14 days with either imipramine (100 mg single oral dose) or desipramine (100 mg single oral dose) was studied in two groups of six healthy men (Spina et al. 1997). Imipramine clearance was decreased and its elimination impaired in the presence of ketoconazole, whereas desipramine metabolism was unaffected. Although the changes in imipramine were modest (about 20%), individuals at high risk such as children, elderly, or individuals with cardiac disease, may be susceptible to adverse effects.

Terbinafine (Lamisil) also inhibits the metabolism of antidepressants metabolized by CYP2D6. A 74-year-old man taking terbinafine for onychomycosis developed nortriptyline toxicity and doubling of serum nortriptyline levels within a week of the addition of the antifungal agent (van der Kuy et al. 1998). An even greater inhibition of metabolism has been observed with the combination of desipramine and terbinafine, with fivefold increases in tricyclic plasma levels reported (O'Reardon et al. 2002, van der Kuy et al. 2002). Similar interactions have been reported for imipramine and terbinafine (Madani et al. 2002, Teitelbaum et al. 2001). The protease inhibitor ritonavir inhibits CYP3A and impairs the metabolism of trazodone (Greenblatt et al. 2003). A single-dose four-way crossover study was conducted in 10 healthy volunteers who received a single 50 mg dose of trazodone or placebo while taking 4 doses of 200 mg of ritonavir or placebo. The ritonavir condition was associated with impaired trazodone clearance, prolonged elimination half life, and increased C_{max}. In addition, the combination was associated with greater sedation, fatigue, and psychomotor impairment. Three subjects reported nausea, dizziness, or hypotension, and one developed syncope. All protease inhibitors are substrates and inhibitors of 3A4. Protease inhibitors include ritonavir, indinavir, lopinavir, nelfinavir, amprenavir, and saquinavir. Ritonavir and nelfinavir also inhibit 2D6, which may lead to other pharmacokinetic interactions with antidepressants. Further complicating the matter is the role of P-glycoprotein (P-gp) in the pharmacokinetics of protease inhibitors. P-gp serves as a pump in the gastrointestinal tract, the liver, the kidney, and the BBB, and alterations may be involved in drug interactions involving the protease inhibitors (de Maat et al. 2003). The nonnucleoside reverse transcriptase inhibitors (delavirdine, efavirenz, nevirapine) are also substrates for 3A4 (among others). Delavirdine inhibits 3A4; efavirenz may induce or inhibit 3A4, and inhibits 2C9/19; nevirapine induces 3A4 and 2B6. The nucleoside reverse transcriptase inhibitors (abacavir, didanosine, lamivudine, stavudine, zalcitabine, zidovudine) do not induce or inhibit cytochromes.

MECHANISM

Rifampin is a potent inducer of oxidative metabolism, whereas fluconazole and related antifungals (ketoconazole, itraconazole) inhibit the metabolism of some drugs (especially those metabolized by CYP3A4, CYP2C19, and CYP2C9). Terbinafine inhibits CYP2D6. The non-nucleoside reverse transcriptase inhibitors (delavirdine, efavirenz, nevirapine) are also substrates for 3A4 (among others). Delavirdine inhibits 3A4; efavirenz may induce or inhibit 3A4, and inhibits 2C9/19; nevirapine induces 3A4 and 2B6. The nucleoside reverse transcriptase inhibitors (abacavir, didanosine, lamivudine, stavudine, zalcitabine, zidovudine) do not induce or inhibit cytochromes.

CLINICAL IMPLICATIONS

When rifampin is discontinued after concurrent therapy with nortriptyline or related antidepressants, the dosage of the antidepressant must be lowered. When fluconazole, ketoconazole, or itraconazole are prescribed concurrently with antidepressants, serum levels of the antidepressant should be monitored, and clinicians should observe patients for signs and symptoms of toxicity. The same is true when terbinafine is prescribed with tricyclic antidepressants. Some quinolones, such as sparfloxacin and grepafloxacin, may produce additive prolongation of the QT_C interval and should not be used with tricyclic antidepressants. HIV therapy with protease inhibitors and some non-nucleoside reverse transcriptase inhibitors may lead to pharmacokinetic interactions with co-administered drugs.

Barbiturates

EVIDENCE OF INTERACTION

Several reports suggest that barbiturates decrease the plasma levels of antidepressants. One patient who had been receiving 100 mg of phenobarbital for 14 days had a 50% decrease in desipramine levels (Hammer et al. 1967). In a study of nortriptyline pharmacokinetics in identical twins, concurrent barbiturate treatment resulted in a 30% reduction in nortriptyline levels (Alexanderson et al. 1969). That study also found lower steady-state nortriptyline plasma levels in subjects treated with antidepressant plus barbiturate than with antidepressant alone. In another single case, amobarbital 200 mg at bedtime for 5 days reduced nortriptyline plasma levels (Burrows et al. 1971). In a report of three patients taking nortriptyline who had amobarbital added, statistically significant decreases in serum nortriptyline levels were seen only after 10 days of concurrent drug therapy (Silverman et al. 1972). Protriptyline levels also may be decreased with the co-administration of barbiturates (Moody et al. 1977).

MECHANISM

Barbiturates induce hepatic enzymes and enhance antidepressant metabolism.

CLINICAL IMPLICATIONS

The role of barbiturates in clinical psychopharmacology is limited. Given their high abuse potential, lethality in overdoses, and enzyme induction, they are of limited usefulness in depressed patients. Benzodiazepine anx-iolytics and hypnotics are safer and easier to use. Should barbiturates be used, however, plasma levels of antidepressants should be monitored.

Bupropion and Tricyclics

EVIDENCE OF INTERACTION

The metabolism of desipramine, imipramine, nortriptyline, and other tri-cyclic antidepressants may be impaired when administered to patients taking bupropion. Although bupropion was approved by the FDA in 1985, and introduced to the U.S. market in 1989, reports of a potential pharmacokinetic interaction with other antidepressants did not begin to appear until 1997. Mujeeb and Preskorn published a report of imipramine levels over an 8-year period for a 64-year-old woman who had taken the tricyclic antidepressant alone (in doses of 150 or 200 mg/day) and with bupropion (225 mg/day). In another report, a 62-year-old woman with depression was treated with trimipramine to which bupropion was added at a dose of 150 mg twice daily. The plasma levels of the tricyclic antidepressant increased from 305 ng/mL to 565 ng/mL and resulted in generalized seizures and unresponsiveness (Enns 2001). The only other report of the interaction is of an 83-year-old woman who was treated with nortriptyline 75 mg at bedtime with a plasma level of 96 ng/mL and was also prescribed bupropion 150 mg twice daily. Using the combination, she had a 200% increase in nortriptyline level and developed confusion, lethargy, and falling episodes (Weintraub 2001). The manufacturer's product information cautions about the concomi-tant use of bupropion and desipramine, because with the combination, the latter agent may have serum levels twice that seen with monotherapy.

MECHANISM

Bupropion inhibits 2D6.

CLINICAL IMPLICATIONS

Dosage adjustments may be required when starting or stopping this combination.

Cholestyramine

An in vitro study found that cholestyramine (Questran) bound amitrip-tyline, desipramine, doxepin, imipramine, and nortriptyline (Bailey et al. 1992). Lower antidepressant serum levels and clinical deterioration has been reported (Geeze et al. 1988, Spina et al. 1994). Patients should take their antidepressant dose 2 hours before or 4 hours after cholestyramine.

Digoxin

EVIDENCE OF INTERACTION

Two reports were published of digoxin toxicity occurring after the addition of trazodone (Dec et al. 1984, Rauch et al. 1984). In one patient, the serum digoxin concentration rose from 0.8 to 2.8 ng/mL after 11 days of trazodone therapy. In a canine model, however, no elevation of serum digoxin level was found during combined digoxin–trazodone therapy.

MECHANISM

Not established.

CLINICAL IMPLICATIONS

Insufficient evidence exists to establish this as an important interaction. Clinicians may wish to closely monitor digoxin levels if trazodone is administered concurrently.

Disulfiram

Maany and associates (1982) described two cases of patients who developed acute organic brain syndrome while receiving disulfiram in combination with amitriptyline. The symptoms included confusion, hallucinations, disorientation, and memory loss. MacCallum (1969) reported that, in his experience, amitriptyline potentiated the effect of disulfiram, allowing the use of smaller doses of the latter drug. The effects of amitriptyline on disulfiram metabolism have not been studied but it has been suggested that the increase of the effects of disulfiram may be due to the increase in the rate of buildup of acetaldehyde. Alternatively, amitriptyline may potentiate the actions of ethanol, which could result in a more severe disulfiram interaction.

Disulfiram markedly inhibited the metabolism of imipramine and desipramine (Ciraulo et al. 1985). Two subjects who had been detoxicated from ethanol within 2 weeks received imipramine alone (12.5 mg intravenously) and again following 4 weeks of disulfiram treatment (500 mg daily). One of the subjects also received desipramine (12.5 mg intravenously) under the same conditions. For imipramine, the total AUC increased 32.5% and 26.8% after disulfiram administration. The elimination half-lives were also increased 18.3% and 13.6%. Disulfiram resulted in a decrease of 24.5% and 21.3% in total body clearance of imipramine. Similar findings were found in the desipramine subject, in whom disulfiram treatment resulted in a 32.3% larger AUC, an increase of 19.8% in elimination half-life, and a decrease in total body clearance of 24.3%. This interaction could lead to toxicity due to systemic availability of the antidepressant after oral administration, an increase in the time required to reach steady-state, and an increase in plasma levels above the therapeutic range. This may explain the toxicity described by Maany and associates (1982).

Estrogens

EVIDENCE OF INTERACTION

Some studies suggest that an interaction occurs between estradiol or conjugated estrogens and imipramine.

In one study, 30 women with a diagnosis of primary depression were given either placebo, imipramine plus placebo, or ethinyl estradiol in doses either 25 or 50 μmg/day orally (Khurana 1972). Side effects occurred more commonly with the imipramine–estradiol combination and included tremor, hypotension, and drowsiness. Serum levels of antidepressants were not measured.

Another study examining oral contraceptives and clomipramine was unable to find evidence of increased toxicity (Beaumont 1973). The lower estrogen doses administered in that study probably account for the absence of untoward effects.

A study of 10 women on long-term, low-dose estrogen oral contraceptive steroids found that after a single oral dose of imipramine 50 mg, absolute systemic bioavailability increased, resulting in decreased apparent oral clearance without a change in oral elimination half-life when compared with controls (Abernethy et al. 1984a). After intravenous imipramine 12.5 mg, elimination half-life was prolonged in the contraceptive users, but clearance and volume of distribution were similar to those of control subjects. These findings suggest that lower doses of imipramine should be used when patients are taking oral contraceptives.

MECHANISM

Estrogenic compounds may impair the N-oxidation and demethylation of imipramine. Ethinyl estradiol inhibits the metabolism of ethylmorphine and hexobarbital in rats (Tephly et al. 1968). Furthermore, other steroids, such as norethindrone (a progestogen), inhibit the metabolism of antipyrine in women (Field et al. 1979) and imipramine in mice (Bellward et al. 1974).

CLINICAL IMPLICATIONS

Several clinical situations occur in which estrogens are used, including oral contraception, menopause, atrophic vaginitis, dysmenorrhea, dysfunctional bleeding (although the cyclic use of progestin is usually preferred), acne, hirsutism, osteoporosis, breast cancer, and suppression of postpartum lactation. Many of these clinical problems are also associated with depression, so that the combination of an estrogen and antidepressant is not uncommon. Although the potential for increased toxicity should be kept in mind, if side effects are carefully monitored and the imipramine dosage increased slowly, this drug combination is safe to use.

Ethanol (*See also section on* Selective Serotonin Reuptake Inhibitors and Ethanol)

EVIDENCE OF INTERACTION

Cyclic antidepressants may interact with alcohol to produce (a) enhanced sedation and impairment of psychomotor skills, (b) enhanced metabolism of the antidepressant, and/or (c) delayed absorption of alcohol from the gut.

Impairment of psychomotor skills has been evaluated with amitriptyline, nortriptyline, doxepin, clomipramine, trazodone, zimelidine, and bupropion. In one study, amitriptyline 0.8 mg/kg orally was administered the night before and the morning of alcohol consumption (to produce a blood alcohol level of 80 mg/100 mL), the morning of the test only, or not at all (placebo on two occasions). Both amitriptyline-treated groups showed impairment of driving skills (Landauer et al. 1969). Another study investigated the effect of 5 days of treatment with amitriptyline (100 mg daily in 2 divided doses) or placebo. Despite the production of blood alcohol levels similar to those in the previous study, no differences in driving performance were found between the amitriptyline and the placebo groups (Patman et al. 1969).

A study of nortriptyline–alcohol interactions showed that nortriptyline (40 to 100 mg during 24 hours prior to ethanol) tended to improve scores on an audio feedback test given when the subject had a blood alcohol level of 50 mg/100 mL. The short period of drug administration limits the clinical significance of this finding (Hughes et al. 1963). Doxepin has been studied in two experiments. In the first, 22 subjects received doxepin ($12–25$ mg/m^2) plus alcohol to the point of intoxication (producing an average blood alcohol level of 73.6 mg/100 mL). This group had better scores on a driving test than a group of 12 control subjects who received alcohol alone (Milner et al. 1978). The second study compared doxepin to amitriptyline, nortriptyline (all were given 30 and 60 mg/day for 7 days), and clomipramine (30 and 75 mg/day for 7 days each). These agents were probably not equipotent, so the comparison once again suffers.

Despite this shortcoming, the important observation was made that the impairment effect diminishes with time. Impairment of psychomotor skills was seen after 7 days of treatment with amitriptyline or doxepin (when blood alcohol levels were 0.47%), but not after an additional 7 days (at twice the dose) (Seppala et al. 1975). Dorian et al. (1983) found that acute ethanol ingestion decreased apparent oral clearance of amitriptyline, impaired memory, and increased body sway.

Single doses of trazodone 100 mg, amitriptyline 50 mg, or placebo were administered alone or with ethanol 0.5 mL/kg to six healthy volunteers in a double-blind crossover study (Warrington et al. 1986). Both trazodone and amitriptyline impaired performance on critical flicker fusion frequency, choice reaction time, and manual dexterity. The antidepressants also increased drowsiness and reduced "clear-headedness," aggression, and inhibition. Ethanol alone, at mean blood concentrations that did not exceed 30 mg/100 mL, had similar pharmacodynamic effects. Ethanol, in combination with either antidepressant, caused a greater impairment in manual dexterity than was seen with the antidepressant alone. Blood alcohol levels were not altered by trazodone or amitriptyline. The time to reach maximum trazodone concentration was prolonged by ethanol co-administration, but all other pharmacokinetic parameters for trazodone and amitriptyline were not significantly affected by ethanol.

In another study, zimelidine 200 mg/24 hours was administered for 10 days to 12 healthy men, and ethanol 0.5 and 1.0 g/kg or placebo drinks were administered with either placebo capsules or zimelidine in the last 3 treatment days (Linnoila et al. 1985). Although the higher dose of ethanol increased plasma zimelidine and norzimelidine concentrations, no significant interactions were noted on a battery of tests measuring skilled performance.

Another study examined the interaction of ethanol with bupropion (Hamilton et al. 1984). In 12 healthy volunteers, bupropion (100 mg) reversed alcoholic-induced sedation, impairment of auditory vigilance, and some of the drug's effects on the electroencephalogram. The subjective sense of inebriation was not reversed by bupropion.

Amitriptyline may enhance alcohol-induced euphoria (Hyatt et al. 1987). Three men with alcohol abuse/dependence used amitriptyline in doses of 200 to 500 mg in combination with ethanol to "stay high cheaply." They reported that when taking amitriptyline, they required smaller amounts of ethanol to become intoxicated.

The second type of alcohol–antidepressant interaction is the enhanced metabolism of the tricyclic antidepressant. In a study of recently detoxified inpatient alcoholics ($N = 11$) and depressed nonalcoholic controls

($N = 12$) treated with imipramine (50 mg three times a day orally), the former group had lower plasma levels of imipramine and 2-hydroxyimipramine, as well as a lower total (imipramine, desipramine, and their two hydroxy metabolites) than did control subjects. Alcoholics were noted to have persistent depression, whereas the control group had significant improvement in depression (as measured by the Beck Depression Inventory) (Ciraulo et al. 1982). A follow-up study by the same investigators (Ciraulo et al. 1988a) found that alcoholics had a threefold greater intrinsic clearance of unbound imipramine than nonalcoholic controls and an approximately twofold decrease in elimination half-life. Desipramine clearance was affected to a greater extent than imipramine, although intravenous clearance was significantly greater in alcoholics. 2-Hydroxyimipramine, a metabolite of imipramine, also was cleared more rapidly in alcoholics (Ciraulo et al. 1990a).

In a study of amitriptyline in 10 alcoholic and 11 nonalcoholic depressed patients, alcoholics had lower steady-state nortriptyline levels (a metabolite of amitriptyline) (Sandoz et al. 1983). Plasma levels of amitriptyline, hydroxyamitriptyline, and hydroxynortriptyline were not different between groups. These findings are puzzling, because most studies indicate that demethylation is induced by chronic ethanol consumption. The large intersubject differences in a small sample may account for a failure to find differences in amitriptyline levels. Furthermore, alcoholics received a mean dose 25 mg greater than nonalcoholics.

The final type of interaction is a delay in ethanol absorption when desipramine is given concurrently (Hall et al. 1976).

MECHANISM

The mechanisms for the pharmacokinetic (metabolic) interaction are easiest to identify. The chronic administration of ethanol to humans causes a proliferation of the smooth endoplasmic reticulum, increases microsomal protein and cytochrome P450, and often results in the augmentation of the drug-metabolizing capability of the liver. Although alcoholics are often cigarette smokers, the antidepressant studies (Ciraulo et al. 1982, Ciraulo et al. 1988a) controlled for this factor.

The delayed absorption of alcohol in the presence of desipramine is most likely due to impaired gastric emptying, secondary to the anticholinergic effect of desipramine.

Impairment of psychomotor skills and enhanced high, when certain tricyclic antidepressants and alcohol are given concomitantly, are most likely results of receptor site interactions, although specifics are not known.

CLINICAL IMPLICATIONS

Studies of psychomotor alterations during combined antidepressant treatment and alcohol consumption present conflicting data, which are difficult to interpret in light of an obvious clinical interaction. It is our impression that most, if not all, tricyclic antidepressants enhance the sedative effects and psychomotor impairment induced by ethanol. Perhaps the less sedating agents (e.g., nortriptyline) interact to a lesser degree. Certainly, bupropion and SSRIs show little interaction with ethanol.

With tricyclic antidepressants and ethanol, patients often say they feel intoxicated after fewer drinks. We advise patients to reduce or discontinue the consumption of alcoholic beverages during antidepressant treatment. For those who continue to drink, tolerance to the interaction often develops.

With regard to the finding of lower plasma levels of imipramine and desipramine in chronic alcoholics, as compared with depressed control subjects, higher doses of tricyclic antidepressants may be needed to achieve the therapeutic plasma levels early in abstinence. Depression, anxiety, and phobias are prominent symptoms among alcoholics and may require treatment with antidepressants. Some studies indicate a possible role for desipramine (Mason et al. 1991) and imipramine (Nunes et al. 1993) in depressed alcoholics.

Grapefruit Juice

Grapefruit juice inhibits CYP1A2 and 3A3/4, resulting in an increase in the clomipramine to desmethyl–clomipramine ratio, which may be associated with improved therapeutic effect in obsessive-compulsive disorder (OCD; Oesterheld et al. 1997).

High-Fiber Diet

High fiber diets may decrease the absorption of antidepressants (Stewart 1992).

Histamine$_2$-Blocking Agents

EVIDENCE OF INTERACTION

Several reports have established that cimetidine may impair the metabolism of tricyclic antidepressants, leading to elevated plasma levels and toxicity.

Anticholinergic toxicity developed in one patient who was taking cimetidine 1,200 mg/day upon initiation of moderate doses of imipramine 125 mg/day. Steady-state concentrations of imipramine increased from 187 to 341 ng/mL and elimination half-life from 22.8 to 43.7 hours (Miller et al. 1983a). Another patient taking both cimetidine and nortriptyline had an average 42% higher nortriptyline serum concentration on the drug combination (Miller et al. 1983b).

In a study of six subjects given imipramine 12.5 mg intravenously or 50 mg orally, alone and with cimetidine, imipramine clearance was reduced 41%, whereas bioavailability was increased (from 40% to 75%) with concurrent cimetidine. Such an interaction could lead to important increases in imipramine plasma levels with chronic treatment (Abernethy et al. 1984b).

Another clinical study examined the interaction of cimetidine with either imipramine or nortriptyline (Henauer et al. 1984). Cimetidine decreased the clearance of imipramine and increased bioavailability. Cimetidine did not increase the bioavailability of nortriptyline, although peak levels and the AUC level versus time curve was increased for 10-hydroxynortriptyline, its active metabolite.

Cimetidine 600 mg twice daily, but not ranitidine 150 mg twice daily, increased serum doxepin levels in a study in healthy volunteers (Sutherland et al. 1987). Cimetidine also impaired the metabolism of nefazodone.

MECHANISM

Cimetidine impairs the hepatic metabolism of antidepressants. Although cimetidine-induced alterations of hepatic blood flow also are a possible mechanism of interaction, this is a less likely explanation.

CLINICAL IMPLICATIONS

Considerable evidence suggests that some antidepressants, such as imipramine, have a minimal plasma level required for optimal response and that other antidepressants, such as nortriptyline, have an optimal therapeutic range ("therapeutic window"). If cimetidine therapy were to be discontinued during chronic imipramine therapy, it is possible that levels of the antidepressant would drop below the minimal therapeutic concentration. On the other hand, if a patient had been stabilized on imipramine, and cimetidine was then added, toxicity could result. Symptoms of tricyclic antidepressant toxicity include tachycardia, large pupils, injected sclera, elevated temperature with dry skin, urinary retention, decreased gut motility, and CNS symptoms, such as anxiety, agitation, psychosis, disorientation, memory impairment, myoclonus, and seizures. The clinical implications of altered metabolite levels are not known.

The most reasonable clinical course is to substitute ranitidine, famotidine, or nizatidine for cimetidine. Ranitidine does not impair oxidative metabolism to the same extent as cimetidine (Abernethy et al. 1984a). Famotidine and nizatidine do not appear to have clinically significant interactions. Alternatively, plasma levels of antidepressants and their active metabolites should be monitored during the concurrent administration of cimetidine and antidepressants.

Levodopa

EVIDENCE OF INTERACTION

An absorption interaction between imipramine and levodopa has been reported in both animals and humans. Imipramine-treated rats retained approximately 30% of single dose of 14C-levodopa in their stomachs for 2 hours, compared with retention in rats that had not received imipramine (Morgan et al. 1975).

A similar interaction was found in humans (Morgan et al. 1975). The absorption of a single dose of 14C-levodopa 500 mg was studied in 4 male subjects after 3 days of administration of imipramine 25 mg 4 times a day and placebo. On the morning of sampling, subjects took one 25-mg tablet of imipramine 2 hours prior to receiving radioactively labeled levodopa through a nasogastric tube (which was also used to obtain samples of gastric juice). Polyethylene glycol also was administered as a marker compound to assess the degree of gastric emptying; it demonstrated that gastric emptying was impaired during imipramine treatment. In addition, total gastric juice radioactivity (from labeled levodopa) was 11% of the initial dose at 6 hours during imipramine treatment, whereas it was less than 0.1% on placebo. Plasma concentrations of radioactivity were significantly lower at 45 and 105 minutes in the levodopa–imipramine group. Although this study showed an impaired rate of absorption of levodopa, it did not establish a difference in the completeness of absorption between groups (24 hours cumulative urinary excretion of radioactivity was not significantly different between groups).

MECHANISM

The anticholinergic activity of imipramine impairs gastric motility, thus reducing the rate of absorption of other drugs. Some evidence suggests that levodopa is metabolized in the stomach and the gastrointestinal tract, thus producing the potential for a decrease in absolute amount of drug absorbed whenever transit time is slowed (Rivera-CalimLim et al. 1970).

CLINICAL IMPLICATIONS

The rate of absorption is not critical for drugs taken on a chronic basis. The combination of these agents may be commonplace in light of the frequent coexistence of depression and parkinsonism (Mindham 1970). There appears to be no evidence that the pharmacokinetic interaction is of clinical significance, and it is likely that effects on both cholinergic and catecholamine systems are either synergistic or additive in the treatment of parkinsonism.

Lithium (*See* Chapter 4)

Methadone

EVIDENCE OF INTERACTION

One study followed five men in a methadone maintenance program who had higher desipramine serum levels while taking methadone than while taking the antidepressant alone (Maany et al. 1989). The combination of methadone 0.5 mg/kg daily and desipramine 2.5 mg/kg daily increased serum antidepressant levels from 72.6% to 168.9%, compared with monotherapy.

MECHANISM

Methadone probably impairs the hydroxylation of desipramine.

CLINICAL IMPLICATIONS

The pharmacokinetic interactions of methadone with antidepressants are not well studied, although methadone probably impairs the metabolism of several cyclic antidepressants. Clinicians should monitor patients taking methadone and cyclic antidepressants for adverse effects. Serum antidepressant levels may be helpful in guiding the dosage in these patients.

Methylphenidate

EVIDENCE OF INTERACTION

Three clinical studies from the same group of investigators have suggested that methylphenidate increases the plasma levels of imipramine and its metabolite desmethylimipramine (Perel 1969, Wharton et al. 1971, Zeidenberg et al. 1971).

In their first report, the researchers indicated that the blood levels of parent drug and metabolite increased when methylphenidate was added to imipramine 150 mg every day. A follow-up study examined patients taking either 450 mg of imipramine alone daily or 150 mg of imipramine plus 20 mg of methylphenidate. One patient received dextroamphetamine 5 mg twice a day in place of methylphenidate. Blood levels were found to be highly variable from patient to patient, as was the effect of methylphenidate. In five patients, the ratios of imipramine concentrations at steady-state after 450 mg daily compared with imipramine 150 mg plus methylphenidate were 1.2, 1.2, 4.1, 2.7, and 1.6, indicating that methylphenidate increased plasma levels of imipramine, but the extent of the effect was highly variable.

The third study by the same group of investigators studied seven patients with "recurrent refractory psychotic depression." Six patients were treated with imipramine in varying doses (from 75 to 225 mg daily) and one with nortriptyline 25 mg three times daily for 3 weeks and then methylphenidate 10 mg twice daily for 10 to 21 days, followed by the original dose of tricyclic antidepressant given alone. Of the seven patients treated with the combination, five had "prompt, striking, complete clinical remission." The plasma levels of imipramine and desmethylimipramine rose following the addition of methylphenidate. Imipramine binding was not affected.

MECHANISM

Methylphenidate inhibits the metabolism of imipramine, leading to elevated plasma levels and increased therapeutic effect. Methylphenidate may possess some antidepressant activity in its own right, which may account for the dramatic improvement in cases of refractory depression.

CLINICAL IMPLICATIONS

Combined treatment with imipramine and methylphenidate may offer little advantage over merely increasing the imipramine dosage to obtain higher plasma levels. For those patients who require an immediate mood response, some clinicians administer methylphenidate when tricyclic antidepressant therapy is initiated. Due to unpredictable alterations in tricyclic drug plasma levels, we advise against this practice. In some cases of refractory depression, the addition of a stimulant to an antidepressant may be helpful (Feighner et al. 1985). A study in children indicated that the combination of methylphenidate and desipramine led to more complaints of nausea, dry mouth, tremor, and higher ventricular rates when compared to monotherapy (Pataki et al. 1993).

Monoamine Oxidase Inhibitors

EVIDENCE OF INTERACTION

Schuckit et al. (1971) reviewed the English language literature and found 25 case reports of morbidity in patients managed on combined therapy. After eliminating those cases in which a suicide attempt was made, other centrally acting drugs were taken, or the drugs were given parenterally, six of seven cases were reviewed in depth (one was omitted because of inadequate clinical details). The patients were all women between the ages of 37 and 66. All received imipramine; the monoamine oxidase inhibitors (MAOIs) included iproniazid (one case), tranylcypromine (two cases), isocarboxazid (two cases), and pargyline (one case). In four of the six cases, the MAOI was used first, and in all six, adverse effects were noted within 36 hours of the patient's beginning the combination. Symptoms included flushing, sweating, dizziness, tremor, fever, restlessness, confusion, hypotension, dyspnea, hallucinations, convulsions, and coma. All six patients recovered. It was the conclusion of Schuckit et al. that these symptoms could not be attributed clearly to the drug combination rather than to an idiosyncratic drug reaction. They also pointed out that there was a similarity between the reported symptoms and those seen with tricyclic antidepressant overdose alone.

Other clinical data are available from the British literature. In a study of 149 outpatients, ages 19 to 70, receiving various tricyclic antidepressant-MAOI combinations, uncomfortable side effects developed in seven patients, but no serious reactions were noted (Gander 1965). Several other British investigators have reported similar findings (Randell 1965, Sargent 1965, 1971). Schuckit et al. (1971) reviewed the medical records of 50 patients receiving a tricyclic antidepressant (usually 75 to 100 mg of imipramine) in combination with an MAOI (an average dose of 30 mg of isocarboxazid "or its equivalent"). In four cases, side effects developed that may or may not have been attributed to the combination; these side effects cleared spontaneously despite continued therapy. In a prospective group of 10 patients receiving a combination of amitriptyline 150 mg daily and tranylcypromine 30 to 40 mg daily, no significant side effects were noted.

Later studies appear to confirm the safety of the drug combination. Davidson et al. (Davidson 1982, 1984) studied 19 treatment-resistant depressed patients and randomly assigned them to either electroconvulsive therapy (ECT) or combined amitriptyline (average dose of 71 mg/day) and phenelzine (average dose of 34 mg/day) for 3 to 5 weeks. No serious toxicity was noted in patients on the drug combination, although dosage was limited in four patients because of side effects. The issue of efficacy was raised by this study, which found ECT superior to drug treatment.

In a larger outpatient study ($N = 135$), trimipramine alone proved to be more efficacious than combinations of that drug with phenelzine or isocarboxazid or isocarboxazid alone. Side effects were minor, with trimipramine alone causing more tremor, and MAOI either alone or in combination causing more insomnia (Young et al. 1979).

In one study, 30 newly hospitalized patients with research diagnostic criteria of major or minor depressive disorder were randomly assigned to open treatment using amitriptyline alone (average daily dose of 165 mg), tranylcypromine (average daily dose of 30 mg), or the combination (80 and 13 mg, respectively, average daily dose) (White et al. 1980). Using the Hamilton and Zung depression scales, the study found that all three groups showed improvement (over 82% of all patients), with no one treatment group showing superior results; it also found no significant differences in side effects among the three groups.

On the other hand, there is one report of three deaths in patients receiving the combination of clomipramine and MAOI, reportedly in "therapeutic" doses (although at least one patient received clomipramine intravenously) (Beaumont 1973). Another report described fatal disseminated intravascular coagulation in a 34-year-old man when clomipramine (10 mg twice daily) was added to tranylcypromine (Tackley et al. 1987).

MECHANISM

The mechanism for the interaction (whether it is sympathetic overstimulation or increased efficacy in depressed patients) appears to be the result of the increased availability of norepinephrine, serotonin, and other neurotransmitters. MAOIs prevent the intraneuronal degradation of norepinephrine, increasing the amount of neurotransmitter available for release. Tricyclic antidepressants inhibit the reuptake of norepinephrine and serotonin into the presynaptic neuron. The combined effects may lead to enhanced clinical effect or toxicity, depending upon which drug combinations are used and the route of administration (see the Clinical Implications section, next).

CLINICAL IMPLICATIONS

It is apparent from available data that the dangers of combined therapy have been exaggerated. The question of efficacy remains unanswered. Several uncontrolled trials have been held on the combination in refractory depression. Sethna (1974) studied 12 patients who had been refractory to treatment with MAOIs, tricyclic antidepressants, and ECT (9 patients) who were "practically free of depression or anxiety." Winston et al. (1971) and Gander (1965) reported similar findings. These studies may be criticized on the basis of being open studies with mixed types of depressions, probably including some form of chronic anxiety or atypical depression. Controlled studies supporting the advantage of the combination over the use of each drug alone are not available.

Nevertheless, some patients refractory to conventional treatments may benefit from combined treatment (Ananth et al. 1977), and the following guidelines are suggested:

- It is preferable to use amitriptyline, trimipramine, or nortriptyline, because clinical experience and controlled studies have established their safety. Imipramine, desipramine, clomipramine, and SSRI should be avoided (also see the section on SSRI). Experience with trazodone is limited, but there is one case of safe combination with phenelzine (Zetin 1984). No published studies with nefazodone exist, but it is pharmacologically similar to trazodone. Nor are there any published studies of bupropion combined with MAOIs, but the manufacturer indicates that animal studies have indicated a possible toxicity with the combination and warns against concurrent use. Carbamazepine, which has a tricyclic structure, has been used successfully with tranylcypromine, but not isoniazid (Joffe et al. 1985, Wright et al. 1982).
- Although some clinicians avoid tranylcypromine in favor of phenelzine, controlled studies support the safety of both drugs.
- An oral route of administration should be used.
- Both drugs should be started simultaneously. Tricyclics should *never* be added to an MAOI regimen.
- Doses should be lower than the usual therapeutic dose for either drug.

Clinicians must always be vigilant when MAOIs are used for medical conditions (e.g., furazolidone [Furoxone]). Moclobemide, a member of a new class of reversible inhibitors of MAO (RIMA), may pose less risk of drug interactions. This remains controversial, however, because although one report suggested no interaction between moclobemide and fluoxetine or fluvoxamine (Dingemanse 1993a, Dingemanse 1993b), another report described an interaction between clomipramine and moclobemide in a 76-year-old woman in whom confusion, fever, somnolence, muscle stiffness, myoclonus, and convulsions developed after she was switched from clomipramine 50 mg per day to moclobemide 300 mg per day (Spigset et al. 1993). The postmarketing surveillance of patients receiving concomitant or sequential treatment with SSRI and moclobemide, and a prospective analysis of combined treatment or medication switches without a drug-free washout period, showed no adverse consequences (Delini-Stula 1995), although these data must be considered preliminary. At present, moclobemide is not available in the United States, but is marketed in Canada and the United Kingdom.

Propafenone (Rythmol)

EVIDENCE OF INTERACTION

In a 68-year-old man, toxic levels of desipramine developed at doses he had tolerated well previously when the antiarrhythmic propafenone was given in doses of 150 mg twice daily and 300 mg at bedtime (Katz 1991).

MECHANISM

Propafenone inhibits cytochrome P450-2D6.

CLINICAL IMPLICATIONS

Clinicians should use lower doses of those antidepressants that are metabolized through the 2D6 isoenzyme when propafenone is given concurrently. Antidepressant plasma levels should be monitored.

Propoxyphene

Case reports indicate that doxepin levels may be doubled (Abernethy et al. 1982) and nortriptyline levels increased by about 16% when propoxyphene is co-administered (Jerling et al. 1994a).

Phenylbutazone

EVIDENCE OF INTERACTION

Consolo et al. (1970) have reported that the absorption of phenylbutazone was delayed in patients taking desipramine. Four patients received 400 mg of phenylbutazone 30 minutes after 50 mg of oral desipramine. Combined treatment delayed absorption so that peak plasma levels of phenylbutazone were not attained even 10 hours following the dose (without desipramine, peaks were attained at 4 to 6 hours). Urine excretion of oxyphenylbutazone (the major metabolite of phenylbutazone) did not differ between groups, indicating that although the rate of absorption was delayed and peak decreased, the total drug absorbed did not differ between groups. These same investigators examined chronic treatment in eight female patients. These patients received a single oral dose of 400 mg of phenylbutazone and, following 10 days of blood sampling, received desipramine (25 mg, 3 times per day) for 7 days. When the two drugs were given 30 minutes apart, a delay in absorption was apparent. When 14 hours separated the administration of the two drugs, a delay in absorption was not apparent, but plasma levels were lower in the combined group.

MECHANISM

Desipramine possesses significant anticholinergic activity that inhibits gastric emptying. Any agent that delays transit time will impair the rate of absorption. This effect requires that the drugs be administered within a short time of each other. The observation that lower levels were achieved on combined drugs, compared with the phenylbutazone group, may indicate that some drug metabolism occurs in the gut.

CLINICAL IMPLICATIONS

A minimal therapeutic level of 100 μmg/mL is required for the therapeutic activity of phenylbutazone. It is conceivable that co-administration of desipramine could interfere with achieving adequate plasma levels. Appropriate dose adjustments should be made. All antidepressants with anticholinergic activity interact similarly. Rat data indicate a similar interaction may occur with oxyphenylbutazone, cortisol, and, to a slight extent, salicylic acid (Consolo et al. 1969).

Quinidine and Quinine

EVIDENCE OF INTERACTION

Both quinidine and quinine may impair desipramine 2-hydroxylation (Steiner et al. 1988). Ten subjects were administered 800 mg of quinidine for 2 days and a single 25-mg oral dose of desipramine was then given. Urinary levels of 2-hydroxydesipramine decreased by 96% in rapid hydroxylators (previously determined by debrisoquin hydroxylation) and 68% in slow hydroxylators. After treatment with 750 mg of quinine for 2 days, urinary levels of 2-hydroxydesipramine in rapid hydroxylators were 54% lower than during the control period, whereas in slow hydroxylators no difference was observed. 2-Hydroxylation of imipramine is also inhibited by quinidine, although demethylation may not be affected (Brosen et al. 1989, Skjelbo et al. 1992).

MECHANISM

Quinidine and quinine inhibit the hepatic hydroxylation of desipramine, probably by affecting CYP2D6.

CLINICAL IMPLICATIONS

The addition of quinidine or quinine to desipramine may impair the metabolism of the antidepressant and lead to toxicity. Plasma levels of desipramine should be monitored and appropriate dosage adjustments made. Many other antidepressants and other psychotropics undergo hydroxylation and may be affected similarly.

Reserpine

EVIDENCE OF INTERACTION

When high doses of reserpine 7 to 10 mg/day were added to imipramine or desipramine (75 mg/day average dose), an initial period of manic excitement was noted, followed by dramatic improvement in depression in previously treatment-resistant cases (Poldinger 1963).

Another study using considerably higher doses of imipramine 300 mg/day in 15 nonresponders found that the addition of 7.5 to 10 mg of reserpine resulted in all but one patient showing initial improvement lasting 2 to 12 days. A return of depressive symptoms occurred in eight patients, whereas in six, the improvement lasted throughout a 6-month follow-up. All patients experienced a "conspicuous vasodilation" as well as an increase of intestinal peristalsis, which was accompanied by profuse diarrhea in one patient (Haskovec et al. 1967).

In another open study of 10 patients unresponsive to imipramine treatment (225 mg/day), 10 mg of reserpine was added for 2 days, and depression-rating scales were used to assess clinical change (Carney et al. 1969). A significant decrease in Hamilton Depression Scale scores (18.3 before treatment, 10.2 after treatment) was noted; however, on a global clinical assessment, only two patients became symptom free, and six of the 10 showed slight or no improvement. Because this was an open trial, which involved admitting outpatients to the hospital, the positive effects of the hospital milieu may have influenced the Hamilton scores. On the other hand, in one patient a manic episode did develop, which suggests (in light of other manic episodes with this drug combination) that the interaction is important for some patients.

MECHANISM

Reserpine rapidly depletes catecholamine and serotonin from intraneuronal storage sites. Most of the catecholamine is deaminated intraneuronally by monoamine oxidase (unless this enzyme has been inhibited). Although the action of imipramine and other tricyclic antidepressants on the noradrenergic synapse is complex, it is generally thought that these agents increase the availability of norepinephrine in the synaptic cleft. In reserpine-treated test animal brains, an increase in deaminated metabolites occurs (the intraneuronal action of MAO) and a decrease in O-methylated metabolites occurs (from the action of catechol-O-methyltransferase (COMT) in the synapse). When reserpine is combined with desipramine, the opposite occurs. The combination appears to produce a shift in norepinephrine metabolism from deamination to O-methylation in animals, and some evidence suggests that this may occur in humans (Haskovec et al. 1967). This would indicate that norepinephrine is being released into the synapse (the site of action of COMT), thus causing a potentiation of the action of the antidepressant. This action would expectedly be rapid, short-lived, and probably corresponds to the brief manic phase seen in some patients.

CLINICAL IMPLICATIONS

Reserpine is an antihypertensive agent that is administered alone or with other drugs in many combination products. It also has been used to treat psychosis and tardive dyskinesia. It is not possible to determine from available data whether the combination of high-dose reserpine and a tricyclic antidepressant is effective in treating refractory depressions. We would not recommend such a combination, because evidence supporting its efficacy is scant. Side effects range from uncomfortable (e.g., diarrhea, cutaneous vasodilation) to dangerous (e.g., mania).

Alseroxylon, deserpidine, rescinnamine, and syrosingopine are related to reserpine and also may interact with antidepressants, although this has not been studied. All available tricyclic antidepressants and several newer antidepressants probably have the potential for interaction with reserpine, but clinical studies are lacking.

S-Adenosylmethionine

EVIDENCE OF INTERACTION

A 71-year-old woman taking S-adenosylmethionine 100 mg intramuscularly had her clomipramine dose increased from 25 mg daily to 75 mg daily and, within 48 to 72 hours, became anxious, agitated, and confused (Iruela et al. 1993). She became stuporous, with tachycardia, tachypnea, diarrhea, myoclonus, rigidity, tremors, hyperreflexia, shivering, diaphoresis, and hyperthermia. Intravenous dantrolene reduced rigidity, but did not alter her level of consciousness. The symptoms gradually diminished over 4 days.

MECHANISM

S-Adenosylmethionine increases central serotonin and norepinephrine. The combination with clomipramine resulted in a serotonin syndrome.

CLINICAL IMPLICATIONS

S-Adenosylmethionine is a donor of methyl groups in transmethylation reactions in the body. It is widely used in Europe as an antidepressant, although it is only available in parenteral form. The combination of S-adenosylmethionine with serotonergic antidepressants may predispose to the serotonin syndrome.

SSRI (See SSRI section, Antidepressants)

Sulfonylureas

EVIDENCE OF INTERACTION

Two women with type II diabetes mellitus had hypoglycemic reactions when a tricyclic antidepressant was added to a medication regimen containing a sulfonylurea (True et al. 1987). Eleven days after starting doxepin (from 25 to 75 mg daily dose), the first woman, a 71-year-old woman taking tolazamide 1 g/day had a fall in blood sugar from 300 to 400 to 75 mg/dL. She presented to the emergency department in an unresponsive state and was admitted. Her blood glucose fell to 35 mg/dL 12 hours following admission. She responded to fluid, electrolyte, and dextrose and was discharged taking doxepin 75 mg/day and tolazamide 100 mg/day (blood sugar 163 mg/dL).

The second woman was given nortriptyline 125 mg/day while taking chlorpropamide 250 mg/day (as well as hydrochlorothiazide and potassium chloride for hypertension). A week after starting nortriptyline, her blood glucose fell from between 180 and 218 to 50 mg/dL, requiring glucagon treatment. Chlorpropamide was discontinued, and the patient's blood glucose stabilized at 90 to 120 mg/dL.

Another report described a patient with type I diabetes in whom hypoglycemia developed when amitriptyline 25 mg was given (Sherman et al. 1988).

MECHANISM

Unknown.

CLINICAL IMPLICATIONS

Hypoglycemia has been reported with nortriptyline and imipramine, although not with maprotiline (Grof et al. 1984, Shrivastava et al. 1983). Clinicians should be aware that the prescription of some antidepressants may lead to hypoglycemia, especially for patients on sulfonylureas. Decreases in the dosage of the hypoglycemic medication and blood glucose monitoring may be necessary.

Sympathomimetic Amines

EVIDENCE OF INTERACTION

The intravenous administration of direct-acting sympathomimetic amines to subjects taking tricyclic antidepressants has produced conflicting data. Intravenous injections of adrenaline and noradrenaline to six human subjects taking protriptyline 20 mg 3 times a day for 4 days showed a ninefold potentiation of the pressor effects of noradrenaline and a threefold potentiation of adrenaline (Svedmyr 1968). Boakes et al. (1973) have found a similar response in subjects treated with imipramine. Subjects given imipramine 25 mg 3 times a day for 5 days showed two- to threefold potentiation of the pressor effects of phenylephrine (200 mg/min, systolic pressure increased from 143 to 173 mm Hg, diastolic increased from 89 to 108 mm Hg), a four- to eightfold increase with noradrenaline (9 mg/min, systolic pressure increased from 131 to 174 mm Hg, diastolic increased from 84 to 99 mm Hg), and a two- to fourfold increase with adrenaline (18 mg/min, systolic pressure increased from 123 to 153 mm Hg, diastolic increased from 60 to 72 mm Hg). No significant increases were seen with isoprenaline (used as an inhalant to treat bronchial asthma).

Another study compared blood pressure responses to norepinephrine in subjects receiving trazodone and imipramine (Larochelle et al. 1979). Trazodone did not potentiate a pressor response to norepinephrine, whereas imipramine did. Desipramine and amitriptyline also increased pressor responses to norepinephrine (Mitchell et al. 1970).

MECHANISM

Cyclic antidepressants may exert their effect by inhibiting the reuptake of norepinephrine from the synaptic cleft or by affecting presynaptic receptor sensitivity, thereby decreasing or blocking feedback inhibition and resulting in increased noradrenergic activity. The exogenous administration of either noradrenaline or direct-acting sympathomimetic amines results in increased sympathetic tone.

CLINICAL IMPLICATIONS

Sympathomimetic amines given orally for such problems as cold symptoms may have the potential to increase sympathetic response; however, oral routes of administration have not been used in drug interaction studies. It is our clinical impression that for most healthy patients, the oral combination poses no risk. Similarly, no evidence suggests increased toxicity in asthmatics who inhale sympathomimetics while taking tricyclic antidepressants. The intravenous administration of levarterenol increases sympathetic response, and a rise in blood pressure and heart rate should be expected. Some question arises as to whether local anesthetics containing noradrenaline might produce similar problems, although we expect that this is quite uncommon. Some dentists feel that the use of local anesthetics containing norepinephrine or levonordefrin is dangerous for patients taking cyclic antidepressants (Goulet et al. 1992). Yagiela et al. (1985) recommended that the maximum amount of norepinephrine that patients on cyclic antidepressants receive is 0.05 mg per session (5.4 mL of local anesthetic with epinephrine 1:100,000). Care must be taken to avoid injection into a blood vessel.

Testosterone

EVIDENCE OF INTERACTION

One report exists of paranoid ideation developing in four men who were taking imipramine (75 to 150 mg daily) and methyltestosterone (15 mg daily) (Wilson et al. 1974). Testosterone supplementation was recently shown to improve depressive symptoms for a subset of male patients with low or borderline testosterone levels suffering from refractory depression. A randomized, double-blind, placebo-controlled trial studied 23 patients with a low or borderline serum testosterone level (range 100 to 350 ng/dL; normal range is 270 to 1,070 ng/dL). These patients met the DSM IV criteria for current major depressive disorder and were being treated with antidepressant medications prior to and during the trial. They received either testosterone gel (1% gel, 10g/d) or placebo for 8 weeks. The investigators reported significantly greater improvement in HAM-D scores in the testosterone-treated group when compared with the placebo-treated group in both the vegetative and affective symptoms subscales of the HAM-D Scale. Overall, the testosterone gel was well tolerated. One patient in the study experienced an exacerbation of benign prostatic hyperplasia (BPH), which may be attributed to testosterone supplementation; this patient was withdrawn from the study. The mechanism of testosterone's antidepressant action is not known (Pope et al. 2003).

Triiodothyronine (T3)

EVIDENCE OF INTERACTION

The observation that imipramine toxicity was enhanced in the presence of hyperthyroidism led Prange et al. (1969) to question whether small amounts of thyroid hormone might enhance the therapeutic effect of antidepressant treatment. Later, animal findings showed that T3 enhanced the activity of imipramine in the pargyline-DOPA mouse activation test (a screening test for the antidepressant activity of drugs) (Prange et al. 1976). In the first study, 20 euthyroid patients (16 women, 4 men) with retarded depression were studied to determine the effect of combined imipramine–T3 treatment. All patients had retarded depression (most were unipolar). Treatment consisted of 150 mg of imipramine plus 25 μmg of T3 or placebo starting on the 5th day of drug treatment. Several patients receiving T3 improved 8 hours after the initial dose, and as a group, the T3 patients improved more quickly than the placebo group (Hamilton Depression Scale scores 8 at 17.4 days for the T3 group and at 24.8 days for the placebo group). Subsequent studies by the same investigators demonstrated that women with nonretarded depressions responded to T3 augmentation, but that T3 added no advantage to the imipramine treatment of men (Prange et al. 1976). Coppen et al. (1972) found that 14 days of 25 μmg of T3 given with imipramine was superior to imipramine alone, but the number of subjects was so small that the study results are difficult to interpret. In fact, the response was dramatic—mean Hamilton scores for depressed female patients receiving the T3-imipramine combination fell from 22 to 0.

Another study by Feighner and associates (Feighner et al. 1972) evaluated the response of primary depressive subjects to imipramine 200 mg plus placebo ($N = 12$; 4 female and 8 male subjects) or imipramine 200 mg plus T3 ($N = 9$; 2 male and 7 female subjects) and found no enhancement of antidepressant activity. The reason for the difference from previous studies is not clear, but the following points have been raised as possible explanations: (a) a relatively small N with a large number of males; (b) failure to delay the start of the study to eliminate positive responders to hospitalization alone; (c) the use of a higher dose of imipramine (200 versus 150 mg) than previous studies; and (d) a heterogeneous population of depressed patients (the criteria for primary depression were used).

Positive results using an amitriptyline–T3 combination have been reported by Wheatley (1972) in a double-blind study of 52 depressed outpatients. He found that patients who received 40 μmg of T3 with amitriptyline 100 mg improved faster than those who received the antidepressant with either placebo or a lower dose of T3 (20 μmg). Women did better than men, and patients with high thyroid indices did better than those with low indices. An open study with clomipramine found similar results (Tsutsui et al. 1979).

Prange et al. (1976) suggested that T3 corrects refractoriness in approximately 50% of patients. Preliminary studies seem to support this impression. Earle (1970) found that 14 of 23 patients unresponsive to tricyclic antidepressants (12 taking imipramine 150 mg daily) showed rapid improvement in depressive symptoms when T3 (25 μmg/day) was added. It is uncertain whether these patients would have improved if the dose of antidepressant was increased without the addition of T3, because we now know that 150 mg may be an inadequate dose of imipramine. Ogura et al. (1974), in a study of 44 depressed (unipolar and bipolar) outpatients, found that the addition of T3 to an antidepressant regimen resulted in improvement in depression in 66% of patients. A double-blind study of Goodwin et al. (1982) investigated the response of 12 treatment-resistant depressed patients (6 male, 6 female patients; unipolar, $N = 4$; bipolar II, $N = 4$; bipolar I, $N = 4$) to a combination of T3 with either imipramine ($N = 8$) or amitriptyline ($N = 4$). Significant differences were found when scores on the 15-point modified Bunney-Hamburg Scale for patients on tricyclic antidepressants alone were compared with scores after 4 weeks of the combination. Nine of the 12 patients had a decrease in depression ratings that was significant at least at the $p < 0.02$ level. Eight patients achieved ratings below 5 while taking the combination. Both male and female subjects, as well as imipramine or amitriptyline patients, showed a potentiation of antidepressant response with the addition of T3.

In a randomized, double-blind, placebo-controlled study, Joffe et al. (1993b) found that both liothyronine 37.5 μmg and lithium (mean level 0.68 nmol/L in responders) improved antidepressant response when added to the drug treatment of 50 patients who previously failed to respond to an adequate trial of either desipramine ($N = 46$) or imipramine ($N = 5$), at a minimum tricyclic dose of 2.5 mg/kg for 5 weeks. Of the 50 completers, 10 of 17 responded to the addition of liothyronine and 9 of 17 responded to lithium, while only 3 of 16 responded to placebo. One possible complicating factor in this study was the greater number of women in the liothyronine group than the lithium group (although this difference did not reach statistical significance), because some authorities believe that women are better responders to thyroid augmentation than are men.

In a crossover study comparing triiodothyronine to placebo, Gitlin et al. (1987) found no significant differences, although their study has been criticized on the basis of small sample size and a crossover design that ignores the possibility that the addition of thyroid could produce a long-lasting effect that would carry over into the placebo period.

Another negative study was reported by Thase et al. (1989), who administered triiodothyronine 25 mg to 20 patients who had previously failed to respond to imipramine. Although 25% responded to adjunctive therapy, the same number of historical control subjects responded to continued imipramine treatment. A study by Targum et al. (1984) found that thyroid augmentation was useful only for those patients with an increased thyroid-stimulating hormone response to thyroid-releasing hormone, which suggests that subtle thyroid abnormalities may be present in at least some patients who do not respond to antidepressants.

An initial report describing three cases of triiodothyronine augmentation of fluoxetine suggested that nonresponse to the SSRI antidepressants may be reversed by thyroid supplementation (Joffe 1992).

MECHANISM

The mechanism by which T3 either accelerates or potentiates clinical response to antidepressants is unknown, but several interesting hypotheses have been proposed (Goodwin et al. 1982, Prange et al. 1969). A generalized thyroid defect has never been associated clearly with mood disorders; however, some evidence suggests a link. Whybrow et al. (1972) showed that in depressed patients not selected for thyroid dysfunction, response to imipramine was positively correlated with pretreatment chemical indices of thyroid function. In addition to these data, Prange et al. (1969) found that, as a group, the 20 depressed patients they studied had slow normal ankle reflex time (an index of thyroid function), which increased after T3-antidepressant treatment. Perhaps small doses of T3 in some way lead to a change in thyroid activity, which is necessary for recovery from a depressive episode. Joffe et al. (1990) suggested that T3 augmentation suppresses endogenous T4 production, and that an increase in the T3 to T4 ratio is an important factor in antidepressant augmentation.

Thyroid hormones increase β-adrenergic receptors in the heart (Williams et al. 1977), and it is possible that they do so in the brain as well (Goodwin et al. 1982). Further evidence of a receptor site interaction is found in the data of Frazer et al. (1974), who demonstrated that the addition of T3 to imipramine-treated rats altered the effect of tricyclic antidepressants on the postsynaptic generation of cyclic adenosine monophosphate (cAMP).

CLINICAL IMPLICATIONS

The addition of triiodothyronine to patients who have not responded to an adequate trial of antidepressant therapy is a reasonable therapeutic strategy, although one study of psychiatrists in the northeastern United States found that it was rarely used as a first step in nonresponsive patients (Nierenberg 1991). Thyroid is usually added as liothyronine (Cytomel), in doses of 25 to 75 μmg. One report suggested that triiodothyronine was superior to thyroxine in the augmentation of antidepressants (Joffe et al. 1990). A response to the addition of thyroid usually occurs within 3 weeks. No long-term studies address the issue of optimal length of triiodothyronine supplementation. Possible adverse consequences of thyroid augmentation include cardiovascular effects (tachycardia, atrial irritability, altered ventricular function, high output failure), anxiety, insomnia, and increased sweating.

Section 2.2   SSRI Drug Interactions

SSRIs (Table 2.5) are a chemically diverse group of antidepressants that are more specific in their inhibition of serotonin reuptake than the older antidepressants. Their most important characteristic, relevant to the study of pharmacokinetic drug interactions, is their inhibition of the cytochrome P450 system. Through its actions on the parent drug and/or metabolites, cytochrome P450-2D6 is responsible for the metabolism of many psychotropic drugs, including amitriptyline, clomipramine, imipramine, desipramine, nortriptyline, perphenazine, and thioridazine. Hydroxylation of the secondary and tertiary amine antidepressants is a function of 2D6 (e.g., desipramine to 2-OH-desipramine), whereas conversion of tertiary to secondary amines is mediated by 1A2 and 3A3/4 (e.g., imipramine to desipramine). 2D6 is also involved in the metabolism of other drugs, such as β-adrenergic blocking agents (carvedilol, metoprolol, timolol, propafenone), antiarrhythmic drugs (encainide, flecainide, mexiletine), and codeine. Cytochrome P450-3A4 metabolizes triazolam, alprazolam, and midazolam, as functions in the initial demethylation step of tricyclic antidepressants. Cytochrome P450-1A2 also contributes to the metabolism of imipramine and theophylline, among other drugs. Some evidence suggests that sertraline may be less potent than other SSRIs in its ability to inhibit CYP2D6 (von Moltke et al. 1994).

Pharmacodynamic interactions may occur with the SSRIs because of their potent serotonergic actions. When given with other pro-serotonergic drugs such as tryptophan or lithium, they may lead to a serotonin syndrome characterized by diarrhea, nausea, headache, hyperthermia, myoclonus, tremor, hyperreflexia, ataxia, seizures, agitation, confusion, excitability, and delirium (Nierenberg et al. 1993, Sternbach 1991a). The serotonin syndrome has long been recognized as a possible consequence of the combination of MAOI antidepressants and other drugs, such as tryptophan, meperidine, or lithium. More recently, however, reports have been published of a serotonergic syndrome occurring with the combination of SSRI with tramadol, lithium, tryptophan, or

(text continues on page 96)

TABLE 2.5. PHARMACOLOGY OF SSRI

	Fluoxetine (Prozac®)	Fluvoxamine (Luvox®)	Paroxetine (Paxil®)	Sertraline (Zoloft®)	Citalopram (Celexa®)	Escitalopram (Lexapro®)
Time to peak plasma level after oral dose	6–8 hr	5 hr	5 hr	4,5–8.4 hr post-dose	2–4 hr	5 hr
Protein binding	94.5%	77%	93–95%	98%	50%	56%
Elimination half-life	Parent 1–3 days acute 4–6 days chronic Metabolite 4–16 days (acute or chronic)	15 hr	21 hr	26 hr (parent) 62–104 hr (metabolite)	33 hr	27–32 hr
Active metabolite	Norfluoxetine	No	No clinically important metabolites	Desmethylser-traline	Desmethyl-citalopram (DCT)	5-DCT(1/3 concentration of parent, 1/7 potency at 5HT re-uptake)

MAOIs. Some reports exist of serotonergic syndromes occurring when strongly serotonergic tricyclic drugs, such as clomipramine, are given alone (Lange-Asschenfeldt et al. 2002, Lejoyeux et al. 1992, Lejoyeux et al. 1993).

Another interesting pharmacodynamic interaction with the SSRIs is enhanced downregulation of β-adrenergic receptors that occurs when they are co-administered with some tricyclic antidepressants (TCA). This interaction may result in the potentiation of therapeutic response.

Anticonvulsants

EVIDENCE OF INTERACTION

Fluoxetine

Several cases have been reported of toxic phenytoin levels developing shortly after the addition of fluoxetine 20 mg daily (Jalil 1992, Shader et al. 1994, Woods et al. 1994) or 40 mg daily (Darley 1994), as well as a decline in phenytoin levels after fluoxetine discontinuation (Shad et al. 1999). In a study of the interaction of fluoxetine and carbamazepine, six healthy volunteers were administered carbamazepine 400 mg daily for 3 weeks, followed by 7 days of combined therapy with fluoxetine 20 mg daily (Grimsley et al. 1992, Grimsley et al. 1991). As a result, the plasma versus time AUC for carbamazepine and its major metabolite carbamazepine-10,11-epoxide increased by 27% and 31%, respectively. Other studies produced contradictory findings. Spina et al. (1993c) administered fluoxetine 20 mg daily ($N = 8$) or fluvoxamine 100 mg daily ($N = 7$) to epileptic patients on chronic carbamazepine therapy. They found no change in steady-state carbamazepine levels. Another study examined the effect of fluoxetine and norfluoxetine on carbamazepine-10,11-epoxide formation in perfused rat liver, in vitro human liver microsomes, and 14 patients (Gidal et al. 1993). No effect on carbamazepine clearance was observed in perfused rat liver, and the inhibition of carbamazepine-10,11-epoxide formation occurred only at concentrations 20 times those found clinically. Patients receiving carbamazepine monotherapy and those receiving carbamazepine with fluoxetine had similar ratios of carbamazepine to the epoxide metabolite. Despite the contradictory findings in clinical studies, several case reports have described toxicity when carbamazepine and fluoxetine were combined (Dursun et al. 1993, Pearson 1990). In one of these patients, symptoms were consistent with a serotonin syndrome (agitation, diaphoresis, hyperreflexia, shivering, incoordination), but other patients had symptoms consistent with carbamazepine toxicity (slurred speech, vertigo, tinnitus, blurred vision, diplopia, tremor). Case reports indicated increased carbamazepine plasma levels as high as 63% above baseline, although the changes in plasma levels have been highly variable.

A case report described a possible interaction between valproate and fluoxetine (Sovner et al. 1991). A 57-year-old woman with atypical bipolar disorder and severe mental retardation was taking divalproex sodium (Depakote) in daily doses of up to 3,500 mg/day, with levels of 100 to 120 mg/L. Prior to initiation of fluoxetine 20 mg daily, she was taking 3,000 mg of divalproex sodium, with a level of 93.5 mg/L. Two weeks after the addition of fluoxetine, her valproic acid level was 152 mg/L, although clinical toxicity did not develop.

Fluvoxamine

Some studies indicate that high doses of fluvoxamine (100 to 300 mg daily) may impair carbamazepine metabolism (Bonnet et al. 1992, Fritze et al. 1991, Spina et al. 1993c). One week after the initiation of fluvoxamine (100 mg/day), a patient who had been taking carbamazepine (600 mg/day) had an increase in plasma CBZ levels, from 8 to 19 mcg/mL, and developed toxicity (Martinelli et al. 1993). Toxicity was also reported in three patients taking the combination (Fritze et al. 1991). On the other hand, in the study cited above (Spina et al. 1993c), no interaction was reported. Fluvoxamine may inhibit phenytoin metabolism and has induced toxicity (Mamiya et al. 2001).

Paroxetine

Paroxetine did not affect the metabolism of phenytoin, carbamazepine, or valproate in 20 patients with epilepsy who were well controlled on monotherapy (Andersen et al. 1991). One study, however (Kaye et al. 1989), reported that phenytoin (300 mg/day for 14 days) decreased paroxetine AUC and half-life by 27% and 28%, respectively.

Sertraline

Sertraline in doses of 200 mg daily for 17 days led to a slight, but nonsignificant, increase in plasma versus time AUC for phenytoin and a 14% decrease for carbamazepine (Harvey et al. 1996a, b). There is a report of two elderly men who were taking phenytoin and had increased plasma levels of the anticonvulsant after the addition of modest doses of sertraline (25 to 75 mg/day) (Haselberger et al. 1997). Carbamazepine may reduce sertraline plasma levels, requiring doses of 300 mg/day for antidepressant efficacy (Khan et al. 2000, Pihlsgard et al. 2002). Another study found no alteration of carbamazepine metabolism at sertraline doses of 50 to 200 mg/day for 10 to 20 days (Preskorn et al. 1997).

MECHANISM

The inhibition of metabolism can be explained at least partially, based on the known effects of SSRIs on the cytochrome P450 system. Multiple pathways are involved in the metabolism of carbamazepine and phenytoin, but 3A3/4 is important for the former, and 2C9 and 2C19 for the latter anticonvulsant. Phenytoin induces 3A4 and 2B6.

CLINICAL IMPLICATIONS

Several reports document the impaired metabolism of phenytoin, carbamazepine, and perhaps valproate when administered with fluoxetine and also with other SSRIs. The data are far from consistent however, with some studies indicating no interaction. Until more information is available, careful monitoring of anticonvulsant serum levels and frequent evaluation of clinical signs and symptoms of drug toxicity are warranted when these medication combinations are used.

Antidepressants (*See also* Monoamine Oxidase Inhibitors)

EVIDENCE OF INTERACTION

SSRIs interact with other antidepressants through pharmacokinetic and pharmacodynamic mechanisms (Ciraulo et al. 1990). They impair oxidative metabolism and thus result in higher plasma levels of antidepressants metabolized via this route. The effects on the cytochrome system are shown in Table 2.2.

Pharmacodynamic interactions include CNS toxicity and augmentation of antidepressant action. With respect to the pharmacokinetic interactions of SSRIs with other antidepressants, it is well established that fluoxetine inhibits CYP2D6, 2C19, and 3A4 (norfluoxetine). Vaughan (1988) described a 31-year-old woman who was being treated with nortriptyline. At doses of 125 mg/day and 175 mg/day, her plasma levels of nortriptyline were 77 and 88 ng/mL, respectively. The nortriptyline dose was reduced to 100 mg daily, and fluoxetine 20 mg daily was started. After 2 weeks of combined therapy, the patient reported decreased energy, sedation, and psychomotor retardation. A plasma nortriptyline level done 10 days after the onset of symptoms was 162 ng/mL, a level generally considered above the therapeutic range. Nortriptyline was discontinued, and symptoms resolved in 3 weeks. Another woman received fluoxetine 20 mg, lithium 1200 mg, and desipramine 150 mg daily for 3 days until the fluoxetine was discontinued when a skin rash developed. Decreased energy, drowsiness, and psychomotor retardation also developed in the patient; desipramine was increased to 350 mg/day but symptoms persisted. A plasma desipramine level was 632 ng/mL. A previous level of the same dose of desipramine, prior to fluoxetine, was 133 ng/mL (Vaughan 1988).

In another report, a 33-year-old man had been taking fluoxetine 40 mg daily and desipramine 150 mg daily for 5 weeks (Goodnick 1989). Although his depression improved, the patient reported dry mouth, tinnitus, memory impairment, and decreased alertness. Fluoxetine was discontinued, and plasma desipramine levels were followed. The levels were 938.0 ng/mL, 595.9 ng/mL, and 47.8 ng/mL at 2, 9, and 49 days after discontinuation, respectively.

A third report described a 75-year-old woman who was being treated with desipramine 300 mg daily, l-tryptophan 2 g at bedtime, and multivitamins when fluoxetine 20 mg daily was added to the regimen (Bell et al. 1988). Desipramine levels prior to the fluoxetine had been 150 ng/mL, 109 ng/mL, and 131 ng/mL. Five days after fluoxetine was started, her desipramine level was 212 ng/mL. Four days after fluoxetine was increased to 40 mg daily, her desipramine level was 419 ng/mL. Increased levels were associated with clinical deterioration. After the desipramine dose was reduced to 200 mg and the fluoxetine discontinued, desipramine levels declined and symptoms improved.

Since those initial clinical case reports appeared, others have been published (Aranow et al. 1989, Preskorn et al. 1990). One study attempted to quantify the alterations in metabolism (Bergstrom et al. 1992). In that study, six subjects were given desipramine 50 mg and six subjects were given imipramine 50 mg, on three separate occasions—alone, 3 hours after a single 60-mg oral dose of fluoxetine, and 3 hours after the eighth dose of fluoxetine given 60 mg daily. With daily fluoxetine dosing, desipramine concentrations were approximately 10 times higher and clearance was tenfold lower. Imipramine concentrations were about three times higher and clearance four times lower with daily fluoxetine. Even after a single 60-mg dose, an approximate 50% decline occurred in the clearance of the two tricyclic antidepressants. Amitriptyline elimination half-life also may be impaired by fluoxetine (Muller et al. 1991). The combination of amitriptyline (150 mg/day) and fluoxetine (40 mg/day) for 6 days resulted in death (Preskorn et al. 1997).

A possible interaction between fluoxetine and bupropion has also been reported (van Putten et al. 1990). In that case, a 42-year-old man was started on bupropion 1 day after stopping fluoxetine 60 mg daily. Over the next 2 weeks, he had myoclonus, agitation, psychosis, and delirium. Because norfluoxetine has a long half-life and is a potent enzyme inhibitor, it may have elevated bupropion levels to cause toxicity. Another report also details catatonia developing when bupropion was given following fluoxetine therapy (Preskorn 1991).

Fluvoxamine increased plasma levels of imipramine and desipramine in four patients in whom adverse effects developed (Spina et al. 1992). Another report described a 40% increase in plasma imipramine level (Maskall et al. 1993). Subsequent studies have found that the effect of fluvoxamine on imipramine metabolism is greater than the effect on desipramine metabolism (Spina et al. 1993, 1993a). Fluvoxamine also impaired the metabolism of trimipramine (Seifritz et al. 1994), clomipramine (Bertschy et al. 1991), and mirtazapine (Anttila et al. 2001, Demers et al. 2001). The inhibitory effects of fluvoxamine last for 1 to 2 weeks after discontinuation of the antidepressant (Hartter et al. 1993).

Sertraline (50 mg/day) when added to desipramine (200 mg/day) led to an increase in desipramine plasma levels from 44 ng/mL to 108 ng/mL, resulting in dysphoria and tremors in a 50-year-old woman (Barros et al. 1993). Another patient had an increase in desipramine level from 152 ng/mL to 240 ng/mL 1 month after sertraline (50 mg/day) was added to desipramine (Lydiard et al. 1993). Sertraline and its metabolite desmethylsertraline may be less potent inhibitors of desipramine metabolism than fluoxetine and norfluoxetine (von Moltke et al. 1994). In a study of 18 healthy volunteers who were extensive metabolizers of dextromethorphan (a 2D6 probe drug) (Preskorn et al. 1994), the average maximum desipramine concentration increased from 51.2 ng/mL to 193.3 ng/mL after 21 days of treatment with fluoxetine (20 mg daily), compared with an increase from 24.5 ng/mL to 32.8 ng/mL after sertraline 50 mg daily. Furthermore, 3 weeks after discontinuation, the inhibition of desipramine hydroxylation was still apparent (due to persistent levels of norfluoxetine), whereas the effects of sertraline abated within 1 week. The dosages of the antidepressants used in this study may not have been therapeutically equivalent. Other studies suggest that sertraline may increase nortriptyline (Solai et al. 1997), desipramine, and imipramine levels (Kurtz et al. 1997).

Paroxetine and its M2 metabolite are inhibitors of 2D6, and these agents significantly reduced desipramine clearance in one study (Brosen et al. 1993) and increased desipramine plasma levels fivefold in another (Harvey et al. 1996a, b). Paroxetine had similar effects on nortriptyline (Leucht et al. 2000) and amitriptyline (Laine et al. 2001). Sertraline metabolism was not affected by desipramine (Harvey et al. 1996a, b).

Citalopram had no effect on amitriptyline, nortriptyline, or maprotiline plasma levels when co-administered (Baettig et al. 1993).

In addition to a pharmacokinetic interaction, a potentially significant receptor site interaction has also been reported. The combination of SSRI and cyclic antidepressants has been used to augment antidepressant response. Although it was once thought that fluoxetine and desipramine could lead to a more rapid and greater downregulation of β-adrenergic receptors than that seen with desipramine alone (Nelson et al. 1991, Rothschild 1994), recent studies do not support a more rapid antidepressant response using the combination (Nelson et al. 2004). Animal studies have found greater β-receptor downregulation. Male Sprague-Dawley rats were given intraperitoneal injections of desipramine (5 mg/kg once a day), fluoxetine (10 mg/kg once or twice a day), or a combination for either 4 or 14 days (Baron et al. 1988). After 4 days, there was a 27% decline in cerebral cortical β-adrenergic receptor density using the combination treatment, whereas no change was observed using either drug alone. After 14 days of treatment, desipramine resulted in a 14% decrease. Although both drugs alone resulted in a decrease in isoproterenol-stimulated cAMP accumulation, the combination produced greater decrements. To the extent that β-adrenergic receptor downregulation is related to antidepressant response, the combination may, theoretically at least, provide enhanced antidepressant response.

In a clinical study, inpatients with unipolar nonpsychotic major depression were randomized to fluoxetine 20 mg, desipramine adjusted to adequate plasma levels, or the combination (Nelson et al. 2004). The combination was more effective than either drug alone, although no difference was observed in the time to onset of antidepressant effect (the sample size may have been too small to detect a difference). The combination was particularly effective when response, defined as 50% improvement from baseline, was used as the outcome measure. This study, along with others (Charney et al. 1986), challenges the association of rapid downregulation of β-receptors and onset of clinical improvement, although it supports the superior efficacy of the combination.

MECHANISM

The evidence suggests that several SSRIs impair oxidative metabolism, through varying effects on the cytochrome P450 system. Differences in the subtypes of cytochrome P450 that are affected by the various SSRIs are well studied, but still incomplete. Tables 2.2 and 2.3 can be used as a general guide to allow clinicians to anticipate, and therefore avoid, drug interactions; however, caution should be exercised whenever adding or discontinuing SSRIs in a patient taking other medications, because our knowledge of the P450 subfamilies is still growing. It appears that 2D6 is responsible for the hydroxylation of secondary and tertiary amines, whereas demethylation may be mediated by 1A2 and 3A3/4. Effects on 2B6, which is responsible for bupropion metabolism, are not well studied.

With respect to enhanced antidepressant response, it is hypothesized that the serotonergic system plays a role in the regulation of β-adrenergic receptors. For example, lesions of serotonergic terminals or the inhibition of serotonin synthesis prevents or reverses the β-adrenergic downregulation secondary to desipramine (Baron et al. 1988). It is also possible, however, that aside from controlled trials (e.g., Nelson et al. 2004), in some instances the combination treatment merely results in higher cyclic antidepressant brain levels.

CLINICAL IMPLICATIONS

The co-administration of SSRI with cyclic antidepressants that are hydroxylated through cytochrome P450-2D6 may lead to higher plasma levels of the latter. In some cases, initial demethylation may also be affected, but data are limited. Unless appropriate dosage reductions are made, toxicity may result. Because fluoxetine and its major metabolite norfluoxetine have long elimination half-lives (2 to 3 and 7 to 9 days, respectively), switching from fluoxetine to another antidepressant may require smaller than usual initial doses of the new medication. Recovery from enzyme inhibition will take several weeks after fluoxetine therapy, 1 to 2 weeks for fluvoxamine, and shorter times for paroxetine and sertraline.

The serotonin syndrome occasionally seen with the combination of SSRI and other antidepressants usually resolves rapidly—often within a day of stopping the offending agents (Weiner et al. 1997).

The combination of fluoxetine and desipramine may provide the more effective treatment of some types of depression, when compared to monotherapy. The clinical importance of the interaction awaits additional study. The mechanism is not fully understood, because a pharmacokinetic interaction cannot be ruled out. It is possible that the combination treatment merely led to high CNS desipramine levels. Greater downregulation of β-adrenergic receptors has also been suggested as a mechanism underlying enhanced antidepressant response.

Barbiturates

EVIDENCE OF INTERACTION

In mice, fluoxetine (0.3 to 10 mg/kg) caused a dose-dependent increase in sleep time and hexobarbital brain levels (Fuller et al. 1976). Hexobarbital half-life was increased from 18 minutes in control mice to 95 minutes in the fluoxetine-treated group.

Phenobarbital may reduce serum levels of paroxetine (Greb et al. 1989a, Greb et al. 1989b).

MECHANISM

Fluoxetine and other SSRIs may inhibit barbiturate metabolism. Data on SSRIs as object drugs are limited, but one study suggests that phenobarbital may enhance the metabolism of paroxetine.

CLINICAL IMPLICATIONS

Fluoxetine and other SSRIs probably will inhibit the metabolism of other barbiturates in addition to hexobarbital. Furthermore, the barbiturates may reduce serum levels of SSRIs, although little data are available. Clinicians should monitor serum levels of barbiturates during combined treatment and observe patients for barbiturate toxicity or decreased antidepressant response.

Benztropine

EVIDENCE OF INTERACTION

In five patients taking either fluoxetine or paroxetine, in combination with an antipsychotic and benztropine, delirium developed (Roth et al. 1994). In two patients, delirium was evident 2 days after benztropine (0.5 mg twice daily in one case, three times daily in the other) was started. The other patients had been stabilized on an antipsychotic and benztropine, but delirium developed shortly after either fluoxetine or paroxetine was added.

MECHANISM

The mechanism is unknown.

CLINICAL IMPLICATIONS

Although data are limited to one series of cases, clinicians should monitor for altered mental status when using benztropine with SSRIs. Symptoms appear to develop rapidly within a few days of adding benztropine. In the reported cases, benztropine doses were moderate (1 to 3 mg daily).

β-Adrenergic Blocking Agents

EVIDENCE OF INTERACTION

A 54-year-old man was treated with metoprolol (Lopressor) 100 mg daily for 1 month prior to the addition of fluoxetine 20 mg daily. Within 2 days of starting fluoxetine, bradycardia (pulse rate fell from 64 to 36 beats/min) and lethargy developed. These adverse effects abated upon discontinuation of the medication and did not reappear when fluoxetine was given with sotalol (Betapace) (Walley et al.

1993). Paroxetine also impairs metoprolol metabolism and prolongs β-blockade (Hemeryck et al. 2000).

An interaction of fluoxetine with propranolol has also been reported (Drake et al. 1994). In a 53-year-old man who had been taking propranolol 80 mg daily and lorazepam 4 mg daily for 2 years without cardiac symptoms, complete heart block and loss of consciousness developed 2 weeks after fluoxetine 20 mg daily was added to his medication regimen. Fluoxetine also impairs carvedilol metabolism, with greater effects on the R(+)-enantiomer, but without significant changes in clinical effect (Graff et al. 2001).

MECHANISM

Fluoxetine and norfluoxetine are potent inhibitors of hepatic metabolism. Although the cytochrome P450-mediated metabolism of propranolol and metoprolol is complex, evidence suggests that cytochrome P450-2D6 is involved to some extent, and 2D6 is inhibited by fluoxetine and its metabolite (Marathe et al. 1994). Sotalol is not metabolized by the liver and undergoes renal excretion, which explains why it does not interact with fluoxetine, whereas metoprolol does. Fluvoxamine inhibits the metabolism of propranolol, but the combination is not associated with clinically significant changes in β-blockade (van Harten 1993). On the other hand, fluvoxamine increases the activity of metoprolol. The actions of atenolol appear to be moderately enhanced by fluvoxamine, despite unchanged atenolol levels (Perucca et al. 1994b). Sertraline does not affect atenolol's actions in healthy subjects (Ziegler et al. 1996).

CLINICAL IMPLICATIONS

β-Adrenergic blocking agents that are extensively metabolized by the liver are likely to interact with SSRIs. No data are available on whether β-blockers interfere with the metabolism of SSRIs. If it is clinically appropriate, sotalol or other β-blockers that do not undergo hepatic metabolism should be substituted for propranolol and metoprolol in patients taking SSRIs. Alternatively, lower doses of propranolol or metoprolol should be used. Sertraline may be a better choice in patients on β-blockers metabolized via CYP2D6.

Buspirone

EVIDENCE OF INTERACTION

A case report described a 35-year-old man who had depression, generalized anxiety, and panic attacks who had been unsuccessfully treated with a number of medications (Bodkin et al. 1989). He was started on buspirone 60 mg daily and, after 2 weeks, had decreased symptoms of anxiety but worsening depression. Trazodone 200 mg/day was added without benefit. Fluoxetine 20 mg/day was then started, and within 48 hours symptoms of anxiety returned. Buspirone was increased to 80 mg/day for 1 week, but still the anxiety symptoms persisted. A satisfactory antidepressant and antipanic effect was obtained with fluoxetine 20 mg and trazodone 250 mg, but the patient remained anxious. Fluvoxamine may increase buspirone levels two- to threefold (Anderson et al. 1996, Lamberg et al. 1998).

A preliminary study was undertaken of buspirone augmentation of fluoxetine or fluvoxamine in 25 treatment-refractory depressed patients (Joffe et al. 1993a). Of 25 patients, 17 improved on the combination with "minimal" side effects. Buspirone augmentation of drug response to SSRI in OCD has been tried with mixed results, with success reported in open trials, and no effect in a controlled study (Grady et al. 1992, Jenike et al. 1991, Markovitz et al. 1990). Paradoxical worsening of obsessive symptoms was noted in a 31-year-old woman 3 days after buspirone 10 mg three times daily was started (Tanquary et al. 1990). In addition, a seizure has been reported in one patient taking the combination (Grady et al. 1992). A 31-year-old woman taking fluoxetine 80 mg/day for OCD had a generalized tonic-clonic (grand mal) seizure 3 weeks after buspirone 30 mg daily was added. Buspirone augmentation of SSRI antidepressant response has also been reported (Bakish 1991, Dimitriou et al. 1998).

MECHANISM

The mechanisms of the interactions are not known.

CLINICAL IMPLICATIONS

The efficacy of buspirone augmentation of antidepressant and antiobsessive effects of SSRI is not established. A definite drug interaction has not been established either, but clinicians should be aware of the possibility of rare adverse effects from the combination, including worsening of psychiatric symptoms, seizures, and a serotonin syndrome (Manos 2000).

Calcium Channel Blockers

EVIDENCE OF INTERACTION

Sternbach (1991b) reported three cases of calcium channel blocker interaction with fluoxetine. In a 79-year-old woman taking sustained release verapamil 240 mg daily, chlorpropamide 250 mg three times daily, bumetanide 1 mg daily, and aspirin, edema (at first pedal, then pretibial with neck vein distension) developed 6 weeks after fluoxetine 20 mg every other day was started. The edema subsided within 2 to 3 weeks after the verapamil dose was lowered to 120 mg daily. In a 45-year-old man, dull, throbbing headaches developed after he began taking fluoxetine 40 mg daily and sustained-release verapamil 240 mg daily; these headaches subsided when he discontinued verapamil (although his migraine headaches, which were the reason for verapamil therapy, returned). A third patient, a 76-year-old woman, became nauseated and flushed on the combination of fluoxetine 20 mg every other day and nifedipine 60 mg daily. When the nifedipine dosage was reduced to 30 mg daily, her symptoms resolved over 2 to 3 weeks.

MECHANISM

The mechanism for this interaction is not established but may involve an impaired metabolism of calcium channel blockers by fluoxetine. All calcium channel blockers marketed in the United States undergo hepatic metabolism, making them susceptible to pharmacokinetic interactions.

Verapamil and diltiazem inhibit oxidative metabolism, but the effects of calcium channel blockers on SSRIs are not known. Nifedipine does not inhibit oxidative metabolism but does increase hepatic blood flow.

CLINICAL IMPLICATIONS

The combination of fluoxetine with calcium channel blockers may increase the adverse effects of the latter, such as edema, headache, nausea, and flushing. This appears to be adequately controlled by a dosage reduction of the calcium channel blocker.

Cyproheptadine (Periactin)

EVIDENCE OF INTERACTION

Prior to the introduction of specific agents for erectile dysfunction, it was common clinical practice to use cyproheptadine, a histamine-1 (H_1) and serotonin antagonist, to counteract the frequent sexual dysfunction in patients taking SSRIs, although the efficacy of the drug for this purpose was never established. Some clinicians instructed patients to take cyproheptadine on a regular basis, whereas others recommended a single dose 2 hours prior to sexual intercourse. Although a wide dosage range was used, the total daily dose usually did not exceed 0.5 mg/kg. Fluoxetine-induced anorgasmia was reversed in one patient by a single 8-mg dose of cyproheptadine and in another by daily doses of 16 mg (McCormick et al. 1990).

As might be anticipated, the reversal of sexual dysfunction has been associated with antagonism of the antidepressant and antibulimic effects of fluoxetine. A 24-year-old woman with a 7-year history of bulimia nervosa was treated with fluoxetine 60 mg daily, with a positive response after 2 weeks of therapy (Goldbloom et al. 1991). One month later, anorgasmia developed, which was treated with cyproheptadine, 2 mg daily and then 4 mg daily. A few days following the increase to 4 mg, the patient reported increased depression, an urge to binge, and chocolate cravings. In the same report, a 32-year-old woman with an 11-year history of bulimia nervosa was treated successfully with fluoxetine 40 mg daily, and after 4 months anorgasmia developed, which responded to cyproheptadine 4 to 8 mg daily. After the addition of the cyproheptadine, she had a recurrence of binge eating and weight gain.

A reversal of antidepressant effect was reported in three men treated with fluoxetine for depression, in whom ejaculatory disturbances developed, and who received cyproheptadine 2 to 6 mg daily (Feder 1991). Reversal of effect occurred rapidly, from several hours after the cyproheptadine to 2 days later. Antagonism of clinical effect has been reported by others (Christensen 1995, Katz et al. 1994).

MECHANISM

The reversal of antidepressant effect is most likely a consequence of the serotonin antagonist activity of cyproheptadine. Reversal of the antibulimic effect is probably due to a combination of antihistaminic and antiserotonin actions.

CLINICAL IMPLICATIONS

Cyproheptadine is most commonly used with SSRIs to treat the serotonin syndrome. The use of cyproheptadine to reverse sexual dysfunction resulting from SSRI therapy has largely been replaced by more specific treatments (e.g., sildenafil, vardenafil, tadalafil). Because the reversal of antidepressant response is possible when using cyproheptadine, it is preferable to begin with low doses and instruct patients to take it 2 hours prior to intercourse. Chronic treatment may be tolerated by some patients, if intermittent use is not effective. Patients with bulimia nervosa may be at high risk for relapse because of the antihistaminic effects on appetite and weight gain, as well as the antiserotonergic effects of cyproheptadine. Specific treatments for erectile dysfunction, such as sildenafil, vardenafil, or tadalafil, are preferable for the treatment of SSRI-induced sexual dysfunction. Alternative antidepressant therapy with agents less likely to produce sexual dysfunction, such as bupropion, should be considered for patients with major depression who are unable to tolerate SSRIs.

Digoxin

Most studies have found that SSRIs do not alter digoxin pharmacokinetics (Bannister et al. 1989, Forster et al. 1991, Kaye et al. 1989, Ochs et al. 1989). A case report has been published of a 93-year-old woman who had an almost fourfold increase in digoxin levels 1 week after fluoxetine (10 mg/day) was begun (Leibovitz et al. 1998).

Ethanol

EVIDENCE OF INTERACTION

Fluoxetine does not affect psychomotor performance or the subjective effects of ethanol, nor does it affect ethanol metabolism (Lemberger et al. 1985). Six healthy men were given fluoxetine capsules (30 or 60 mg) or placebo, with ethanol (45 mL absolute ethanol per 70 kg body weight, equivalent to 4 ounces of whiskey) or ethanol-placebo. Effects were tested after a single fluoxetine dose and after 9 days of fluoxetine administration. Stability of stance, manual coordination, motor performance, and subjective responses were assessed. Subjects achieved peak blood concentrations of ethanol of 50 to 70 mg/dL at 60 to 90 minutes. No differences in ethanol kinetics were seen between groups. Ethanol did not affect the kinetics of fluoxetine or norfluoxetine. Pretreatment with fluoxetine did not affect psychomotor activity following ethanol administration.

In another study, 12 healthy volunteers were given amitriptyline, fluoxetine, and placebo for 7 days, with 28 days intervening drug treatments (Allen et al. 1988). On the 8th day ethanol was given (mean blood alcohol levels via breathalyzer were 78 mg/dL, 77 mg/dL, and 81 mg/dL in the three groups, respectively). Mean plasma levels of the study drugs were as follows: amitriptyline 26.1 ng/mL, nortriptyline 25.6 ng/mL, fluoxetine 115.4 ng/mL, norfluoxetine 102.6 ng/mL. The ethanol–fluoxetine combination had few clinically significant interactions. For example, reaction time and digit symbol substitution did not differ among the groups after ethanol administration. Body sway measured with eyes open, on the other hand, was less in the fluoxetine group 1 hour after ethanol, compared with the amitriptyline or placebo group. Three hours post-ethanol dose, however, only the placebo group showed less sway. The data available with other SSRIs also suggest that SSRIs do not potentiate the psychomotor impairment and CNS depression produced by ethanol alone (Allen et al. 1989, 1988, Hindmarch et al. 1989, 1990, Linnoila et al. 1993, van Harten et al. 1992).

Another type of ethanol–antidepressant interaction is the ability of serotonergic agents to reduce ethanol consumption. Fluoxetine, fluvoxamine, sertraline, zimelidine, norzimelidine, fenfluramine, citalopram, tianeptine, and alaproclate decreased ethanol consumption by rats, whereas amitriptyline, desipramine, and doxepin had no effect (Amit et al. 1984, Daoust et al. 1992, Haraguchi et al. 1990, Hyttel et al. 1985, Lu et al. 1992, Lyness et al. 1992, McBride et al. 1988, Meert 1993, Murphy et al. 1988, Zabik et al. 1985). In a study that may be significant in light of the efficacy of naltrexone in alcoholism treatment, fluoxetine decreased ethanol consumption in rats, but was not as potent in that effect as the opioid antagonist, nalmefene (Hubbell et al. 1991). In two studies, desipramine also decreased ethanol consumption in animal models (Gatto et al. 1990, Murphy et al. 1985).

In a clinical study, zimelidine reduced ethanol consumption in problem drinkers (Naranjo et al. 1984b). In that study, 13 healthy male drinkers (ages 22 to 51 years), who drank an average 6.2 "standard drinks per day" at baseline, were given zimelidine (200 mg daily) or placebo in five, 2-week periods in a double-blind, randomized crossover experiment. Zimelidine decreased the number of drinks consumed and increased the percentage of days abstinent. As a group, no significant differences were observed between the number of drinks consumed on drinking days during zimelidine and placebo (7.23 vs. 6.63). There were, however, interindividual variations, with some subjects drinking less per episode, others having fewer drinking days but consuming the usual quantity, while still others reduced both frequency and quantity. The onset of effect is apparently rapid, as opposed to the 2- to 3-week delay in antidepressant effects. The mechanism for zimelidine's ability to reduce ethanol consumption may be blocking of the positive, reinforcing characteristics of ethanol or accentuation of the aversive effects of ethanol. The neurobiologic basis of this may lie in the serotonergic system. The reduction of ethanol consumption in this study was modest, less than a one-drink reduction per episode, and chemical hepatitis developed in three subjects, which reversed upon discontinuation of zimelidine.

Amit et al. (1985) studied the effects of zimelidine on the ethanol consumption of social drinkers. Healthy male volunteers who were social drinkers (defined as "consuming moderate amounts of alcohol one to three times per week but not having any admitted history of alcoholism") participated in three experimental sessions. One group ($N = 12$) received ethanol (in four equal doses of 0.25 g/kg of body weight at 10-minute intervals) plus zimelidine (200 mg or 300 mg), or placebo at weekly intervals. The other group ($N = 12$) received mixers without alcohol and the same drugs. Subjective self-rating scales and independent observers found no drug effect on alcohol-induced intoxication or euphoria. An open-ended self-report, however, found that 14.5% and 20% more subjects on zimelidine, 200 and 300 mg, respectively, had alcohol-induced euphoria attenuated as compared with placebo. Furthermore, after only one session of ethanol and zimelidine, subjects expressed a decreased desire to drink and a reduction in the actual amount of alcohol consumed the week following the experimental session. The administration of 200 mg of zimelidine plus ethanol resulted in a 35% reduction in alcohol consumption compared with baseline, whereas 300 mg of zimelidine led to a 21.3% reduction. These findings suggest that zimelidine reduced the positive reinforcement of ethanol.

In another study of problem drinkers, fluoxetine 60 mg daily (but not 40 mg daily or placebo) decreased mean daily alcohol drinks from 8.3 to 6.9 (Naranjo et al. 1990). In a study of male alcoholics treated with up to 80 mg of fluoxetine daily or placebo, the active treatment group had a 14% lower alcohol intake during the first week only, with no differences in intake, desire for alcohol, or rating scale scores of psychiatric symptoms during the rest of the 28-day study (Gorelick et al. 1992). Similarly, Kranzler et al. (1995) found that fluoxetine did not reduce relapse frequency or severity in alcohol-dependent patients.

MECHANISM

Ethanol consumption may be reduced through serotonergic-mediated appetite/consumption mechanisms (Gill et al. 1989, Gorelick 1989, 1989, Naranjo et al. 1984a). Some have proposed a role for the renin-angiotensin system (Grupp et al. 1988).

CLINICAL IMPLICATIONS

Depression and alcoholism frequently coexist. Because SSRIs do not appear to interact with ethanol in a clinically important way, they may provide a margin of safety in depressed patients who use ethanol. It should be noted, however, that fatal overdoses have occurred with fluoxetine alone or when it was combined with alcohol (Kincaid et al. 1990, Rohrig et al. 1989).

Animal studies have demonstrated that the SSRIs reduce ethanol consumption. Zimelidine, citalopram, and fluoxetine have produced modest reductions of alcohol intake in problem drinkers. Studies in alcoholics have not demonstrated a lasting or clinically significant effect. We recommend the use of SSRIs in alcoholics with primary depression, because it provides a margin of safety not offered with alternative antidepressants. As noted however, an overdose of SSRIs with ethanol may lead to fatalities or other medical complications (Lazarus 1990). Liver disease may also influence dosage, because impaired metabolism is likely in patients with cirrhosis (Schenker et al. 1988).

Hallucinogens

EVIDENCE OF INTERACTION

A 16-year-old boy who had been taking fluoxetine 20 mg daily for 1 year took two doses of lysergic acid diethylamide (LSD; blotter acid) and developed stupor and a generalized tonic-clonic (grand mal) seizure (Picker et al. 1992). Thirty previous experiences with LSD at lower doses had not produced a seizure in this patient even while he was taking fluoxetine.

Two cases of worsening of the LSD flashback syndrome by SSRI have been reported (Markel et al. 1994). The first patient was an 18-year-old girl who had stopped using LSD 10 months prior to her treatment for depression and panic attacks. During that period of drug abstinence, she had four LSD flashbacks. Two days after starting sertraline 50 mg daily, she had the worst flashback she had ever experienced, which lasted over 15 hours. She was then given paroxetine, which also led to a severe flashback lasting the entire day. After SSRIs were stopped, the patient did not experience any flashbacks during a 6-month follow-up. A second patient in the same report was a 17-year-old boy with prior LSD use in whom severe flashbacks developed 2 weeks after paroxetine was administered.

MECHANISM

The mechanism of the hallucinogenic effect of LSD is not known, although it probably involves sensitization of one or more subtypes of the serotonin receptor. The way in which SSRIs may increase the flashback phenomenon is unknown.

CLINICAL IMPLICATIONS

We have had the opportunity to prescribe SSRIs to many adults and adolescents who have a history of LSD use. Our experience has been that patients who have had dysphoric experiences and/or flashbacks from LSD often have a recurrence of these effects when SSRIs are started. The onset of these unpleasant effects is rapid, appearing most often after the first dose or after the first several doses of the SSRIs. We have not seen seizures with the combination, but our experience of patients who use LSD while taking SSRIs is very limited.

Histamine-2 (H_2) Blocking Agents (Cimetidine)

Limited evidence suggests that cimetidine impairs paroxetine metabolism (Greb et al. 1989a, 1985). Other SSRIs may also be affected, but no data are available.

Lithium (*See* Chapter 4)

L-Tryptophan

EVIDENCE OF INTERACTION

Steiner and Fontaine reported five cases of toxicity with the combination of L-tryptophan and fluoxetine (Steiner et al. 1986). Three men and two women with OCD were treated with fluoxetine in doses of 50 to 100 mg daily for periods ranging from 3 to 9 months. L-Tryptophan was added in doses of 2 to 4 g/day for 7 to 22 days. A toxic syndrome of varying intensity developed in all patients. Symptoms included agitation, restlessness, poor concentration, insomnia, aggressive behavior, chills, headaches, palpitations, worsening OCD symptoms, nausea, abdominal cramps, and diarrhea. Two of the patients had previously been treated with L-tryptophan at twice the dosage without ill effect, and two of the patients had previously taken L-tryptophan with clomipramine without problems.

A second type of interaction has been reported in animal studies. Both fluoxetine and L-tryptophan lower blood pressure in hypertensive rats (Fuller et al. 1979). The combination produces an additive decrement in blood pressure (Sved et al. 1982). Implications for humans with hypertension are not known.

MECHANISM

Fluoxetine is a selective inhibitor of serotonin reuptake into presynaptic nerve terminals, and L-tryptophan is a serotonin precursor. The combination results in enhanced serotonergic activity.

CLINICAL IMPLICATIONS

The case reports cited here were all patients with OCD, an illness that typically requires treatment with higher fluoxetine doses than those used for depression. We have seen patients who have tolerated L-tryptophan while taking 20-mg doses of fluoxetine; nevertheless, clinicians should be aware of possible toxicity using the combination.

The reduction of blood pressure in hypertensive rats treated with fluoxetine and L-tryptophan is an interesting observation, but its significance in humans has not been studied.

Melatonin

EVIDENCE OF INTERACTION

Five healthy male volunteers were given 5 mg of oral melatonin with and without a single 50 mg oral dose of fluvoxamine, separated by 1 week (Hartter et al. 2000). All subjects had increases in serum melatonin, "with an at least ninefold increase in AUC . . . and an at least sixfold increase in C_{max}" (Hartter et al. 2000).

MECHANISM

Melatonin is metabolized to 6-hydroxymelatonin by CYP1A2, and to N-acetylserotonin by CYP1A2 and 2C19 (Hartter et al. 2001). CYP1A2, which is inhibited by fluvoxamine, has the predominant role in melatonin metabolism.

CLINICAL SIGNIFICANCE

Fluvoxamine appears to be the only SSRI that interacts with melatonin. Other agents that alter CYP1A2 activity are likely to affect melatonin metabolism. Although the clinical implications of the interaction are not fully known, it has been suggested that the interaction could be of therapeutic benefit to increase the bioavailability of orally administered melatonin, which is used for sleep induction (Hartter et al. 2001).

Methadone (*See also* Opioids, Tramadol)

EVIDENCE OF INTERACTION

Fluvoxamine inhibits the metabolism of methadone, with resulting 20% to 100% increases of total R- and S-methadone (Bertschy et al. 1994, Bertschy et al. 1996). Fluoxetine increases only R-methadone, which is the active enantiomer, with slight but not significant increases in total plasma methadone levels (Eap et al. 1997).

MECHANISM

Fluvoxamine is a strong inhibitor of CYP1A2 and a weak inhibitor of CYP2D6. Fluoxetine and norfluoxetine strongly inhibit 2D6, with a somewhat lower inhibitory activity of 3A4 and 1A2; these enzymes are involved in methadone metabolism (Eap et al. 1997, Iribarne et al. 1997). One study (Eap et al. 1997) suggests that 2D6 is relatively specific for the metabolism of R-methadone, whereas 1A2 has lower stereoselectivity, although other interpretations are also possible.

CLINICAL SIGNIFICANCE

Depression is common among opioid-dependent patients. SSRIs with minimal effects on the cytochrome system, such as citalopram or escitalopram, should be first-line agents. The interaction has been used therapeutically to increase methadone levels in very rapid metabolizers. A patient who did not achieve effective methadone plasma levels at a dose of 200 mg/day was given fluvoxamine to increase the level and prevent withdrawal symptoms (DeMaria et al. 1999). The combination of fluvoxamine and methadone also has been associated with opioid toxicity (Alderman et al. 1999).

Monoamine Oxidase Inhibitors

EVIDENCE OF INTERACTION

In 1988, the manufacturer of fluoxetine reported that three fatalities occurred when tranylcypromine was prescribed subsequent to fluoxetine. Consequently, they recommended a 5-week washout period between fluoxetine discontinuation and the institution of MAOI therapy. Prior to the dissemination of that warning, a 31-year-old woman who had been taking fluoxetine 20 mg daily for 14 days was switched to tranylcypromine 10 mg daily, 2 days after stopping fluoxetine (Sternbach 1988). She increased the dose of tranylcypromine to 20 mg daily 6 days after the fluoxetine was discontinued. Two to three hours after she took the increased dose, she experienced "uncontrollable shivering, double vision, nausea, confusion . . . anxiety . . . and audible chattering of her teeth." Her blood pressure was 110/80 mm Hg and temperature 37.2°C. Her symptoms cleared 24 hours after tranylcypromine was discontinued. Six weeks later, a fluoxetine challenge in the absence of tranylcypromine was negative. Except for the absence of hyperthermia, the clinical presentation was consistent with a serotonergic syndrome.

Since those reports appeared, additional information on fluoxetine– MAOI interactions has been made available. In a report, Beasley et al. (1993) described eight severe reactions to the drug combination involving seven deaths that were known to the manufacturer of fluoxetine. Five patients died when tranylcypromine was added within a few days after stopping fluoxetine; one died after phenelzine was started shortly after discontinuing fluoxetine. The seventh patient died after tranylcypromine was added to fluoxetine. The clinical presentation of these cases was characteristic of the serotonin syndrome, with hyperthermia, headache, agitation, myoclonus, disorientation, hypertension, delirium, seizures, and ventricular tachycardia. One patient in whom severe symptoms developed but who survived began treatment with tranylcypromine 7 days after stopping fluoxetine. Two days later, toxicity began to develop— slurred speech, nystagmus, confusion, ataxia. She was treated successfully with the discontinuation of tranylcypromine and administration of cyproheptadine.

A case report also was published of sertraline (at first 50 mg daily, which was then reduced to 25 mg daily) added to tranylcypromine 10 mg daily, plus clonazepam 1.5 mg daily, after which adverse effects developed—anergy, decreased libido, chills, restlessness, unsteadiness, constipation, and urinary hesitancy (Bhatara et al. 1993).

Although reports exist of safely combining selegiline (Eldepryl) with sertraline, fluoxetine, or paroxetine in depressed patients with Parkinson disease (Toyama et al. 1994, Waters 1994), the manufacturer of Eldepryl, in a warning letter to physicians in November 1994, reported instances of muscular rigidity, autonomic instability, severe agitation, and delirium when SSRIs were combined with selegiline. Several published reports document an adverse interaction between selegiline and fluoxetine (Dingemanse et al. 1990, Jermain et al. 1992, Montastruc et al. 1993, Shader et al. 1985, Suchowersky et al. 1990).

The reversible inhibitor of monoamine oxidase A, moclobemide, has been linked to a serotonergic syndrome when combined with citalopram and clomipramine, but one group of investigators has used it safely in combination with sertraline or fluvoxamine in the treatment resistant depressions (Dingemanse 1993) (for a more complete discussion of moclobemide, see the section on Monoamine Oxidase Inhibitors). Linezolid (Zyvox and Macrobid) is an antibiotic that has monoamine oxidase inhibiting activity. A case report documents a 56-year-old female who developed serotonin syndrome when linezolid was given soon after the discontinuation of paroxetine (Wigen et al. 2002).

MECHANISM

The serotonergic syndrome is well described. It is believed to be the same mechanism underlying the well-recognized meperidine–MAOI interaction. Symptoms include excitement, diaphoresis, rigidity, hyperthermia, hyperreflexia, tachycardia, hypotension, coma, and death. Animal studies confirm that rats pretreated with tranylcypromine develop a hyperthermic syndrome after fluoxetine (Marley et al. 1984). Pretreatment with parachlorophenylalanine blocks the toxic effects, suggesting that serotonin is responsible for the syndrome. Graham et al. (1988) and Marley et al. (1984) propose that it is the balance between an antidepressant's serotonin and dopamine reuptake blocking potencies that determines the risk of the syndrome. In this model, antidepressants that have marked effects on serotonin reuptake but little effect on dopamine (e.g., fluoxetine, clomipramine) would be a high risk for interactions with MAOIs. Drugs with intermediate ratios (e.g., amitriptyline, imipramine) would be at lower risk, and mianserin, which affects neither dopamine nor serotonin, would be at least risk.

CLINICAL IMPLICATIONS

With the advent of more selective serotonergic agents, overstimulation of the serotonergic system has become a more common clinical problem. A minimum of 5 weeks should separate fluoxetine discontinuation from the administration of a MAOI. This will permit the elimination of both fluoxetine and norfluoxetine. If especially high doses of fluoxetine have been administered, an even longer drug-free period may be necessary (Coplan et al. 1993). With those SSRIs for which the parent drug and metabolite having shorter elimination half-lives than fluoxetine (e.g., sertraline) or no clinically important metabolites (e.g., fluvoxamine), a 2-week drug-free period is recommended. It is important for clinicians to remember that the half-lives of a drug are variable from one patient to another, and the mean values provided by the manufacturer should only serve as a guide to prescribing. Serum SSRI levels may be helpful in assessing adequate washout periods between SSRIs and MAOIs.

Neuroleptics/Antipsychotics (*See* Chapter 3)

Opioids (*See also* Methadone)

EVIDENCE OF INTERACTION

Fluoxetine, like many other antidepressants, can potentiate the analgesic effects of some opioids. Pretreatment with fluoxetine increased and prolonged catalepsy induced by morphine, codeine, and fentanyl. Antinoceptive action was potentiated for morphine and fentanyl, but not codeine or pentazocine (Larson et al. 1977).

A case report described an interaction between pentazocine and fluoxetine (Hansen et al. 1990). A 39-year-old man taking fluoxetine 40 mg daily was given an oral analgesic containing pentazocine 100 mg and naloxone 0.5 mg (Talwin NX). Within 30 minutes, lightheadedness, anxiety, nausea, paresthesia, tremor, ataxia, and elevated blood pressure developed. He was treated with diphenhydramine 50 mg intramuscularly, and symptoms lasted for about 4 hours.

There have been two case reports of SSRI interactions with cough and cold products containing dextromethorphan. In one case a 51-year-old man taking paroxetine took a combination product containing dextromethorphan, doxylamine, pseudoephedrine, and acetaminophen (NyQuil) (Skop et al. 1994). After 2 days of treatment using the combination, nausea, tremor, diaphoresis, confusion, headache, shortness of breath, vomiting, muscular rigidity, frontal release signs, and elevated blood pressure developed. A good response occurred to drug discontinuation and intravenous lorazepam. The other case report described a 32-year-old woman taking fluoxetine 20 mg daily who, on the 17th day of treatment, started a cough syrup containing dextromethorphan (Achamallah 1992). A day later, 2 hours after taking 2 teaspoons of the syrup, she had hallucinations of vivid colors, and she perceived distortions in the shape and dimensions of her surroundings. Her symptoms persisted for 6 to 8 hours, and she described them as similar to her prior experience with LSD 12 years earlier. Interpretation of this case is complicated by reports of flashbacks in former LSD users taking only SSRIs (*see* Hallucinogens, this section). Another report of vivid hallucinations and tremors in a 34-year-old man was attributed to the combination of sertraline and oxycodone (Rosebraugh et al. 2001).

MECHANISM

The combination of an SSRI with pentazocine, dextromethorphan, or other opioids affecting serotonin may lead to serotonergic overstimulation. A pharmacokinetic interaction between SSRI and dextromethorphan is also possible.

With respect to analgesic effects, several studies have indicated that serotonergic activity is important in the analgesic effects of morphine. Depletion of serotonin by drugs such as p-chlorophenylalanine or 5,6-hydroxytryptamine diminishes morphine analgesia. Lesions in the midbrain or medullary serotonin system also block morphine's analgesic effects. Enhanced serotonergic activity by the administration of agonists, uptake inhibitors, or precursors potentiates morphine analgesia.

CLINICAL IMPLICATIONS

SSRIs in combination with opioid drugs that affect serotonin, such as dextromethorphan, meperidine, and perhaps pentazocine, may cause a serotonergic syndrome similar to that seen with the MAOIs and these opioids. This reaction has not been clearly established for SSRIs, and issues related to dose and pharmacokinetic interactions have not been studied. Nevertheless, until more information is available, clinicians may wish to avoid the combination and warn patients about over-the-counter medications that contain dextromethorphan.

Fluoxetine potentiates the analgesic effects of morphine and fentanyl in rats (Kellstein et al. 1988). Clinical studies are lacking, but it should be noted that tolerance occurs to antidepressant potentiation of opioid analgesia (Malec et al. 1980).

Stimulants

Pemoline (Metz et al. 1991), amphetamine (Linet 1989), and methylphenidate (Bussing et al. 1993, Gammon et al. 1993, Salonen et al. 2003) have been used to potentiate SSRI response in depression and attention deficit disorder. Minimal adverse effects have been reported, usually related to stimulant effects (e.g., anxiety, insomnia).

Terfenadine (Seldane)

EVIDENCE OF INTERACTION

A single case report documents a purported link of fluoxetine and ter-fenadine to symptoms of shortness of breath, sinus tachycardia, and atrial premature contractions (Swims 1993). The patient described was taking multiple medications, including a sympathomimetic (isometheptene contained in Midrin), ibuprofen, misoprostol (Cytotec), and ranitidine (Zantac). Symptoms of shortness of breath and irregular heartbeat developed about 1 month after fluoxetine 20 mg daily was added to terfenadine 60 mg twice daily, in addition to the aforementioned medications.

MECHANISM

Terfenadine has been linked to drug interactions when given with drugs that inhibit cytochrome P450-3A4 (e.g., ketoconazole). Although some have dismissed the interaction because fluoxetine itself does not substantially affect 3A4, they have overlooked the fact that norfluoxetine, its major metabolite does inhibit 3A4, the isoenzyme responsible for ter-fenadine metabolism. Other SSRIs and nefazodone also inhibit 3A4.

CLINICAL IMPLICATIONS

Although only one case report of the interaction exists, it is potentially serious, because terfenadine can impair cardiac conduction and cause arrhythmias. We would recommend avoiding the combination of ter-fenadine with any SSRI, nefazodone, or other drug that inhibits cytochrome P450-3A4 (Table 2.3). Astemizole (Hismanal) is also contraindicated in patients taking drugs that inhibit 3A4.

Testosterone

EVIDENCE OF INTERACTION

Testosterone supplementation was recently shown to improve depressive symptoms for a subset of male patients with low or borderline testosterone levels suffering from refractory depression. A randomized, double-blind, placebo-controlled trial in 23 patients with a low or borderline serum testosterone level (range 100 to 350 ng/dL; normal range is 270 to 1,070 ng/dL) who met the DSM IV criteria for current major depressive disorder and were being treated with antidepressant medications prior to and during the trial received either testosterone gel (1% gel, 10g/d) or placebo for 8 weeks. The investigators reported significantly greater improvement in HAM-D scores in the testosterone-treated group when compared to the placebo-treated group in both the vegetative and affective symptoms subscales of the HAM-D Scale. Overall, the testosterone gel was well tolerated. One patient in the study experienced an exacerbation of benign prostatic hyperplasia (BPH), which may be attributed to testosterone supplementation; this man was withdrawn from the study. The mechanism of testosterone's antidepressant action is not known.

Tetrahydrocannabinol

EVIDENCE OF INTERACTION

β-9-Tetrahydrocannabinol-induced aggressive behavior in rats previously deprived of rapid eye movement (REM) sleep was potentiated by fluoxetine and tryptophan, but blocked by parachlorophenylalanine, cyproheptadine, and cinanserin (Carlini et al. 1982).

MECHANISM

Increased serotonergic activity potentiates the aggressive behavior, and drugs that decrease serotonergic activity block the aggression. It is believed that both dopamine and serotonin play a role in this animal model of aggression (Carlini et al. 1982).

CLINICAL IMPLICATIONS

Human studies of this interaction are lacking.

Theophylline

EVIDENCE OF INTERACTION

Several case reports document theophylline toxicity when the drug was given in combination with fluvoxamine (Diot et al. 1991). In a 78-year-old woman taking sustained-release theophylline 400 mg twice daily, theophylline toxicity developed 2 days after fluvoxamine 50 mg was started (van den Brekel et al. 1994). Anorexia, nausea, supraventricular tachycardia, a generalized tonic-clonic (grand mal) seizure, and coma developed, as her theophylline level increased from 74 mmol/L to 197 mmol/L. She recovered, and theophylline was restarted at the previous dose without fluvoxamine, and therapeutic levels were maintained. In another case, theophylline toxicity, with ventricular tachycardia, developed in a 70-year-old man when his fluvoxamine dose was increased from 50 to 100 mg daily (Thomson et al. 1992). A third report (Sperber 1991) described an 11-year-old boy taking sustained-release theophylline 300 mg twice daily whose serum theophylline levels doubled when he was given fluvoxamine (25 mg twice daily, then lowered to 25 mg once daily).

MECHANISM
Fluvoxamine is a potent inhibitor of cytochrome P450-1A2, which metabolizes theophylline.

CLINICAL IMPLICATIONS
Fluvoxamine should be avoided when patients are taking theophylline. Alternative SSRIs that do not inhibit 1A2, such as sertraline, fluoxetine, or paroxetine, may be used. Theophylline toxicity is a serious, sometimes fatal, medical condition. Early signs are nausea (which may be confused with SSRI effects), diarrhea, dizziness, headache, hyperreflexia, and tachycardia. In severe cases, myoclonic jerks, generalized tonic-clonic seizures, and ventricular tachycardia may develop.

Tramadol (Ultram, *See also* Opioids, Methadone)

EVIDENCE OF INTERACTION
Tramadol is a synthetic opioid analgesic that acts by directly binding to the μ-opioid receptor and by reuptake inhibition of serotonin and norepinephrine. Several case reports have documented toxicity developing with the combination of an SSRI and tramadol.

A 42-year old woman taking sertraline (100 mg/day for over 1 year) developed confusion, agitation, psychosis, "sundowning," diaphoresis, tremor, and chest pain shortly after the addition of 300 mg/day of tramadol (Mason et al. 1997). Another case of sertraline interaction with tramadol has been reported in an elderly woman (Sauget et al. 2002).

A serotonin syndrome also has been reported when the analgesic was combined with citalopram (Mahlberg et al. 2004). In that case, a 70-year-old woman who was taking citalopram (20 mg/day for 3 years) was given tramadol (50 mg/day) for pain relief following abdominal surgery. She developed "tremors, restlessness, fever, confusion, and visual hallucinations" (Mahlberg et al. 2004). Symptoms resolved after the discontinuation of tramadol, but returned a year later when she was again given tramadol in a lower dose (20 mg/day). This patient had heterozygous genotypes for CYP2D6 and CYP2C19, which may have impaired metabolism of both drugs. Serotonin syndrome has also been reported when tramadol was combined with venlafaxine (Prescire Int, 2004), with venlafaxine or mirtazapine (Houlihan 2004), and with paroxetine (Egberts et al. 1997, Lantz et al. 1998). The serotonin syndrome was associated with manic symptoms in one case report (Gonzalez-Pinto et al. 2001).

MECHANISM

Several SSRIs inhibit CYP2D6, which is involved in tramadol metabolism. Increased serotonergic tone also may be a result of additive or synergistic pharmacodynamic effects.

CLINICAL IMPLICATIONS

The use of tramadol with SSRIs should be undertaken with caution. The highest risk appears to be in patients who have impaired metabolism, from either a genetic predisposition or concomitant drug therapy. Discontinuation of tramadol results in rapid symptom alleviation. Some case reports have used cyproheptadine for treatment of the serotonin syndrome.

WARFARIN

EVIDENCE OF INTERACTION

Data on the interactions of SSRIs with warfarin are contradictory. With respect to fluoxetine, studies in rats and humans have yielded conflicting results (Rowe et al. 1978). Rats were pretreated with fluoxetine (10 mg/kg) or saline 15 minutes prior to the oral administration of warfarin. The plasma half-life of warfarin in the fluoxetine group was 22.8 hours, compared with 8 hours in the saline group. In the same report, the warfarin half-life in three healthy male volunteers did not change with pretreatment of a single oral dose of fluoxetine 30 mg 3 hours prior to warfarin, fluoxetine 30 mg daily for 1 week, or when warfarin was given alone (36 hours, 33 hours, and 33 hours, respectively). Warfarin-induced prolongation of prothrombin time was not affected by fluoxetine. Similarly, the addition of fluoxetine (20 mg/day for 21 days) in six patients stabilized on warfarin did not alter bleeding (Ford et al. 1997).

On the other hand, case reports continue to appear suggesting an interaction between fluoxetine and warfarin. In one case, bruising developed in a woman taking fluoxetine after warfarin was added (Claire et al. 1991). In another case, a 47-year-old man who had been stabilized on warfarin had an increase in INR (a measure of anticoagulant activity) 10 days after fluoxetine 20 mg daily was added (Woolfrey et al. 1993). That same report identified another patient, a 72-year-old woman, whose INR became elevated 10 days after starting fluoxetine 20 mg daily. An 83-year-old man had an elevation of INR almost 5 days after beginning fluoxetine (10 mg/day) and died of a cerebral hemorrhage (Dent et al. 1997).

The plasma versus time AUC for warfarin was increased by multiple doses of sertraline, and prothrombin time was increased 8.9% in one study (Wilner et al. 1991).

In a separate study, paroxetine did not increase plasma warfarin concentrations, but the combination was associated with bleeding (van Harten 1993).

Two weeks of therapy with fluvoxamine increased warfarin concentrations by 65% and resulted in increased prothrombin times (van Harten 1993). Fluvoxamine (50 mg/day) was associated with an increased INR when it was substituted for citalopram (Limke et al 2002), which does alter warfarin pharmacokinetics (Priskorn et al. 1997). On the other hand, one case report indicated that when citalopram was added to acenocoumarol (an anticoagulant that is not marketed in the United States), INR increased to 15 and was associated with gingival bleeding (Borras-Blasco et al. 2002).

MECHANISM

Three potential mechanisms exist for SSRI interactions with warfarin. The first is the possibility that highly protein-bound SSRIs (e.g., fluoxetine, sertraline, paroxetine) could displace warfarin from binding sites, transiently increasing its effects.

The second type of interactions is that involving drug metabolism. As described by Harvey et al. (1996a, 1996b), the metabolism of warfarin is complex. Warfarin is a racemic mixture, with the (S)-enantiomer providing most of the anticoagulant action. The cytochrome responsible for the metabolism of (S)-warfarin is 2C9. The inactive (R)-warfarin is hydroxylated through the 1A2 and 3A4 isoenzymes, and (R)-warfarin inhibits 2C9, even though that enzyme is not involved in its metabolism. The effects of SSRIs on 2C9 are not well studied, making it impossible at this time to predict the effects of different SSRIs on metabolism of the (S)-enantiomer. The interaction with fluvoxamine, however, may be understood on the basis of its inhibition of 1A2, which results in increased levels of the inactive (R)-enantiomer. This enantiomer, in turn, inhibits the metabolism of the active (S)-enantiomer by influencing 2C9 activity.

A third possibility is that fluoxetine itself has anticoagulant effects in some patients (Aranth et al. 1992, Yaryura-Tobias et al. 1991).

CLINICAL IMPLICATIONS

In a small human sample given clinically relevant doses of fluoxetine, no alterations were seen in warfarin half-life or prothrombin time. Animal studies, however, using very large fluoxetine doses, showed impaired clearance of warfarin. Fluoxetine, sertraline, and paroxetine are highly protein bound, and a potential exists for a protein-binding interaction with warfarin. Isolated case reports continue to appear suggesting the possibility of increased anticoagulant effect in some patients on fluoxetine and warfarin. The possibility of bleeding as an adverse effect of fluoxetine alone also has been raised by case reports (Aranth et al. 1992, Yaryura-Tobias et al. 1991). A metabolic drug interaction may be most likely with fluvoxamine. Until additional information on the effects of specific SSRIs on warfarin metabolism is available, clinicians should be aware of a potential interaction. A protein-binding interaction would be of most concern when adding a highly protein-bound SSRI to warfarin, because this could transiently increase free warfarin and enhance the anticoagulant effect. It should be emphasized that this is a transient effect. Interactions involving impaired metabolism usually take longer to develop, as steady-state levels of the SSRI are reached. The frequency of these types of interactions between SSRI and warfarin is not known.

Section 2.3 Monoamine Oxidase Inhibitors

Monoamine oxidase (MAO) is an enzyme that is located principally on the outer mitochondrial membrane. This enzyme acts via a pathway of oxidative deamination to inactivate over 15 different monoamines formed in the human body, some of which serve very important roles as neurotransmitters, neuromodulators, or hormones (Baker et al. 1999, Murphy et al. 1984). Several substrate-selective MAOIs were developed in the late 1960s, which provided the first evidence for two forms of the enzyme. MAO-A selectively deaminates serotonin and norepinephrine, whereas MAO-B selectively degrades benzylamine and phenylethylamine. Dopamine is metabolized by both MAO-A and MAO-B, but is considered by some authorities to be the preferred substrate for MAO-B in humans. Specificity of a substrate for the enzyme is dependent on concentration, so that specificity is relative rather than absolute.

The purpose of this chapter is to discuss the interactions of several prescribed and over-the-counter medications, with MAOI antidepressant drugs—phenelzine (Nardil), tranylcypromine (Parnate), and isocarboxazid (formerly marketed as Marplan, but no longer available in the United States). Selegiline, an MAOI that is approved for treatment of Parkinson disease, has antidepressant activity at higher therapeutic doses. Other MAOIs are not used to treat depression, such as pargyline (formerly marketed in the United States as an antihypertensive, Eutonyl), procarbazine (marketed as Matulane, an antineoplastic agent), isoniazid (an antituberculosis agent), and furazolidone (marketed as Furoxone, a synthetic antimicrobial), which are all nonselective inhibitors of MAO-A and MAO-B. These nonselective MAOIs irreversibly inactivate the monoamine oxidase A and B enzymes. Irreversible inhibition is sometimes referred to as "suicide enzyme inhibition," because irreversible covalent bonds are formed at the active site of the enzyme. This action has clinical importance because it accounts for the long duration of the pharmacodynamic effect of these drugs, although many of them, such as phenelzine and tranylcypromine, have short elimination half-lives.

Intestinal MAO is primarily type A, whereas MAO in the brain is mainly (70% to 75%) type B; however, little is known about the regional brain differences of these two MAO subtypes in humans.

Surprisingly few studies exist of the pharmacokinetics of phenelzine or tranylcypromine, the two most widely prescribed MAOI antidepressants in this country. Phenelzine was once thought to undergo acetylation as its primary metabolic step, but more recent studies have challenged that assertion; new data suggest that oxidative metabolism to phenylacetic acid and its ring-hydroxylated metabolite may be the major pathway of degradation. Tranylcypromine is rapidly absorbed with peak plasma levels occurring within 1 to 2 hours, and it has an elimination half-life of less than 2 hours. A single 10-mg dose can produce MAO inhibition lasting 1 week. After 4 weeks of treatment, tyramine sensitivity lasts for several days, but the occasional patient may maintain sensitivity for several weeks.

Phenelzine and tranylcypromine are thought to act at different sites on the MAO enzyme, with phenelzine inactivating the flavin group, whereas tranylcypromine acts at the sulfhydryl group. Return of MAO activity is more rapid after tranylcypromine is discontinued than after phenelzine is stopped, which may reflect slow reversibility, rather than complete irreversibility, of its action on the enzyme.

The actions of MAOIs on cytochrome systems are not well studied, however tranylcypromine is a competitive inhibitor of CYP2C19 and 2D6 and a noncompetitive inhibitor of 2C9, although these actions do not appear to be clinically relevant at therapeutic doses (Salsali et al. 2004). Selegiline (Eldepryl, often referred to in the research literature as *l*-deprenyl) is an MAOI marketed for the treatment of Parkinson disease. At low doses, it is an irreversible selective inhibitor of MAO-B, but it loses its selectivity as dosage is increased, and in some cases, especially with chronic dosing, may be nonselective even at a 10-mg dose. For all practical purposes, clinicians in the United States do not at present have a truly selective MAOI to treat depression. Selegiline is a substrate for CYP2B6, IA2, 2C8, 2C19, but probably not 2D6, although data are contradictory (Salonen et al. 2003).

Moclobemide is a reversible MAO-A inhibitor, which is available in Canada and the United Kingdom, but not in the United States. It is rapidly absorbed after an oral dose, with maximum plasma concentrations occurring between 0.5 to 2 hours. It is not highly bound, so protein binding interactions do not occur. The reversibility of its MAO inhibition leads to a smaller increase in blood pressure in response to tyramine, especially in healthy volunteers, but in depressed patients the increase may produce clinical symptoms. Moclobemide is much less likely to produce hypertension in response to ingested tyramine than is tranylcypromine. The former drug produces a two- to four-fold enhancement of the pressor response to tyramine, whereas the latter causes a 30-fold increase. Some studies have indicated that moclobemide does not interact with SSRIs or tricyclic antidepressants, although a serotonergic syndrome has been reported when it was given shortly after clomipramine was stopped, and fatalities have resulted when it was taken in overdose with clomipramine or citalopram. Moclobemide is oxidatively metabolized, and it is a potent inhibitor of cytochrome P450-2D6, making it susceptible to pharmacokinetic interactions.

Despite the introduction of new MAOIs in other countries, clinicians in the United States are limited to the older agents. The two most important types of interactions with these MAOIs are the hypertensive crisis due to interactions with sympathomimetic drugs or tyramine and a serotonergic syndrome due to the combination of MAOIs with SSRIs or those opioids that have serotonergic effects (Blackwell 1991). Some pharmacokinetic interactions also occur with the MAOIs, but these are not well studied. Major interactions are summarized in Table 2.6.

Amantadine

EVIDENCE OF INTERACTION

A possible interaction between phenelzine and amantadine has been noted in the clinical literature (Jack et al. 1984). Amantadine hydrochloride is a dopaminergic agent frequently used as adjunctive therapy in the treatment of Parkinson disease and as a treatment of the neuroleptic-induced parkinsonian side effects of antipsychotic medication. A 49-year-old woman was administered haloperidol and amantadine hydrochloride in progressively increasing dosage, up to 15 and 300 mg/day, respectively. Haloperidol was discontinued, and phenelzine was started because of treatment refractoriness, with the daily dose increased to 60 mg over 3 days. The patient's blood pressure increased from a baseline of approximately 140/90 mm Hg to

(text continues on page 128)

TABLE 2.6.   MAOI DRUG INTERACTIONS[a]

Drug	Interaction
Antiasthmatics	Oxtriphylline, a theophylline derivative, and albuterol when given to patients on phenelzine may lead to apprehension, tachycardia, and palpitations. One case report describes the onset of hypomania following the addition of isoetharine (an inhaled β-adrenergic agonist) to phenelzine.
Antibiotics	Sulfisoxazole, when added to phenelzine may result in ataxia, vertigo, tinnitus, muscle pain, parestheslec.
Anticholinergics	Atropine and scopolamine are potentiated by MAOI.
Antidepressants	Although the danger of this combination may have been exaggerated, there are several reports indicating that combined therapy may lead to a potentially fatal interaction. Commonly described symptoms are diaphoresis, tremor, fever, confusion, agitation, dyspnea, hallucinations, hypotension, and convulsions. Coma and death may ensue. Recent studies suggest that the combination may be safe when certain guidelines are followed. Both drugs should be started simultaneously in lower than usual doses and only via the oral route. Amitriptyline, trimipramine, and nortriptyline appear to be the safest. Imipramine, desipramine, clomipramine, and selective serotonin reuptake inhibitors should be avoided.
Antihypertensives	Reserpine given with MAOI may result in autonomic excitation, delirious agitation, and hypertension. Clonidine administered with MAOI may lead to hypertensive reaction, but clinical experience is lacking. Some experts believe propranolol should not be used with MAOI to avoid hypertensive reactions, but low doses have been safely used. MAOI potentiates the hypotensive action of thiazides. The antihypertensive effects of guanethidine are blocked by MAOI.
Atracurium	A case report described a 61-year-old woman with narcolepsy taking tranylcypromine (<20 mg b.i.d.). She developed hypertension (systolic 350 mm Hg) 2 minutes after induction with etomidate (0.3 mg/kg) intravenous infusion followed by atracurium (0.8 mg/kg). Over 3 minutes, systolic pressure declined to 180 mm Hg and by 15 minutes was 150/90 mm Hg. Because etomidate has been used without incident in patients taking tranylcypromine, this report suggests that atracurium may be the agent responsible for the adverse reaction (Sides 1987).
Barbiturates	Tranylcypromine may prolong barbiturate-induced hypnosis.

(continued)

TABLE 2.6. MAOI DRUG INTERACTIONS (CONTINUED)

Drug	Interaction
Benzodiazepines	The combination is widely used without serious interactions. Two case reports exist describing generalized edema when chlordiazepoxide was given with phenelzine or tranylcypromine, but this could develop with an MAOI alone. One group reports a number of patients developing a disinhibited state when given this combination. Chorea has also been reported.
Buspirone	The manufacturer has reported four cases of elevated blood pressure with this drug combination. Many patients taking the combination, however, do not experience blood pressure alterations.
Ethanol	Alcoholic beverages with high tyramine content may produce a hypertensive reaction in patients on MAOI. Pargyline may produce a disulfiram-like reaction when ethanol is ingested.
Ginseng	May cause headache, tremulousness or hypomanic symptoms when taken by patients on phenelzine (Jones et al. 1987).
Hypoglycemic agents	Enhanced hypoglycemic response have been reported in some patients receiving MAOI with insulin or sulfonylurea hypoglycemics.
Lithium	The combination may be useful in treatment of refractory depressions.
Narcotic analgesics	Hypo- and hypertension, excitement, diaphoresis, rigidity, hyperreflexia, hyperthermia, tachycardia, coma, and death have been reported with meperidine-MAOI combinations. Dextromethorphan may also cause a hypertensive, hypermetabolic reaction with MAOI (i.e. a serotonin syndrome). Morphine, codeine, and fentanyl are less likely to interact when used in reduced dosages.
Neuroleptics	The combination may lead to enhanced anticholinergic side effects, and extrapyramidal symptoms. Clinical use includes protection against MAOI-tyramine hypertensive crisis and treatment of anhedonic schizophrenics. A combination of tranylcypromine and trifluoperazine is marketed outside the United States and is considered by many to be safe.
Protein dietary supplement	There is a case report of a patient on MAOI (phenelzine) who, following ingestion of a powdered protein diet supplement, experienced a hypertensive crisis. This product and similar ones contain yeast, yeast spirulina, or yeast extract (Zetin et al. 1987).

(continued)

TABLE 2.6.   MAOI DRUG INTERACTIONS (CONTINUED)

Drug	Interaction
Succinylcholine	Phenelzine may reduce cholinesterase levels and lead to prolonged apnea during electroconvulsive therapy or surgical procedures. Other MAOI do not appear to have this effect.
Sympathomimetics indirect (amphetamine, methamphetamine, cyclopentamine, ephedrine, pseudoephedrine, guanethidine, L-dopa, α-methyldopa, dopamine, mephentermine, phentermine, metaraminol, methylphenidate, phenylpropanolamine, reserpine, tyramine)	Both direct and indirect sympathomimetic amines may interact with MAOI although the latter are more dangerous. Concomitant use may lead to hypertension, agitation, fever, convulsion, and coma. On the other hand, recent case reports suggest that dextroamphetamine, methylphenidate, and phentermine may have a role when coprescribed with MAOI in treatment-resistant depressions.
Direct (epinephrine, norepinephrine, phenylephrine, isoproterenol, methoxymine)	
Tryptophan	Occasionally used as a hypnotic in patients taking MAOI or to potentiate antidepressant effect. It may cause delirium, myoclonus, or hypomania.
Verapamil	Verapamil blocks phenelzine-induced hypomania (Dubovsky et al. 1985).

[a]Modified from Ciraulo et al.: Drug interactions with monoamine oxidase inhibitors. In: Shader, RI (ed.): *MAOI Therapy* Audio Visual Medical Marketing, New York, 1988b, p. 63. For references not listed, please see text.

160/110 mm Hg. Prior to the administration of phenelzine and amantadine, the patient had never had elevated blood pressure.

MECHANISM

It is well known that a hypertensive reaction can occur secondary to the combination of L-dopa or dopamine and phenelzine, and this case report may be the first documented reaction between another dopaminergic agent (amantadine) and phenelzine.

CLINICAL IMPLICATIONS

Although the evidence is limited to one case, it is possible that elevated blood pressure may result from an interaction between amantadine and phenelzine. This is probably an uncommon drug combination, but if these medications are used together, monitoring of blood pressure is indicated.

Antibiotics

EVIDENCE OF INTERACTION

A probable adverse interaction between the MAOI phenelzine and sulfisoxazole, a sulfonamide antimicrobial agent has been reported (Boyer et al. 1983). A 37-year-old woman was being treated with phenelzine 15 mg three times daily for depression. Three weeks after beginning phenelzine therapy, the patient was prescribed a 10-day course of oral sulfisoxazole, 1 g every 6 hours, for a urinary tract infection. Approximately 1 week after starting the antibiotic concurrently with phenelzine, the patient felt extremely weak walking up steps, fell, and was momentarily unable to stand. For the following 72 hours (during the remainder of her sulfisoxazole course), the patient also experienced ataxia, vertigo, tinnitus, muscle pain, and paresthesia. The symptoms started to resolve immediately after discontinuation of sulfisoxazole and were entirely absent 10 days after their first presentation.

MECHANISM

Phenelzine interacts with several compounds by inhibiting the hepatic enzymes responsible for drug metabolism. The role of acetylation as the primary degradation pathway for phenelzine has recently been challenged, although it is the major metabolic pathway for sulfisoxazole. Irrespective of this dispute, it is still likely that the combination of sulfisoxazole and phenelzine impaired this patient's acetylation capacity, resulting in higher than usual plasma levels and side effects of one or both medications (Boyer et al. 1983).

CLINICAL IMPLICATIONS

Although the authors of the report underscore the fact that one case does not conclusively establish the existence of a predictable adverse reaction between sulfisoxazole and phenelzine, because sulfisoxazole is frequently prescribed, it is important for clinicians to be aware of the possibility of toxicity when these drugs are administered concurrently.

Anticholinergics

EVIDENCE OF INTERACTION

Several authors emphasize the potential dangers of co-prescribing MAOI medications with anticholinergic drugs, especially atropine and scopolamine, which are both potentiated by MAOI (Davidson et al. 1984, Walker et al. 1984).

MECHANISM

Although MAOIs possess little anticholinergic activity as measured by in vitro laboratory measures, patients often report symptoms such as dry mouth, constipation, and urinary hesitancy (especially with phenelzine), suggesting that these drugs may act indirectly to enhance anticholinergic activity.

CLINICAL IMPLICATIONS

Because the anticholinergic properties of atropine and scopolamine are potentiated by MAOIs, it may be advisable to discontinue an MAOI prior to elective surgery. The dosages of antihistamines, antiparkinsonian agents, and other anticholinergic agents often must be reduced.

Anticonvulsants (*See* Chapter 5)

Antihypertensives (*See also* β-Adrenergic Blockers)

EVIDENCE OF INTERACTION

Some serious complications have been reported with antihypertensive–MAOI combinations, including α-methyldopa, clonidine, reserpine, and guanethidine (Davidson et al. 1984, Davies 1960). Despite animal studies that suggest possible adverse interactions between pargyline and methyldopa, only one case report exists in the human literature describing hallucinosis as a result of the combination. A hypertensive woman who was being treated with pargyline at a dosage of 25 mg given four times daily, developed hallucinations approximately 1 month after initiating concomitant treatment with methyldopa at a dosage of 250 to 500 mg daily. This is unusual in light of several other patients who received the combination with no unusual reactions or toxic effects (Paykel 1966).

Although reserpine has rarely been used in hypertensive patients requiring treatment for depression, case reports document central excitation and hypertension as a consequence of combined therapy. This reaction, however, appears to be less likely if reserpine is administered prior to the monoamine oxidase inhibitor. One case report described a chronically depressed woman treated first with nialamide alone at a dosage of 100 mg given three times daily, followed by the addition of reserpine on the third day of treatment at a dosage 0.5 mg given three times daily. The woman became hypomanic approximately 24 hours after initiating the reserpine, which progressed to frank mania (Gradwell 1960). Other case reports have documented disturbance of affect and memory associated with autonomic excitation, delirious agitation, and disorientation. It has also been reported that the antihypertensive effects of guanethidine can be antagonized by nialamide. Five hypertensive patients whose blood pressure had been controlled well with guanethidine in a dosage of 25 to 35 mg daily were then given single 50-mg doses of nialamide, which caused mean blood pressure readings to rise from about 140/85 to 165/100 mm Hg (Fann et al. 1971).

MECHANISM

Methyldopa may cause the sudden release of accumulated catecholamines, which are presumed to be at higher levels in individuals being treated with MAOIs. This sudden release of accumulated catecholamines could be responsible for a hypertensive crisis. Because reserpine depletes intracellular catecholamines by causing their release from bound stores, the acute administration of reserpine to a patient taking an MAOI can lead to a hypertensive crisis. The initial release of norepinephrine and serotonin can produce dangerous elevations of temperature as well as blood pressure. The mechanism of the interaction of guanethidine and MAOIs is not fully understood, but may involve antagonism of guanethidine-induced catecholamine depletion.

CLINICAL IMPLICATIONS

Although the concurrent use of pargyline and methyldopa has been reported to be a safe combination in general, it may be prudent whenever possible to avoid giving methyldopa after pargyline to prevent any possible sudden release of accumulated stores of catecholamines. There appears to be little documentation about the use of methyldopa and other MAOIs. Reserpine has depressive effects and should be avoided in patients requiring treatment for depression. Guanethidine should be avoided in patients taking MAOIs.

Aspartame

EVIDENCE OF INTERACTION

The acute ingestion of aspartame, particularly when combined with carbohydrates, can increase the level of tyrosine in the brain. A 22-year-old woman who used about 10 packets of an artificial sweetener that contained aspartame was given a trial of tranylcypromine 10 mg/day to treat her "tricyclic-resistant" depression (Ferguson 1985). After being on the regimen of 10 mg/day of tranylcypromine for approximately 2 weeks, the patient noticed severe throbbing headaches and felt flushed and sweaty when consuming aspartame. On each of five separate occasions, the headaches stopped within a few hours after she stopped consuming the artificial sweetener. Unfortunately, the patient refused to have her blood pressure checked at these times. However, the patient's headaches were sufficiently unpleasant, and the correlation between the ingestion of the aspartame sweetener and the headaches were so closely linked that the patient changed her sweetener to saccharin, which did not produce headaches.

MECHANISM

Elevated CNS levels of tyrosine may occur in patients who consume carbohydrate loads and aspartame.

CLINICAL IMPLICATIONS

This is the only case report of an aspartame–MAOI adverse reaction and, given the wide use of aspartame, it is probably not a common clinical problem.

Barbiturates/Sedative-Hypnotics

EVIDENCE OF INTERACTION

Several case reports and warnings exist in the clinical literature regarding the augmentation of barbiturate and sedative-hypnotic effects when combining these medications with MAOIs (Becker et al. 1974, Donlon 1982). Clinical experience suggests that considerable caution should be exercised when barbiturates are used with MAOIs, although the MAOIs are almost devoid of sedative effects. MAOIs prolong the hypnotic activity of barbiturates (Domino et al.: 1962). A 20-year-old woman taking 10 mg of tranylcypromine three times daily became extremely agitated, necessitating seclusion and treatment with amobarbital sodium 250 mg intramuscularly for sedation. Approximately 3 hours after the barbiturate injection, the patient was found vomiting, semi-comatose, with widely dilated pupils, and blood pressure of 82/64 mm Hg. The patient remained semi-comatose for approximately 36 hours and then gradually responded to supportive treatment.

MECHANISM

Tranylcypromine may inhibit the metabolism of amobarbital. In animals, premedication with tranylcypromine prolongs the duration of amobarbital hypnosis by at least 2 1/2 times (Domino et al. 1962).

CLINICAL IMPLICATIONS

Clinicians should generally be aware of the potential toxicity resulting from the administration of MAOIs and barbiturate sedative-hypnotic medications.

Benzodiazepines

EVIDENCE OF INTERACTION

One review article reported that a number of patients have developed disinhibited states attributable to the combination of MAOIs and benzodiazepines. As part of this syndrome, these patients became irresponsible, socially indiscreet, and inappropriately happy (Davidson et al. 1984). Two cases were reported of generalized edema occurring when chlordiazepoxide was given with a MAOI (Goonewardene et al. 1977, Pathak 1977) and one case of chorea (MacLeod 1964).

MECHANISM

Unknown.

CLINICAL IMPLICATIONS

Although MAOIs and benzodiazepines can usually be safely combined, disinhibited states may sometimes occur. Benzodiazepines themselves, can produce a disinhibition reaction. With respect to generalized edema, phenelzine, tranylcypromine, and possibly other MAOIs may produce this adverse reaction when administered alone.

β-Adrenergic Blockers

EVIDENCE OF INTERACTION

The use of propranolol with MAOI has resulted in severe hypertensive crises (Risch et al. 1982). Some clinicians assert that lower doses of propranolol can be well tolerated in combination with phenelzine (Davidson et al. 1984). Bradycardia developed in two patients taking nadolol (Corgard) or metoprolol (Lopressor) when phenelzine was added to their treatment (Reggev et al. 1989).

MECHANISM

The hypertensive response apparently results from β-receptor blockade, in the presence of unopposed α-adrenergic activity. Phenelzine may impair the metabolism of some β-blockers.

CLINICAL IMPLICATIONS

When β-blockers are used with MAOIs, doses should be reduced and blood pressure and pulse rate monitored.

Buspirone

The manufacturer reported six cases of elevated blood pressure with the combination of a MAOI and buspirone. Some patients, however, appear to tolerate the combination well (for a detailed discussion, see Ciraulo et al. 1990c).

Dietary Amines

One of the most worrisome adverse drug reactions involving MAOIs is the tyramine-induced hypertensive crisis or the "cheese reaction." The interaction between MAOIs and tyramine, an indirect-acting sympath-omimetic amine, which is plentiful in the typical diet, can potentially produce a serious and sometimes fatal increase in blood pressure (hypertensive crisis). The knowledge that tyramine was responsible for the "cheese reaction" led to dietary precautions that have greatly improved the safety of MAOI usage. Tables 2.5 through 2.7 list the tyramine content of common foods and beverages (Shulman et al. 1989).

Foods with a high tyramine content must be avoided. These foodstuffs would include most unpasteurized cheeses containing strong, aromatic chemical structures including cheddar, camembert, and blue cheese (Folks 1983, Nies et al. 1982, Sullivan et al. 1984). Yeast extracts, pickled herring, aged and unpasteurized meats and sausages also must be avoided (Gelenberg 1982). Limited amounts of foodstuffs with moderate tyramine content are allowable, and these include avocados, meat extracts, certain ales and beers, as well as most white wines and champagne. One documented hypertensive crisis resulted from avocados (used in guacamole) and MAOIs.

Some controversy exists regarding the consumption of alcohol with MAOIs. Some clinicians recommend that red wines be avoided, but white wines, vodka, gin, rye, or scotch are allowable because they are low in tyramine content (Murphy et al. 1984). Shader (Shader 1986) reported that, in his experience, patients taking MAOIs can safely drink up to 4 ounces of white wine or distilled spirits. One author (Jenike 1983) noted that there is no tyramine in most alcoholic beverages and suggested that patients can drink gin, vodka, and whiskey without danger of an interaction with an MAOI. He further stated that the fermentation of most beers does not ordinarily involve the processes that produce tyramine, although he noted that some imported beers have caused hypertensive reactions in patients taking MAOIs. Most, but not all, white wines are free of tyramine. Substantial variability exists in the tyramine content of different brands of beer and wine (Tables 2.7, 2.8, 2.9). In addition to tyramine interac-

(text continues on page 136)

TABLE 2.7. TYRAMINE CONTENT OF MISCELLANEOUS FOODS

Food	Tyramine Concentration μg/g	Tyramine Content per Serving, mg
Fish		
Pickled herring brine	15.1	—
Lump fish roe	4.4	0.2 mg/50 g
Sliced schmaltz herring in oil	4.0	0.2 mg/50 g
Pickled herring	Nil	Nil
Smoked carp	Nil	Nil
Smoked salmon	Nil	Nil
Smoked white fish	Nil	Nil
Meat and Sausage (/30 g)		
Salami	188	5.6
Mortadella	184	5.5
Air-dried sausage	125	3.8
Chicken liver (day 5)	51	1.5
Bologna	33	1
Aged sausage	29	0.9
Smoked meat	18	0.5
Corned beef	11	0.3
Kielbasa sausage	6	0.2
Liverwurst	2	0.1
Smoked sausage	1	<0.1
Sweet Italian sausage	1	<0.1
Pepperoni sausage	Nil	Nil
Chicken liver	Nil	Nil
Pate (/30 g)		
Salmon mousse	22	0.7
Country style	3	0.1
Peppercorn	2	0.1
Fruit		
Banana peel	51.7	1.424 mg/peel
Avocado	Nil	Nil
Ripe avocado	Nil	Nil
Banana	Nil	Nil
Raisins (California seedless)	Nil	Nil
Figs (California Blue Ribbon)	Nil	Nil
Yeast Extracts		
Marmite concentrated yeast extract	645	6.45 mg/10 g
Brewer's yeast tablets (Drug Trade Co.)	—	191.27 μg/400 mg
Brewer's yeast tablets (Jamieson)	—	66.72 μg/400mg
Brewer's yeast flakes (Vegetrates)	—	9.36 μg/15 g
Brewer's yeast debittered (Maximum Nutrition)	—	Nil

(continued)

TABLE 2.7. TYRAMINE CONTENT OF MISCELLANEOUS FOODS (CONTINUED)

Food	Tyramine Concentration μg/g	Tyramine Content per Serving, mg
Other		
Sauerkraut (Krakus)	55.47	13.87
Beef bouillon mix (Bovril)	—	231.25 μg/package
Beef bouillon (Oetker)	—	102 μg/cube
Soy Sauce	18.72	0.2 mg/10 mL
Beef gravy (Franco American)	0.85	<0.1 mg/30 mL
Chicken gravy (Franco American)	mL	<0.1 mg/30 mL
Chicken bouillon mix (Maggi)	0.46	Nil
Vegetable bouillon mix	Nil	Nil
Yogurt	Nil	Nil
Fava beans	Nil	Nil

Reprinted from Shulman KI, Walker SE, MacKenzie S, Knowels S: Dietary restriction, tyramine, use of monamine oxidate inhibitors. J Clin Psychopharmacol 9(6):397–402, copyright Williams & Wilkins, 1989.

tion with ethanol, pargyline may inhibit acetaldehyde metabolism, leading to disulfiram-like reaction (Collins et al. 1975).

Generally, foods that have low or no tyramine content are permissible in the MAOI diet; these include bananas, pasteurized cheeses, or any of the distilled spirits (in moderation). Most authorities believe that greater than 10 mg of tyramine must be ingested to produce a hypertensive reaction in a patient taking MAOIs. After the discontinuation of MAOI usage, many clinicians suggest that at least 2 weeks may be required for sufficient synthesis of new MAO enzyme so that restriction of tyramine-rich foods should last a minimum of 2 weeks after stopping a MAOI. (DeCastro 1985, Rabkin et al. 1985, Smookler et al. 1982). Tyramine challenge produces smaller increases in blood pressure in patients taking the reversible MAOI moclobemide compared with irreversible MAOIs. This may be because tyramine is able to displace moclobemide from its MAO binding site (Table 2.10).

"Ecstasy" (3,4-Methylenedioxymethamphetamine)

EVIDENCE OF INTERACTION

One case report documents an 18-year-old woman taking phenelzine 60 mg daily and lithium (serum level 0.7 to 0.9 mEq/L) who ingested juice that allegedly contained 3,4-methylenedioxymethamphetamine (MDMA) (Kaskey 1992). Within 15 minutes, increased muscular

(text continues on page 139)

TABLE 2.8.   TYRAMINE CONTENT OF CHEESES

Type	Tyramine Content, μg	Tryramine Content per Serving, mg[a]
English stilton	1156.91	17.3
Blue cheese	997.79	15.0
3-yr-old white	779.74	11.7
Extra-old	608.19	9.1
Old cheddar	497.20	7.5
Danish blue	389.47	5.5
Danish blue	294.67	4.4
Mozzarella	168.08	2.4
Cheese spread, Handisnack	133.81	2.0
Swiss gruyere	125.17	1.9
Muenster, Canadian	101.69	1.5
Old Coloured, Canadian	77.47	1.2
Feta	75.78	1.1
Parmesan, grated (Italian)	74.57	1.1
Gorgonzola (Italian)	55.94	0.8
Blue cheese dressing	39.20	0.6
Medium (Black Diamond)	37.64	0.6
Mild (Black Diamond)	34.75	0.5
Swiss Emmenthal	23.99	0.4
Beric (M-C) with rind	21.19	0.3
Cambozola blue vein (germ)	18.31	0.3
Parmesan, grated (Kraft)	15.01	0.2
Brie (d'OKA) without rind	14.65	0.2
Farmers, Canadian plain	11.05	0.2
Cream cheese (plain)	9.04	0.1
Cheeze Whiz (Kraft)	8.46	0.1
Brie (d'OKA) with rind	5.71	0.1
Brie (M-C) without rind	2.82	<0.1
Sour cream (Astro)	1.23	<0.1
Boursin	0.93	<0.1
Havarti, Canadian	Nil	Nil
Ricotta	Nil	Nil
Processed cheese slice	Nil	Nil
Bonbel	Nil	Nil
Cream cheese (Philadelphia)	Nil	Nil

[a]Based on a 15 g (single slice) serving.
Reprinted from Shulman Kl, Walker SE, MacKenzie S, Knowles S: Dietary restriction, tyramine, and the use of monoamine oxidase inhibitors. J Clin Psychopharmacol 9:307 402, copyright Williams & Wilkins, 1989.

TABLE 2.9. TYRAMINE CONTENT OF BEER, WINE, AND DISTILLED SPIRITS

Tyramine Content of Beer

		Tyramine Concentration, µg/mL	Tyramine Content per Serving, mg[a]
Amstel	Amstel	4.52	1.54
Export Draft	Molson	3.79	1.29
Blue Light	Labatts	3.42	1.16
Guinness Extra Stout	Labatts	3.37	1.15
Old Vienna	Carling	3.32	1.13
Canadian	Molson	3.01	1.03
Miller Light	Carling	2.91	0.99
Export	Molson	2.78	0.95
Heineken	Holland	1.81	0.62
Blue	Labatts	1.80	0.61
Coors Light	Molson	1.45	0.49
Carlsberg Light	Carling	1.15	0.39
Michelob	Anheuser Busch	0.98	0.33
Genesee Cream	Genesee	0.86	0.29
Stroh's	Stroh's	0.78	0.27

Tyramine Content of Wines

Wine	Color	Type	Country	Tyramine Concentration, µg/mL	Tyramine Content per Serving, mg[b]
Rioja (Siglo)	Red	—	Spain	4.41	0.53
Ruffino	Red	Chianti	Italy	3.04	0.36
Blue Nun	White	—	Germany	2.70	0.32
Retsina	White	—	Greece	1.79	0.21
La Colombaia	Red	Chianti	Italy	0.63	0.08
Brolio	Red	Chianti	Italy	0.44	0.05
Beau-Rivage	White	Bordeaux	France	0.39	0.05
Beau-Rivage	Red	Bordeaux	France	0.35	0.04
Maria Christina	Red	—	Canada	0.20	0.02
Cinzano	Red	Vermouth	Italy	Nil	Nil
Le Piazze	Red	Chianti	Italy	Nil	Nil

(continued)

TABLE 2.9. TYRAMINE CONTENT OF BEER, WINE, AND DISTILLED SPIRITS (CONTINUED)

Type	Other Tyramine Concentration, µg/mL	Tyramine Content per Serving, mg
Harvey's Bristol Cream	2.65	0.32 mg/4 oz.
Dubonnet	1.59	0.19 mg/4 oz.
London distilled dry gin (Beefeater)	Nil	Nil
Vodka	Nil	Nil
Rare blended scotch whiskies	Nil	Nil

[a]Based on a 341-mL serving (one bottle).
[b]Based on a 120-mL (4-ounce) serving.
Reprinted from Shulman KI, Walker SE, MacKenzie S, Knowles S: Dietary restriction, tyramine, and the use of monoamine oxidase inhibitors. J Clin Psychopharmacol 9:397–402, Copyright Williams & Wilkins, 1989.

tension and tremor developed, and she became comatose with decorticate-like posturing. She had a temperature of 100.5°F and a blood pressure of 150/100 mm Hg. She recovered within 5 hours. Another case of an MAOI–MDMA interaction also has been reported (Smilkstein et al. 1987).

MECHANISM

MDMA may increase central serotonergic effects.

CLINICAL IMPLICATIONS

An evaluation of interactions of therapeutic agents with illicit drugs is complex. Although patients may believe they are taking MDMA, it is often surreptitiously adulterated or substituted with other drugs, especially stimulants. A theoretical basis certainly exists for suspecting that MDMA would lead to a serotonin syndrome in patients taking MAOIs, although one of us (DAC) has seen patients use MDMA while on MAOI without adverse effects. Caution would dictate that patients who continue to use illicit drugs or who are at high risk for relapse to drug use should not be treated with MAOIs.

Ethanol

EVIDENCE OF INTERACTION

The hypertensive crisis associated with the concurrent usage of some red wines or imported beers (those that have high tyramine contents) with MAOIs is well known (Table 2.7). A fatal malignant hyperthermic

TABLE 2.10. DIETARY RESTRICTIONS WITH MAOI THERAPY (SEE TABLES 2.7, 2.8, 2.9 FOR TYRAMINE CONTENT OF SPECIFIC FOODS)

Contraindicated	Moderate Restrictions	Relative Restrictions	Unnecessary to Restrict
Aged cheese (English Stilton, Blue Cheese, 3-year old white, Old Cheddar and others)	Bottled or canned beer (highest contents have 1–1.5 mg tyramine per serving)	Red or white wine (most have less than 0.5 mg tyramine per serving)	Bananas
			Chocolate
			Fresh/mild cheeses
Marmite yeast	Pizza (caution patients about different types of cheeses that may be used)	Banana peel or overripe bananas (1.4 mg tyramine per peel)	Fresh meat
Sauerkraut			Pickled/smoked fish
Some aged/cured meats (salami contains 5.6 mg, mortadella 5.5 mg, air-dried sausage 3.8 mg tyramine/30 g)		Distilled spirits (most do not contain tyramine, but some MAOI inhibit acetaldehyde metabolism creating a potential for a disulfiram-like effect)	Yeast extracts, except Marmite
Tap beer			Chicken liver (little evidence unless not fresh; by day 5 contains 1.5 mg tyramine/30 g, while undetectable at day 1)
Improperly stored meats or fish			
Soy sauce (tyramine content is highly variable)			
Soybean			
Tofu			
Fava beans (reactions not related to tyramine content, which is negligible)			

Reprinted with permission from *Pharmacotherapy of Depression*, DA Ciraulo and RI Shader (Eds.). Totowa, N.J.: Humana Press, 2004; p. 88.

reaction as a result of ingestion of tranylcypromine combined with white wine and cheese has also been described (Mirchandani et al. 1985). In a comprehensive review of psychotropic drugs and alcohol (Weller et al. 1984), the authors underscored the fact that alcohol increases central amine synthesis and release, which may account for the observed potentiation of the sedative effects of alcohol when used with MAOIs. The authors also indicated that some MAOIs (e.g., pargyline) inhibit alcohol dehydrogenase, thus delaying the clearance of alcohol from the body and potentially lengthening the individual's duration of intoxication.

MECHANISM

The fermentation of wine does not usually produce tyramine, but contamination with other than the usual fermenting organisms has resulted in appreciable amounts of tyramine in Chianti and could occur in any red wine (Jenike 1983). On a pharmacodynamic level, MAOI generally will cause an accentuation or prolongation of the usual actions of alcohol, such as sedation, associated with its usage (Blackwell et al. 1984).

CLINICAL IMPLICATIONS

Differing views exist with regard to the combination of MAOIs and "safe" alcoholic beverages. In view of the possibility of tyramine-mediated hypertensive crises, potentiation of alcohol sedative properties, and lengthening of intoxication periods, patients should be cautioned against the combined use of alcohol and MAOIs (Weller et al. 1984). Some clinicians suggest that patients taking a MAOI should not drink fermented beverages (including beer and wine), and if they drink distilled spirits, quantities should be limited because MAOIs potentiate the effects of alcohol (Domino et al. 1984). Other clinicians suggest that it is incorrect to state that alcohol is contraindicated with MAOIs, because virtually no tyramine (the agent responsible for the hypertensive events) is present in most alcoholic beverages, especially gin, vodka, whiskey, and most white wines. Instructions to avoid imported beer and red wine while permitting distilled spirits is consistent with this approach, which may increase medication compliance (Jenike 1983). Each clinician must decide which approach suits the specific circumstances of the individual patient.

Hypoglycemic Drugs

EVIDENCE OF INTERACTION

MAOIs potentiate hypoglycemic agents (Becker et al. 1974, Gelenberg 1982, Nies et al. 1982). Dangerous hypoglycemia has been reported to occur in patients receiving both insulin and MAOI treatment (Davidson et al. 1984). Enhanced hypoglycemic responses have been documented in diabetics on tolbutamide when also treated with mebanazine (Adnitt 1968, Adnitt et al. 1960, Cooper 1966).

MECHANISM

Several mechanisms have been proposed to explain the potentiation of hypoglycemic agents by MAOIs. MAOIs lower blood glucose and interfere with the adrenergically mediated compensatory reaction to hypoglycemia. Another contributing factor may be that the insulin resistance said to occur during depression is reversed with adequate drug treatment.

CLINICAL IMPLICATIONS

Clinicians may wish to monitor blood glucose frequently in patients taking MAOIs and hypoglycemic agents. Cyclic antidepressants may also interact with hypoglycemic drugs (see the section on Cyclic Antidepressants).

Lithium (*See* Chapter 4)
Local Anesthetics with Vasoconstrictors (Dental)

EVIDENCE OF INTERACTION

The clinical literature is replete with warnings regarding the combining of MAOIs and local anesthetics that contain vasoconstrictors (Davidson et al. 1984, Nies et al. 1982, Risch et al. 1982). Although direct-acting sympathomimetic compounds (norepinephrine, epinephrine, etc.) do not cause the serious hypertensive reactions that the indirect-acting sympathomimetic compounds cause, nevertheless several anecdotal case reports have indicated that when these compounds are used as vasoconstrictors in combination with dental anesthesia, they may interact with MAOIs to produce hypertension (Risch et al. 1982).

MECHANISM

The mechanism may involve a postsynaptic "denervation hypersensitivity" caused by the chronic administration of MAOIs.

CLINICAL IMPLICATIONS

When dental anesthesia is necessary, it may be preferable to use lidocaine or mepivacaine without epinephrine or any other sympathomimetic substances. Levonordefrin has less of a hypertensive effect than epinephrine, yet still provides the vasoconstrictor effect and may be a suitable alternative for patients taking MAOIs. The most recent reviews of dental anesthesia emphasize that greater risks are involved when patients taking tricyclic agents are given sympathomimetic vasoconstrictors as compared with patients taking MAOIs (Goulet et al. 1992).

Monoamine Oxidase Inhibitors

EVIDENCE OF INTERACTION

A potential problem may occur in switching from one MAOI to another. For many years, clinicians believed that switching from tranylcypromine to phenelzine was not a major problem because MAO activity recovered more rapidly after tranylcypromine discontinuation (5 days) than after phenelzine discontinuation. Unfortunately, the time required for the recovery of MAO activity is highly variable and unpredictable among patients. Regardless of the order of switch, hypertensive MAOI–MAOI reactions have been observed in several patients when inadequate washout periods have occurred.

MECHANISM

The mechanism is unknown, but may involve the metabolism of tranylcypromine to compounds that are indirect-acting sympathomimetic amines.

CLINICAL IMPLICATIONS

Patients should not be switched directly from one MAOI to another (Davidson et al. 1984). The minimum recommended interval of time between two different MAOIs is 1 week, but more conservative clinicians recommend that the first MAOI be discontinued for 2 to 3 weeks before starting a second MAOI. Although the period of washout after moclobemide, a reversible MAOI, should be shorter, clinical experience is limited.

Narcotic Analgesics

EVIDENCE OF INTERACTION

Many anecdotal case reports described patients who had toxic reactions when placed on MAOI and a narcotic analgesic (Gelenberg 1981, Janowsky et al. 1981, Meyer et al. 1981, Vigran 1964). Hypertensive crises also have been reported when MAOIs and dextromethorphan were combined (Janowsky et al. 1985, Nierenberg et al. 1993). Although hypertension has been described in the MAOI–meperidine interactions, hypotension is a more common occurrence. Other signs and symptoms of this interaction include excitement, sweating, rigidity, neuromuscular irritability, and hyperreflexia. In the extreme case, signs and symptoms have included respiratory depression, agitation, hyperactivity, disorientation, cyanosis, coma, extensor plantar responses, hypertension, tachycardia, hyperthermia, and occasionally death (Meyer et al. 1981). This has been referred to as "the serotonin syndrome" (Sternbach 1991a). Selegiline, an MAOI that is selective for MAO-B at low doses, also reacts with meperidine (Zornberg et al. 1991).

MECHANISM

The mechanism of the MAOI–meperidine and MAOI–dextromethorphan interactions probably involves the alteration of cerebral serotonin levels. In addition, opioid analgesics may be potentiated by MAOIs via an inhibition of hepatic metabolism (Janowsky et al. 1981), although a pharmacodynamic mechanism is also possible.

CLINICAL IMPLICATIONS

The use of meperidine or dextromethorphan in patients treated with MAOIs must be avoided. This prohibition also applies to the reversible MAOIs, such as moclobemide, and to the somewhat selective MAO-B inhibitor selegiline. This restriction does not apply to the larger issue of using non-meperidine narcotics in patients who are also on MAOI therapy. Should narcotics be necessary in a patient taking a MAOI, authorities recommend beginning narcotic therapy from one fifth to one half the usual dosage and titrating the dosage very carefully on the basis of response. Patients should be carefully observed for 15 to 20 minutes after the dose for change in vital signs or level of consciousness. Meperidine should not be used; acceptable narcotic medications would include codeine, oxycodone (Gratz et al. 1993), fentanyl, alfentanil, or morphine, which have not caused this very serious reaction. They will, however, have their usual opiate effects potentiated.

Neuroleptics/Antipsychotics

EVIDENCE OF INTERACTION

A number of clinical investigators have noted that MAOI treatment may inhibit phenothiazine metabolism, potentiate hypotensive or extrapyramidal reactions, and prolong the central anticholinergic side effects of phenothiazine medication (Donlon 1982, Tollefson 1983). One study found that the combination of MAOIs with neuroleptics was useful in the treatment of anhedonic schizophrenics (Hedberg et al. 1971).

MECHANISM

MAOIs retard dealkylation, demethylation, and hydroxylation. MAOIs may also alter the action of other drugs by pharmacodynamic or receptor site interactions.

CLINICAL IMPLICATIONS

There may be additive hypotensive effects and enhanced anticholinergic reactions with the combined use of MAOIs and phenothiazine medications. The clinician should be prepared to monitor for these effects and make appropriate dosage adjustments. The combination product of tranylcypromine and trifluoperazine is widely used outside the United States.

Steroids

EVIDENCE OF INTERACTION

Fludrocortisone has offered effective relief from the problem of MAOI-induced orthostatic hypotension (Rabkin et al. 1984, Rabkin et al. 1985). Some studies indicate that up to 25% of patients taking phenelzine or tranylcypromine will experience orthostatic hypotension.

MECHANISM

The mechanism by which steroids increase blood pressure is not completely understood. Hypotheses include (a) salt retention, leading to edema within arteriole walls; (b) sensitization of blood vessels to the effects of catecholamines and angiotensin; (c) elevation of renin substrate; (d) antidiuretic hormone effects.

CLINICAL IMPLICATIONS

Although a variety of conservative measures may be taken, such as decreasing dosage, increasing salt intake, and wearing custom-fitted support hose, fludrocortisone can also counteract orthostatic hypotension induced by MAOI treatment.

Because orthostatic hypotension often can limit the use of MAOI therapy, doses of fludrocortisone between 0.3 and 0.6 mg/day may allow MAOI treatment to continue even when orthostatic symptoms develop. Often after 4 to 6 weeks, the patient will no longer need the fludrocortisone. It should be noted, however, that the prescription of fludrocortisone is not without risk, particularly with elderly patients or those individuals with limited cardiac or renal function, because it can cause edema, hypervolemia, and even congestive heart failure.

Succinylcholine

EVIDENCE OF INTERACTION

Phenelzine may reduce cholinesterase levels and lead to prolonged apnea during electroconvulsive therapy or surgical procedures. Four patients undergoing treatment with phenelzine had low serum pseudocholinesterase levels, and apnea developed in one for more than 1 hour following a modified electroconvulsive treatment (Bodley et al. 1969). In the other three patients, serum pseudocholinesterase levels returned to normal after the withdrawal of phenelzine therapy.

MECHANISM

Low serum pseudocholinesterase levels appeared to be responsible for increased levels of succinylcholine, with resultant prolonged apnea.

Some authorities believe that with appropriate dosage adjustments, succinylcholine may be used in patients taking MAOIs who require ECT or surgery. In actual practice, irreversible MAOIs are often discontinued 10 to 14 days prior to elective procedures requiring succinylcholine. Tranylcypromine does not inhibit pseudocholinesterase.

Sympathomimetic Amines

EVIDENCE OF INTERACTION

Both indirect-acting sympathomimetics (more dangerous) as well as direct-acting (less dangerous) sympathomimetics may cause a hypertensive crisis when administered with MAOIs. The following indirect-acting vasopressors produce their pressor effects through the release of bound intraneuronal stores of norepinephrine and dopamine: amphetamine, methamphetamine cyclopentamine, ephedrine, pseudoephedrine, L-dopa, dopamine, mephentermine, phentermine, metaraminol, methylphenidate, phenylpropanolamine, and tyramine. The indirect-acting agents generally are believed to be more dangerous than direct-acting amines, with the indirect agents ephedrine, pseudoephedrine, and phenylpropanolamine being especially hazardous.

Several case reports described the co-administration of MAOIs and amphetamines (Feighner et al. 1985, Kline et al. 1981, Krisko et al. 1969). Some have documented the occurrence of hypertensive crises, while others suggested that the combination may be used without problems. One report noted that phentermine was prescribed for a 35-year-old man for weight reduction. After a 2-week trial, the patient was given tranylcypromine and, although instructed to discontinue phentermine and wait 7 days before starting tranylcypromine, the patient used both drugs concurrently (Raskin 1984). No documented blood pressure changes occurred using the combined medication. Another example involved a 40-year-old man taking amphetamines for 3 years; he was instructed to discontinue the amphetamines and substitute tranylcypromine. The patient decided to continue taking the amphetamines with tranylcypromine, and no problems occurred with this combination (Raskin 1984).

Another paper reported a case series demonstrating the safety and efficacy of adding a stimulant to a MAOI in the treatment of intractable depression (Feighner et al. 1985). The indirect stimulants used in this case series were methylphenidate and dextroamphetamine, with daily divided dosage ranging 5 to 20 mg/day for dextroamphetamine and 10 to 15 mg/day for methylphenidate. The most common MAOIs administered were tranylcypromine and phenelzine. No hypertensive crises occurred in this series, and the combination proved to be of benefit in treatment-resistant depression.

Earlier case reports, on the other hand, support the commonly held notion that MAOIs and stimulants in combination can cause serious toxicity. One report involved a 41-year-old woman who had progressive agitation, hyperkinesis, fever, coma, opisthotonos, and convulsions after ingesting 10 mg of tranylcypromine plus a combination product containing dextroamphetamine and amobarbital. The woman's temperature was above 109°F for over 30 minutes in a rare "drug fever" resulting from the simultaneous ingestion of tranylcypromine and dextroamphetamine (Krisko et al. 1969).

Another report describes a 49-year-old woman who suffered a subarachnoid hemorrhage following ephedrine and MAOI treatment (Hirsch et al. 1965). This woman was being treated for depression with the MAOI nialamide (100 to 150 mg/day). She experienced episodes of lightheadedness and postural dizziness; oral ephedrine was given to raise her blood pressure. Within 1 hour, a severe vertex headache developed, associated with neck stiffness, diaphoresis, left-sided chest pain, nausea, vomiting and leg-muscle spasms. A systolic blood pressure taken shortly thereafter was 160 mm Hg. A lumbar puncture documented subarachnoid hemorrhage. The toxic syndrome eventually cleared, with no apparent neurologic or psychiatric residual symptoms.

In another series of case reports, drug interactions between L-dopa, tranylcypromine, and carbidopa were studied in four patients with idiopathic parkinsonism (Teychenne et al. 1975). Pressor responses were induced by the combination of L-dopa and tranylcypromine. Because these hypertensive reactions were inhibited by carbidopa, they were probably mediated at a peripheral level.

MECHANISM

Most indirect-acting vasopressors produce their pressor effects through the release of bound intraneuronal stores of norepinephrine and dopamine. Combining MAOI medication with indirect-acting vasopressors increases the pressor effect of neurotransmitters, resulting in hypertensive crises. Similarly, the combination of L-dopa with MAOI prolongs and potentiates the pressor effects of dopamine, although this can be blocked by carbidopa.

The direct-acting vasopressors are believed to be less dangerous than the indirect-acting sympathomimetic amines because they do not release intracellular stores of monoamines, but rather bind to postsynaptic receptors. They also do not depend on monoamine oxidase for metabolic inactivation and are primarily degraded by the extracellular enzyme catecholamine-O-methyl-transferase (Risch et al. 1982). However, in isolated incidences, they can cause a hypertensive effect with MAOIs.

CLINICAL IMPLICATIONS

Since the recognition of the mechanism of action regarding hypertensive crises, careful patient instruction about foodstuffs and drug interactions of prescribed and over-the-counter drugs have made this worrisome side effect a rare problem (Shader et al. 1985a). When patients do experience hypertensive reaction heralded by headache, diaphoresis, and elevation of blood pressure, the prompt intervention with α-blocking drugs such as phentolamine or the calcium channel blocker, nifedipine, will usually lower blood pressure. In general, the administration of a stimulant drug (indirect-acting vasopressor), such as amphetamine, to patients also receiving an MAOI is a potentially worrisome combination. When prescribing both MAOI and stimulant medication, the physician should start the MAOI first, with the addition of dextroamphetamine or methylphenidate in 2.5-mg increments to stabilize blood pressure and enhance clinical response (Feighner et al. 1985). For the most part, these combinations should be used only in treatment-refractory depression that is unresponsive to either medication alone, and by clinicians experienced in their use (Feinberg 2004). The indirect-acting vasopressors are far more dangerous than the direct-acting vasopressors with respect to hypertensive crisis reactions and should be avoided in patients taking MAOIs.

Theophylline

EVIDENCE OF INTERACTION

One case report described an adverse reaction between phenelzine and the theophylline derivative oxtriphylline (Shader et al. 1985b). The patient was a 28-year-old woman who responded well to phenelzine at a daily dosage of 45 mg. When bronchitis developed, she was instructed to use a cough syrup before bedtime that had been previously used safely on other occasions. The patient awoke approximately 2 hours later with tachycardia, palpitations, and a sense of apprehension that remained at a distressing level for more than 4 hours. The patient's cough syrup was a combination of oxtriphylline and guaifenesin. Upon repeated challenge with the same cough syrup, the patient had a similar apprehensive state. Rechallenging the patient with guaifenesin alone did not produce adverse effects, whereas oxtriphylline tablets alone did.

MECHANISM

Oxtriphylline, a choline salt of theophylline, is a xanthine-bronchodilating agent. β-Adrenergic effects may be enhanced when oxtriphylline is given with a MAOI.

CLINICAL IMPLICATIONS

The combination of MAOI and xanthine bronchodilating agents may lead to anxiety, palpitations, and tachycardia in some individuals. Albuterol may lead to similar symptoms. Another antiasthmatic drug, isoetharine (an inhaled β-adrenergic agonist) induced hypomania in a patient also taking phenelzine.

Tryptophan

EVIDENCE OF INTERACTION

The addition of tryptophan to a MAOI has been used successfully for treatment of refractory patients who did not respond to treatment with a MAOI alone (Glassman et al. 1969). Several authors have reported behavioral or neurologic toxicity with this combination, sometimes with acute behavioral and neurologic toxicity observed immediately after tryptophan administration in patients taking MAOIs. One case report involving a 21-year-old man (Thomas et al. 1984) documented marked behavioral changes consistent with a transient hypomanic episode while he was taking 90 mg/day of phenelzine in addition to 6 g of L-tryptophan. In another series of patients (Pope et al. 1985), the authors described 8 cases of delirium, agitation, and myoclonus apparently attributable to the combination of tranylcypromine and L-tryptophan. Similar cases have been reported by other investigators (Alvine et al. 1990, Levy et al. 1985). Goff (Goff 1985) described two cases of hypomania attributed to the combination. Fatalities have been reported with the combination of lithium, phenelzine, and L-tryptophan (Brennan et al. 1988, Staufenberg et al. 1989).

MECHANISM

The cause of the behavioral toxicity with the combination of MAOI and L-tryptophan remains unclear, but is probably due to stimulation of the serotonergic system.

CLINICAL IMPLICATIONS

If patients taking a MAOI also receive L-tryptophan, it would be safer to start at a low dose of L-tryptophan, such as 0.25 or 0.5 g, and gradually titrate the dosage upward. Patients should be monitored for signs and symptoms of the serotonin syndrome and/or a switch to hypomania.

REFERENCES

Abbas S et al.: The use of fluoxetine and buspirone for treatment-refractory depersonalization disorder. J Clin Psychiatry 56: 484, 1995.

Abebe W: Herbal medication: potential for adverse interactions with analgesic drugs. J Clin Pharm Ther 27: 391, 2002.

Abernethy DR et al.: Imipramine-cimetidine interaction: impairment of clearance and enhanced bioavailability. Clin Pharmacol Ther 33: 237, 1983.

Abernethy DR et al.: Ranitidine does not impair oxidative or conjugative metabolism: noninteraction with antipyrine, diazepam, and lorazepam. Clin Pharmacol Ther 35: 188, 1984b.

Abernethy DR et al.: Imipramine-cimetidine interaction: impairment of clearance and enhanced absolute bioavailability. J Pharmacol Exp Ther 229: 702, 1984.

Abernethy DR et al.: Imipramine disposition in users of oral contraceptive steroids. Clin Pharmacol Ther 35: 792, 1984a.

Abernethy DR et al.: Impairment of hepatic drug oxidation by propoxyphene. Ann Intern Med 97: 223, 1982.

Achamallah NS. Visual hallucinations after combining fluoxetine and dextromethorphan. Am J Psychiatry 149: 1406, 1992.

Adnitt PI. Hypoglycemic action of monoamine oxidase inhibitors (MAOI'S). Diabetes 17: 628, 1968.

Adnitt PI et al.: Hypoglycemic action of monoamine oxidase inhibitors (MAOI). Diabetes 17: 628, 1960.

Adson DE et al.: A probable interaction between a very low-dose oral contraceptive and the antidepressant nefazodone: a case report. J Clin Psychopharmacol 21: 618, 2001.

Albers LJ et al.: Paroxetine shifts imipramine metabolism. Psychiatry Res 59: 189, 1996.

Alderman CP et al.: Fluvoxamine-methadone interaction. Aust N Z J Psychiatry 33: 99, 1999.

Alderman CP et al.: Comment: serotonin syndrome associated with combined sertraline-amitriptyline treatment. Ann Pharmacother 30: 1499, 1996.

Alexanderson B et al.: Steady-state plasma levels of nortriptyline in twins: influence of genetic factors and drug therapy. Br Med J 4: 764, 1969.

Allard S et al.: Coadministration of short-term zolpidem with sertraline in healthy women. J Clin Pharmacol 39: 184, 1999.

Allen D et al.: Interactions of alcohol with amitriptyline, fluoxetine and placebo in normal subjects. Int Clin Psychopharmacol 4 Suppl 1: 7, 1989.

Allen D et al.: A comparative study of the interactions of alcohol with amitriptyline, fluoxetine and placebo in normal subjects. Prog Neuropsychopharmacol Biol Psychiatry 12: 63, 1988.

Alvine G et al.: Case of delirium secondary to phenelzine/L-tryptophan combination. J Clin Psychiatry 51: 311, 1990.

Amit Z et al.: Reduction in alcohol intake in humans as a function of treatment with zimelidine: implications for treatment. In: *Research Advances in New Psychopharmacological Treatment for Alcoholism*. In: *Excerpta Medica*. Amsterdam: Elsevier, 1985, p. 189.

Amit Z et al.: Zimeldine: a review of its effects on ethanol consumption. Neurosci Biobehav Rev 8: 35, 1984.

Ananth J et al.: A review of combined tricyclic and MAOI therapy. Compr Psychiatry 18: 221, 1977.

Andersen BB et al.: No influence of the antidepressant paroxetine on carbamazepine, valproate and phenytoin. Epilepsy Res 10: 201, 1991.

Anderson IM et al.: The effect of chronic fluvoxamine on hormonal and psychological responses to buspirone in normal volunteers. Psychopharmacology (Berl) 128: 74, 1996.

Anttila AK et al.: Fluvoxamine augmentation increases serum mirtazapine concentrations three- to fourfold. Ann Pharmacother 35: 1221, 2001.

Aranow AB et al.: Elevated antidepressant plasma levels after addition of fluoxetine. Am J Psychiatry 146: 911, 1989.

Aranth J et al.: Bleeding, a side effect of fluoxetine. Am J Psychiatry 149: 412, 1992.

Avenoso A et al.: Interaction between fluoxetine and haloperidol: pharmacokinetic and clinical implications. Pharmacol Res 35: 335, 1997.

Baettig D et al.: Tricyclic antidepressant plasma levels after augmentation with citalopram: a case study. Eur J Clin Pharmacol 44: 403, 1993.

Bailey DN et al.: Interaction of tricyclic antidepressants with cholestyramine in vitro. Ther Drug Monit 14: 339, 1992.

Baker GB et al.: Metabolism of monoamine oxidase inhibitors. Cell Mol Neurobiol 19: 411, 1999.

Bakish D: Fluoxetine potentiation by buspirone: three case histories. Can J Psychiatry 36: 749, 1991.

Baldessarini RJ et al.: Anticonvulsant cotreatment may increase toxic metabolites of antidepressants and other psychotropic drugs. J Clin Psychopharmacol 8: 381, 1988.

Bannister SJ et al.: Evaluation of the potential for interactions of paroxetine with diazepam, cimetidine, warfarin, and digoxin. Acta Psychiatr Scand Suppl 350: 102, 1989.

Barnes JS et al.: Lack of interaction between tricyclic antidepressants and clonidine at the alpha 2-adrenoceptor on human platelets. Clin Pharmacol Ther 32: 744, 1982.

Baron BM et al.: Rapid down regulation of beta-adrenoceptors by co-administration of desipramine and fluoxetine. Eur J Pharmacol 154: 125, 1988.

Barrett J et al.: SSRI and sympathominetic interaction. Br J Psychiatry 168: 253, 1996.

Barros J et al.: An interaction of sertraline and desipramine. Am J Psychiatry 150: 1751, 1993.

Bauer M et al.: Adverse events and tolerability of the combination of fluoxetine/lithium compared with fluoxetine. J Clin Psychopharmacol 16: 130, 1996.

Bauer M et al.: Paroxetine and amitriptyline augmentation of lithium in the treatment of major depression: a double-blind study. J Clin Psychopharmacol 19: 164, 1999.

Beasley CM, Jr. et al.: Possible monoamine oxidase inhibitor-serotonin uptake inhibitor interaction: fluoxetine clinical data and preclinical findings. J Clin Psychopharmacol 13: 312, 1993.

Beaumont G. Drug interactions with clomipramine (Anafranil). J Int Med Res 1: 480, 1973.

Bebchuk JM et al.: Drug interaction between rifampin and nortriptyline: a case report. Int J Psychiatry Med 21: 183, 1991.

Becker CE et al.: A quick guide to common drug interactions. Patient Care 1: 1974.

Becquemont L et al.: Influence of the CYP1A2 inhibitor fluvoxamine on tacrine pharmacokinetics in humans. Clin Pharmacol Ther 61: 619, 1997.

Bell IR et al.: Fluoxetine induces elevation of desipramine level and exacerbation of geriatric nonpsychotic depression. J Clin Psychopharmacol 8: 447, 1988.

Bellward GD et al.: The effects of pretreatment of mice with norethindrone on the metabolism of 14C-imipramine by the liver microsomal drug-metabolizing enzymes. Can J Physiol Pharmacol 52: 28, 1974.

Belpaire FM et al.: The oxidative metabolism of metoprolol in human liver microsomes: inhibition by the selective serotonin reuptake inhibitors. Eur J Clin Pharmacol 54: 261, 1998.

Berggren D et al.: Postoperative confusion after anesthesia in elderly patients with femoral neck fractures. Anesth Analg 66: 497, 1987.

Bergstrom RF et al.: Assessment of the potential for a pharmacokinetic interaction between fluoxetine and terfenadine. Clin Pharmacol Ther 62: 643, 1997.

Bergstrom RF et al.: Quantification and mechanism of the fluoxetine and tricyclic antidepressant interaction. Clin Pharmacol Ther 51: 239, 1992.

Bertschy G et al.: Probable metabolic interaction between methadone and fluvoxamine in addict patients. Ther Drug Monit 16: 42, 1994.

Bertschy G et al.: Fluoxetine addition to methadone in addicts: pharmacokinetic aspects. Ther Drug Monit 18: 570, 1996.

Bertschy G et al.: [Valpromide-amitriptyline interaction. Increase in the bioavailability of amitriptyline and nortriptyline caused by valpromide]. Encephale 16: 43, 1990.

Bertschy G et al.: Fluvoxamine-tricyclic antidepressant interaction. An accidental finding. Eur J Clin Pharmacol 40: 119, 1991.

Bhatara VS et al.: Possible interaction between sertraline and tranylcypromine. Clin Pharm 12: 222, 1993.

Blackwell B: Monoamine oxidase inhibitor interactions with other drugs. J Clin Psychopharmacol 11: 55, 1991.

Blackwell B et al.: Drug interactions in psychopharmacology. Psychiatr Clin North Am 7: 625, 1984.

Blier P et al.: The safety of concomitant use of sumatriptan and antidepressant treatments. J Clin Psychopharmacol 15: 106, 1995.

Boakes AJ et al.: Interactions between sympathomimetic amines and antidepressant agents in man. Br Med J 1: 311, 1973.

Bodkin JA et al.: Fluoxetine may antagonize the anxiolytic action of buspirone. J Clin Psychopharmacol 9: 150, 1989.

Bodley PO et al.: Low serum pseudocholinesterase levels complicating treatment with phenelzine. Br Med J 3: 510, 1969.

Bonnet P et al.: Carbamazepine, fluvoxamine. Is there a pharmacokinetic interaction? Therapie 47: 165, 1992.

Borba CP et al.: Citalopram and clozapine: potential drug interaction. J Clin Psychiatry 61: 301, 2000.

Borras-Blasco J et al.: Probable interaction between citalopram and acenocoumarol. Ann Pharmacother 36: 345, 2002.

Bostwick JM et al.: A toxic reaction from combining fluoxetine and phentermine. J Clin Psychopharmacol 16: 189, 1996.

Boyer WF et al.: Interaction of phenelzine and sulfisoxazole. Am J Psychiatry 140: 264, 1983.

Brannan SK et al.: Sertraline and isocarboxazid cause a serotonin syndrome. J Clin Psychopharmacol 14: 144, 1994.

Brazier NC et al.: Drug-herb interaction among commonly used conventional medicines: a compendium for health care professionals. Am J Ther 10: 163, 2003.

Brennan D et al.: 'Neuroleptic malignant syndrome' without neuroleptics. Br J Psychiatry 152: 578, 1988.

Breuel HP et al.: Pharmacokinetic interactions between lithium and fluoxetine after single and repeated fluoxetine administration in young healthy volunteers. Int J Clin Pharmacol Ther 33: 415, 1995.

Briant RH et al.: Interaction between clonidine and desipramine in man. Br Med J 1: 522, 1973.

Brosen K et al.: Quinidine inhibits the 2-hydroxylation of imipramine and desipramine but not the demethylation of imipramine. Eur J Clin Pharmacol 37: 155, 1989.

Brosen K et al.: Inhibition by paroxetine of desipramine metabolism in extensive but not in poor metabolizers of sparteine. Eur J Clin Pharmacol 44: 349, 1993.

Brown CS et al.: Possible influence of carbamazepine on plasma imipramine concentrations in children with attention deficit hyperactivity disorder. J Clin Psychopharmacol 10: 359, 1990.

Brown CS et al.: Possible influence of carbamazepine on plasma imipramine concentrations in children with attention deficit hyperactivity disorder. J Clin Psychopharmacol 12: 67, 1992.

Brynne N et al.: Fluoxetine inhibits the metabolism of tolterodine-pharmacokinetic implications and proposed clinical relevance. Br J Clin Pharmacol 48: 553, 1999.

Burrows GD et al.: Antidepressants and barbiturates. Br Med J 4: 113, 1971.

Bussing R et al.: Methamphetamine and fluoxetine treatment of a child with attention deficit hyperactivity disorder and obsessive compulsive disorder. J Child Adol Psychopharmacol 3: 53, 1993.

Cai WM et al.: Fluoxetine impairs the CYP2D6-mediated metabolism of propafenone enantiomers in healthy Chinese volunteers. Clin Pharmacol Ther 66: 516, 1999.

Carlini EA et al.: Effect of serotonergic drugs on the aggressiveness induced by delta 9-tetrahydrocannabinol in rem-sleep-deprived rats. Braz J Med Biol Res 15: 281, 1982.

Carney MW et al.: Effects of imipramine and reserpine in depression. Psychopharmacologia 14: 349, 1969.

Carrillo JA et al.: Pharmacokinetic interaction of fluvoxamine and thioridazine in schizophrenic patients. J Clin Psychopharmacol 19: 494, 1999.

Centorrino F et al.: Serum concentrations of clozapine and its major metabolites: effects of cotreatment with fluoxetine or valproate. Am J Psychiatry 151: 123, 1994.

Charney DS et al.: Desipramine-yohimbine combination treatment of refractory depression. Implications for the beta-adrenergic receptor hypothesis of antidepressant action. Arch Gen Psychiatry 43: 1155, 1986.

Chong SA et al.: Worsening of psychosis with clozapine and selective serotonin reuptake inhibitor combination: two case reports. J Clin Psychopharmacol 17: 68, 1997.

Christensen RC. Adverse interaction of paroxetine and cyproheptadine. J Clin Psychiatry 56: 433, 1995.

Ciraulo DA et al.: Imipramine disposition in alcoholics. J Clin Psychopharmacol 2: 2, 1982.

Ciraulo DA et al.: Pharmacokinetic interaction of disulfiram and antidepressants. Am J Psychiatry 142: 1373, 1985.

Ciraulo DA et al.: Clinical pharmacokinetics of imipramine and desipramine in alcoholics and normal volunteers. Clin Pharmacol Ther 43: 509, 1988a.

Ciraulo DA et al.: Intravenous pharmacokinetics of 2-hydroxyimipramine in alcoholics and normal controls. J Stud Alcohol 51: 366, 1990a.

Ciraulo DA et al.: Drug interactions with monoamine oxidase inhibitors. In: Shader RI (ed.): MAOI Therapy. New York: Audio Visual Medical Marketing, 1988b; p. 63.

Ciraulo DA et al.: Fluoxetine drug interactions: I. Antidepressants and antipsychotics. J Clin Psychopharmacol 10: 48, 1990b.

Ciraulo DA et al.: Question the experts: buspirone and MAOI. J Clin Psychopharmacol 10: 306, 1990c.

Claire RJ et al.: Potential interaction between warfarin sodium and fluoxetine. Am J Psychiatry 148: 1604, 1991.

Collins MA et al.: Tetrahydroisoquinolines in vivo. I. Rat brain formation of salsolinol, a condensation product of dopamine and acetaldehyde, under certain conditions during ethanol intoxication. Life Sci 16: 585, 1975.

Comfort A: Hypertensive reaction to New Zealand prickly spinach in woman taking phenelzine. Lancet 2: 472, 1981.

Consolo S et al.: Effect of desipramine on intestinal absorption of phenylbutazone and other drugs. Eur J Pharmacol 6: 322, 1969.

Consolo S et al.: Delayed absorption of phenylbutazone caused by desmethylimipramine in humans. Eur J Pharmacol 10: 239, 1970.

Cooper AJ: The action of mebanazine, a mono amine oxidase inhibitor antidepressant drug in diabetes. II. Int J Neuropsychiatry 2: 342, 1966.

Coplan JD et al.: Detectable levels of fluoxetine metabolites after discontinuation: an unexpected serotonin syndrome. Am J Psychiatry 150: 837, 1993.

Coppen A et al.: The comparative antidepressant value of L-tryptophan and imipramine with and without attempted potentiation by liothyronine. Arch Gen Psychiatry 26: 234, 1972.

Cruz-Flores S et al.: Valproic toxicity with fluoxetine therapy. Mo Med 92: 296, 1995.

Cupp MJ: Herbal remedies: adverse effects and drug interactions. Am Fam Physician 59: 1239, 1999.

Damkier P et al.: Effect of fluvoxamine on the pharmacokinetics of quinidine. Eur J Clin Pharmacol 55: 451, 1999.

Daniel DG et al.: Coadministration of fluvoxamine increases serum concentrations of haloperidol. J Clin Psychopharmacol 14: 340, 1994.

Daoust M et al.: Tianeptine, a specific serotonin uptake enhancer, decreases ethanol intake in rats. Alcohol Alcohol 27: 15, 1992.

Darley J: Interaction between phenytoin and fluoxetine. Seizure 3:151, 1994.

Davidson J: Adding a tricyclic antidepressant to a monoamine oxidase inhibitor. J Clin Psychopharmacol 2: 216, 1982.

Davidson J et al.: Practical aspects of MAO inhibitor therapy. J Clin Psychiatry 45: 81, 1984.

Davies TS: Monoamine oxidase inhibitors and rauwolfia compounds (letter). Br Med J 739, 1960.

de Jong J et al.: Interaction of olanzapine with fluvoxamine. Psychopharmacology (Berl) 155: 219, 2001.

de Jong JC et al.: Combined use of SSRIs and NSAIDs increases the risk of gastrointestinal adverse effects. Br J Clin Pharmacol 55: 591, 2003.

de Maat MM et al.: Drug interactions between antiretroviral drugs and comedicated agents. Clin Pharmacokinet 42: 223, 2003.

de Maistre E et al.: Severe bleeding associated with use of low molecular weight heparin and selective serotonin reuptake inhibitors. Am J Med 113: 530, 2002.

Deahl M. Betel nut-induced extrapyramidal syndrome: an unusual drug interaction. Mov Disord 4: 330, 1989.

Dec GW et al.: Trazodone-digoxin interaction in an animal model. J Clin Psychopharmacol 4: 153, 1984.

DeCastro RM: MAOIs, the "cheese" reaction, and sleep apnea. J Clin Psychopharmacol 5: 59, 1985.

DeMaria PA, Jr. et al.: A therapeutic use of the methadone fluvoxamine drug interaction. J Addict Dis 18: 5, 1999.

Demers JC et al.: Serotonin syndrome induced by fluvoxamine and mirtazapine. Ann Pharmacother 35: 1217, 2001.

Dent LA et al.: Warfarin-fluoxetine and diazepam-fluoxetine interaction. Pharmacotherapy 17: 170, 1997.

Deshauer D et al.: Seizures caused by possible interaction between olanzapine and clomipramine. J Clin Psychopharmacol 20: 283, 2000.

DeSilva KE et al.: Serotonin syndrome in HIV-infected individuals receiving antiretroviral therapy and fluoxetine. AIDS 15: 1281, 2001.

DeToledo JC et al.: Status epilepticus associated with the combination of valproic acid and clomipramine. Ther Drug Monit 19: 71, 1997.

Dimitriou EC et al.: Buspirone augmentation of antidepressant therapy. J Clin Psychopharmacol 18: 465, 1998.

Dingemanse J: An update of recent moclobemide interaction data. Int Clin Psychopharmacol 7: 167, 1993a.

Dingemanse J et al.: Interaction of fluoxetine and selegiline (letter). Can J Psychiatr Rev Canadienne de Psychiatrie 35: 571, 1990.

Dingemanse J et al.: Pharmacodynamic and pharmacokinetic interactions between fluoxetine and moclobemide. Clin Pharamcol Ther 53: 178, 1993b.

Diot P et al.: [Possible interaction between theophylline and fluvoxamine]. Therapie 46: 170, 1991.

Domino EF et al.: Red wine and reactions. J Clin Psychopharmacol 4: 173, 1984.

Domino EF et al.: Barbiturate intoxication in a patient treated with a MAO inhibitor. Am J Psychiatry 118: 941, 1962.

Donlon PT: Cardiac effects of antidepressants. Geriatrics 37: 53, 1982.

Dorian P et al.: Amitriptyline and ethanol: pharmacokinetic and pharmacodynamic interaction. Eur J Clin Pharmacol 25: 325, 1983.

Dorn JM: A case of phenytoin toxicity possibly precipitated by trazodone. J Clin Psychiatry 47: 89, 1986.

Dorsey ST et al.: Prolonged QT interval and torsades de pointes caused by the combination of fluconazole and amitriptyline. Am J Emerg Med 18: 227, 2000.

Douglas MW et al.: Tolerability of treatments for postherpetic neuralgia. Drug Saf 27: 1217, 2004.

Drake WM et al.: Heart block in a patient on propranolol and fluoxetine. Lancet 343: 425, 1994.

Dresser GK et al.: St. John's Wort induces intestinal and hepatic CYP3A4 and P-glycoprotein in healthy volunteers. Clin Pharmacol Ther 69: P23, 2001.

Dubocovich ML et al.: Cocaine and desipramine antagonize the clonidine-induced inhibition of [3H]-noradrenaline release from the rat cerebral cortex [proceedings]. Br J Pharmacol 67: 417P, 1979.

Dubovsky SL et al.: Phenelzine-induced hypomania: effect of verapamil. Biol Psychiatry 20: 1009, 1985.

DuMortier G et al.: Elevated clozapine plasma concentrations after fluvoxamine initiation. Am J Psychiatry 153: 738, 1996.

Dursun SM et al.: Toxic serotonin syndrome after fluoxetine plus carbamazepine. Lancet 342: 442, 1993.

Eap CB et al.: Fluvoxamine and fluoxetine do not interact in the same way with the metabolism of the enantiomers of methadone. J Clin Psychopharmacol 17: 113, 1997.

Earle BV: Thyroid hormone and tricyclic antidepressants in resistant depressions. Am J Psychiatry 126: 1667, 1970.

Edwards RP et al.: Cardiac responses to imipramine and pancuronium during anesthesia with halothane or enflurane. Anesthesiology 50: 421, 1979.

Egberts AC et al.: Serotonin syndrome attributed to tramadol addition to paroxetine therapy. Int Clin Psychopharmacol 12: 181, 1997.

Eich-Hochli D et al.: Methadone maintenance treatment and St. John's Wort—a case report. Pharmacopsychiatry 36: 35, 2003.

Elliott HL et al.: Pharmacodynamic studies on mianserin and its interaction with clonidine. Eur J Clin Pharmacol 21: 97, 1981.

Elliott HL et al.: Assessment of the interaction between mianserin and centrally-acting antihypertensive drugs. Br J Clin Pharmacol 15 Suppl 2: 323S, 1983.

el-Yazigi A et al.: Steady-state kinetics of fluoxetine and amitriptyline in patients treated with a combination of these drugs as compared with those treated with amitriptyline alone. J Clin Pharmacol 35: 17, 1995.

Enns MW: Seizure during combination of trimipramine and bupropion. J Clin Psychiatry 62: 476, 2001.

Ernst E: The risk-benefit profile of commonly used herbal therapies: ginkgo, St. John's wort, ginseng, echinacea, saw palmetto, and kava. Ann Intern Med 136: 42, 2002.

Facciola G et al.: Cytochrome P450 isoforms involved in melatonin metabolism in human liver microsomes. Eur J Clin Pharmacol 56: 881, 2001.

Fadden JS: Nifedipine and nonresponse to antidepressants. J Clin Psychiatry 53: 416, 1992.

Fann WE et al.: Chlorpromazine reversal of the antihypertensive action of guanethidine. Lancet 2: 436, 1971.

Feder R: Reversal of antidepressant activity of fluoxetine by cyproheptadine in three patients. J Clin Psychiatry 52: 163, 1991.

Fehr C et al.: Increase in serum clomipramine concentrations caused by valproate. J Clin Psychopharmacol 20: 493, 2000.

Feighner JP et al.: Combined MAOI, TCA, and direct stimulant therapy of treatment-resistant depression. J Clin Psychiatry 46: 206, 1985.

Feighner JP et al.: Hormonal potentiation of imipramine and ECT in primary depression. Am J Psychiatry 128: 1230, 1972.

Feinberg SS: Combining stimulants with monoamine oxidase inhibitors: a review of uses and one possible additional indication. J Clin Psychiatry 65: 1520, 2004.

Ferguson JM. Interaction of aspartame and carbohydrates in an eating-disordered patient. Am J Psychiatry 142: 271, 1985.

Field B et al.: Inhibition of hepatic drug metabolism by norethindrone. Clin Pharmacol Ther 25: 196, 1979.

Finch L: The cardiovascular effects of intraventricular 5,6-dihydroxytryptamine in conscious hypertensive rats. Clin Exp Pharmacol Physiol 2: 503, 1975.

Fisher AA et al.: Serotonin syndrome caused by selective serotonin reuptake-inhibitors-metoclopramide interaction. Ann Pharmacother 36: 67, 2002.

Fleishaker JC et al.: A pharmacokinetic and pharmacodynamic evaluation of the combined administration of alprazolam and fluvoxamine. Eur J Clin Pharmacol 46: 35, 1994.

Fogelson DL: Fenfluramine and the cytochrome P450 system. Am J Psychiatry 154: 436, 1997.

Folks DG: Monoamine oxidase inhibitors: reappraisal of dietary considerations. J Clin Psychopharmacol 3: 249, 1983.

Ford MA et al.: Lack of effect of fluoxetine on the hypoprothrombinemic response of warfarin. J Clin Psychopharmacol 17: 110, 1997.

Forster PL et al.: The effects of sertraline on plasma concentration and renal clearance of digoxin. Biol Psychiatry 29: 355, 1991.

Frazer A et al.: The effect of tri-iodothyronine in combination with imipramine on [3H]-cyclic AMP production in slices of rat cerebral cortex. Neuropharmacology 13: 1311, 1974.

Fritze J et al.: Interaction between carbamazepine and fluvoxamine. Acta Psychiatr Scand 84: 583, 1991.

Fuller RW et al.: Antihypertensive effects of fluoxetine and L-5-hydroxytryptophan in rats. Life Sci 25: 1237, 1979.

Fuller RW et al.: Inhibition of drug metabolism by fluoxetine. Res Commun Chem Pathol Pharmacol 13: 353, 1976.

Gammon G et al.: Fluoxetine and methylphenidate in combination for treatment of attention deficit disorder and comorbid depressive disorder. J Child Adol Psychopharmacol 3: 1, 1993.

Gander DR: Treatment of depressive illnesses with combined antidepressants. Lancet 19: 107, 1965.

Gannon RH et al.: Fluconazole-nortriptyline drug interaction. Ann Pharmacother 26: 1456, 1992.

Gatto GJ et al.: Effects of fluoxetine and desipramine on palatability-induced ethanol consumption in the alcohol-nonpreferring (NP) line of rats. Alcohol 7: 531, 1990.

Geeze DS et al.: Doxepin-cholestyramine interaction. Psychosomatics 29: 233, 1988.

Gelenberg AJ: Can MAO inhibitor drugs be taken with analgesics? J Clin Psychopharmacol 1: 160, 1981.

Gelenberg AJ: MAOI inhibitors in sickness and in health. Biol Ther Psychiatry 5: 25, 1982.

Gelenberg AJ: Adverse reactions to MAOIs. Biol Ther Psychiatry 8:4, 1985.

Gidal BE et al.: Evaluation of the effect of fluoxetine on the formation of carbamazepine epoxide. Ther Drug Monit 15: 405, 1993.

Gill K et al.: Serotonin uptake blockers and voluntary alcohol consumption. A review of recent studies. Recent Dev Alcohol 7: 225, 1989.

Gillette DW: Desipramine and ibuprofen. J Am Acad Child Adolesc Psychiatry 37: 1129, 1998.

Gitlin MJ et al.: Failure of T3 to potentiate tricyclic antidepressant response. J Affect Disord 13: 267, 1987.

Glassman AH et al.: Potentiation of a monoamine oxidase inhibitor by tryptophan. J Psychiatr Res 7: 83, 1969.

Glisson SN et al.: Amitriptyline therapy increases electrocardiographic changes during reversal of neuromuscular blockade. Anesth Analg 57: 77, 1978.

Goff DC: Two cases of hypomania following the addition of L-tryptophan to a monoamine oxidase inhibitor. Am J Psychiatry 142: 1487, 1985.

Goldberg MR et al.: Lack of pharmacokinetic and pharmacodynamic interaction between rizatriptan and paroxetine. J Clin Pharmacol 39: 192, 1999.

Goldbloom DS et al.: Adverse interaction of fluoxetine and cyproheptadine in two patients with bulimia nervosa. J Clin Psychiatry 52: 261, 1991.

Goldstein FJ et al.: Elevation in analgetic effect and plasma levels of morphine by desipramine in rats. Pain 14: 279, 1982.

Gonzalez-Pinto A et al.: Mania and tramadol-fluoxetine combination. Am J Psychiatry 158: 964, 2001.

Goodnick PJ: Influence of fluoxetine on plasma levels of desipramine. Am J Psychiatry 146: 552, 1989.

Goodwin FK et al.: Potentiation of antidepressant effects by L-triiodothyronine in tricyclic nonresponders. Am J Psychiatry 139: 34, 1982.

Goonewardene A et al.: Gross oedema occurring during treatment for depression. Br Med J 1: 879, 1977.

Gordon JB: SSRIs and St. John's Wort: possible toxicity? Am Fam Physician 57: 950, 1998.

Gorelick DA: Serotonin uptake blockers and the treatment of alcoholism. Recent Dev Alcohol 7: 267, 1989.

Gorelick DA et al.: Effect of fluoxetine on alcohol consumption in male alcoholics. Alcohol Clin Exp Res 16: 261, 1992.

Gossen D et al.: Influence of fluoxetine on olanzapine pharmacokinetics. AAPS Pharm Sci 4: E11, 2002.

Goulet JP et al.: Contraindications to vasoconstrictors in dentistry: Part III. Pharmacologic interactions. Oral Surg Oral Med Oral Pathol 74: 692, 1992.

Graber MA et al.: Sertraline-phenelzine drug interaction: a serotonin syndrome reaction. Ann Pharmacother 28: 732, 1994.

Gradwell BG: Psychotic reactions and phenelzine. Br Med J 2: 1018, 1960.

Grady TA et al.: Seizure associated with fluoxetine and adjuvant buspirone therapy. J Clin Psychopharmacol 12: 70, 1992.

Graff DW et al.: Effect of fluoxetine on carvedilol pharmacokinetics, CYP2D6 activity, and autonomic balance in heart failure patients. J Clin Pharmacol 41: 97, 2001.

Graham PM et al.: Danger of MAOI therapy after fluoxetine withdrawal. Lancet 2: 1255, 1988.

Gram LF et al.: Imipramine metabolism: pH-dependent distribution and urinary excretion. Clin Pharmacol Ther 12: 239, 1971.

Gratz SS et al.: MAOI-narcotic interactions. J Clin Psychiatry 54: 439, 1993.

Greb WH et al.: Absorption of paroxetine under various dietary conditions and following antacid intake. Acta Psychiatr Scand Suppl 350: 99, 1989a.

Greb WH et al.: The effect of liver enzyme inhibition by cimetidine and enzyme induction by phenobarbitone on the pharmacokinetics of paroxetine. Acta Psychiatr Scand Suppl 350: 95, 1989b.

Greenblatt DJ et al.: Short-term exposure to low-dose ritonavir impairs clearance and enhances adverse effects of trazodone. J Clin Pharmacol 43: 414, 2003.

Grimsley SR et al.: Paroxetine, sertraline, and fluvoxamine: new selective serotonin reuptake inhibitors. Clin Pharm 11: 930, 1992.

Grimsley SR et al.: Increased carbamazepine plasma concentrations after fluoxetine coadministration. Clin Pharmacol Ther 50: 10, 1991.

Grof E et al.: Effects of lithium, nortriptyline and dexamethasone on insulin sensitivity. Prog Neuropsychopharmacol Biol Psychiatry 8: 687, 1984.

Grupp LA et al.: Attenuation of alcohol intake by a serotonin uptake inhibitor: evidence for mediation through the renin-angiotensin system. Pharmacol Biochem Behav 30: 823, 1988.

Gulati OD et al.: Antagonism of adrenergic neuron blockade in hypertensive subjects. Clin Pharmacol Ther 7: 510, 1966.

Gundert-Remy U et al.: Lack of interaction between the tetracyclic antidepressant maprotiline and the centrally acting antihypertensive drug clonidine. Eur J Clin Pharmacol 25: 595, 1983.

Hall RC et al.: The effect of desmethylimipramine on the absorption of alcohol and paracetamol. Postgrad Med J 52: 139, 1976.

Hamilton MJ et al.: The effect of bupropion, a new antidepressant drug, and alcohol and their interaction in man. Eur J Clin Pharmacol 27: 75, 1984.

Hamilton S et al.: Serotonin syndrome during treatment with paroxetine and risperidone. J Clin Psychopharmacol 20: 103, 2000.

Hammer W et al.: Antidepressant Drugs. Milan: Excerpta Medica, 1967.

Hansen TE et al.: Interaction of fluoxetine and pentazocine. Am J Psychiatry 147: 949, 1990.

Hansten PD: Clonidine and tricyclic antidepressants. Drug Inter Newsl 4: 13, 1984.

Haraguchi M et al.: Reduction in oral ethanol self-administration in the rat by the 5-HT uptake blocker fluoxetine. Pharmacol Biochem Behav 35: 259, 1990.

Hardy JL et al.: Reduction of prothrombin and partial thromboplastin times with trazodone. Cmaj 135: 1372, 1986.

Hartter S et al.: Increased bioavailability of oral melatonin after fluvoxamine coadministration. Clin Pharmacol Ther 67: 1, 2000.

Hartter S et al.: Differential effects of fluvoxamine and other antidepressants on the biotransformation of melatonin. J Clin Psychopharmacol 21: 167, 2001.

Hartter S et al.: Inhibition of antidepressant demethylation and hydroxylation by fluvoxamine in depressed patients. Psychopharmacology (Berl) 110: 302, 1993.

Harvey AT et al.: Cytochrome P450 enzymes: interpretation of their interactions with selective serotonin reuptake inhibitors. Part II. J Clin Psychopharmacol 16: 345, 1996.

Harvey AT et al.: Cytochrome P450 enzymes: interpretation of their interactions with selective serotonin reuptake inhibitors. Part I. J Clin Psychopharmacol 16: 273, 1996.

Haselberger MB et al.: Elevated serum phenytoin concentrations associated with coadministration of sertraline. J Clin Psychopharmacol 17: 107, 1997.

Haskovec L et al.: The action of reserpine in imipramine-resistant depressive patients. Clinical and biochemical study. Psychopharmacologia 11: 18, 1967.

Hedberg DL et al.: Tranylcypromine-trifluoperazine combination in the treatment of schizophrenia. Am J Psychiatry 127: 1141, 1971.

Heisler MA et al.: Serotonin syndrome induced by administration of venlafaxine and phenelzine. Ann Pharmacother 30: 84, 1996.

Hemeryck A et al.: Paroxetine affects metoprolol pharmacokinetics and pharmacodynamics in healthy volunteers. Clin Pharmacol Ther 67: 283, 2000.

Henauer SA et al.: Cimetidine interaction with imipramine and nortriptyline. Clin Pharmacol Ther 35: 183, 1984.

Hermann DJ et al.: Comparison of verapamil, diltiazem, and labetalol on the bioavailability and metabolism of imipramine. J Clin Pharmacol 32: 176, 1992.

Hernandez AF et al.: Fatal moclobemide overdose or death caused by serotonin syndrome? J Forensic Sci 40: 128, 1995.

Hiemke C et al.: Fluvoxamine augmentation of olanzapine in chronic schizophrenia: pharmacokinetic interactions and clinical effects. J Clin Psychopharmacol 22: 502, 2002.

Hiemke C et al.: Elevated levels of clozapine in serum after addition of fluvoxamine. J Clin Psychopharmacol 14: 279, 1994.

Hindmarch I et al.: The effects of paroxetine and other antidepressants in combination with alcohol on psychomotor activity related to car driving. Acta Psychiatr Scand Suppl 350: 45, 1989.

Hindmarch I et al.: The effects of sertraline on psychomotor performance in elderly volunteers. J Clin Psychiatry 51 Suppl B: 34, 1990.

Hirsch MS et al.: Subarachnoid hemorrhage following ephedrine and MAO inhibitor. JAMA 194: 1259, 1965.

Hori H et al.: Grapefruit juice-fluvoxamine interaction—is it risky or not? J Clin Psychopharmacol 23: 422, 2003.

Horton RC et al.: Interaction between cyclosporin and fluoxetine. Br Med J 311: 422, 1995.

Houghton GW et al.: Inhibition of phenytoin metabolism by other drugs used in epilepsy. Int J Clin Pharmacol Biopharm 12: 210, 1975.

Houlihan DJ: Serotonin syndrome resulting from coadministration of tramadol, venlafaxine, and mirtazapine. Ann Pharmacother 38: 411, 2004.

Hubbell CL et al.: Opioidergic, serotonergic, and dopaminergic manipulations and rats' intake of a sweetened alcoholic beverage. Alcohol 8: 355, 1991.

Hughes FW et al.: Delayed audiofeedback (DAF) for induction of anxiety. Effect of nortriptyline, ethanol, or nortriptyline-ethanol combinations on performance with DAF. JAMA 185: 556, 1963.

Hui KK: Hypertensive crisis induced by interaction of clonidine with imipramine. J Am Geriatr Soc 31: 164, 1983.

Hullett FJ et al.: Depression associated with nifedipine-induced calcium channel blockade. Am J Psychiatry 145: 1277, 1988.

Hyatt MC et al.: Amitriptyline augments and prolongs ethanol-induced euphoria. J Clin Psychopharmacol 7: 277, 1987.

Hyttel J et al.: Neuropharmacological mechanisms of serotonin reuptake inhibitors. In: Research Advances in New Psychopharmacological Treatment for Alcoholism. In: Excerpta Medica, Amsterdam: Elsevier, 1985; p. 107.

Iribarne C et al.: Involvement of cytochrome P450 3A4 in N-dealkylation of buprenorphine in human liver microsomes. Life Sci 60: 1953, 1997.

Iruela LM et al.: Toxic interaction of S-adenosylmethionine and clomipramine. Am J Psychiatry 150: 522, 1993.

Izzo AA et al.: Interactions between herbal medicines and prescribed drugs: a systematic review. Drugs 61: 2163, 2001.

Jack RA et al.: Possible interaction between pheneizine and amantadine. Arch Gen Psychiatry 41: 726, 1984.

Jalil P: Toxic reaction following the combined administration of fluoxetine and phenytoin: two case reports. J Neurol Neurosurg Psychiatry 55: 412, 1992.

Janowsky EC et al.: What precautions should be taken if a patient on a MAOI is scheduled to undergo anesthesia? J Clin Psychopharmacol 5: 128, 1985.

Janowsky EC et al.: Effects of anesthesia on patients taking psychotropic drugs. J Clin Psychopharmacol 1: 14, 1981.

Jenike MA: Alcohol and antihistamines not contraindicated with MAOIs? Am J Psychiatry 140: 1107, 1983.

Jenike MA et al.: Buspirone augmentation of fluoxetine in patients with obsessive compulsive disorder. J Clin Psychiatry 52: 13, 1991.

Jerling M et al.: The use of therapeutic drug monitoring data to document kinetic drug interactions: an example with amitriptyline and nortriptyline. Ther Drug Monit 16: 1, 1994a.

Jerling M et al.: Fluvoxamine inhibition and carbamazepine induction of the metabolism of clozapine: evidence from a therapeutic drug monitoring service. Ther Drug Monit 16: 368, 1994b.

Jermain DM et al.: Potential fluoxetine-selegiline interaction. Ann Pharmacother 26: 1300, 1992.

Joffe RT: Triiodothronine potentiation of fluoxetine in depressed patients. Can J Psychiatry 37: 48, 1992.

Joffe RT et al.: Lack of pharmacokinetic interaction of carbamazepine with tranylcypromine. Arch Gen Psychiatry 42: 738, 1985.

Joffe RT et al.: An open study of buspirone augmentation of serotonin reuptake inhibitors in refractory depression. J Clin Psychiatry 54: 269, 1993b.

Joffe RT et al.: A comparison of triiodothyronine and thyroxine in the potentiation of tricyclic antidepressants. Psychiatry Res 32: 241, 1990.

Joffe RT et al.: A placebo-controlled comparison of lithium and triiodothyronine augmentation of tricyclic antidepressants in unipolar refractory depression. Arch Gen Psychiatry 50: 387, 1993a.

Joffe RT et al.: Co-administration of fluoxetine and sumatriptan: the Canadian experience. Acta Psychiatr Scand 95: 551, 1997.

Johne A et al.: Decreased plasma levels of amitriptyline and its metabolites on comedication with an extract from St. John's wort (Hypericum perforatum). J Clin Psychopharmacol 22: 46, 2002.

Johnson BA et al.: Development of novel pharmacotherapies for the treatment of alcohol dependence: focus on antiepileptics. Alcohol Clin Exp Res 28: 295, 2004.

Jokinen MJ et al.: The effect of erythromycin, fluvoxamine, and their combination on the pharmacokinetics of ropivacaine. Anesth Analg 91: 1207, 2000.

Jones BD et al.: Interaction of ginseng with phenelzine. J Clin Psychopharmacol 7: 201, 1987.

Joseph AB et al.: Potentially toxic serum concentrations of desipramine after discontinuation of valproic acid. Brain Inj 7: 463, 1993.

Karki SD et al.: Combination risperidone and SSRI-induced serotonin syndrome. Ann Pharmacother 37: 388, 2003.

Kaskey GB: Possible interaction between an MAOI and "ecstasy". Am J Psychiatry 149: 411, 1992.

Katz MR: Raised serum levels of desipramine with the antiarrhythmic propafenone. J Clin Psychiatry 52: 432, 1991.

Katz RJ et al.: Adverse interaction of cyproheptadine with serotonergic antidepressants. J Clin Psychiatry 55: 314, 1994.

Kaye CM et al.: A review of the metabolism and pharmacokinetics of paroxetine in man. Acta Psychiatr Scand Suppl 350: 60, 1989.

Kellstein DE et al.: Contrasting effects of acute vs. chronic tricyclic antidepressant treatment on central morphine analgesia. Pain 20: 323, 1984.

Kellstein DE et al.: Effect of chronic treatment with tricyclic antidepressants upon antinociception induced by intrathecal injection of morphine and monoamines. Neuropharmacology 27: 1, 1988.

Kesavan S et al.: Serotonin syndrome with fluoxetine plus tramadol. J R Soc Med 92: 474, 1999.

Khan A et al.: Lack of sertraline efficacy probably due to an interaction with carbamazepine. J Clin Psychiatry 61: 526, 2000.

Khurana RC: Estrogen-imipramine interaction. JAMA 222: 702, 1972.

Kincaid RL et al.: Report of a fluoxetine fatality. J Anal Toxicol 14: 327, 1990.

Kleijnen J: Evening primrose oil. Br Med J 309: 824, 1994.

Kline NS et al.: Protection of patients on MAOIs against hypertensive crises. J Clin Psychopharmacol 1: 410, 1981.

Klysmer R et al.: Toxic interaction of venlafaxine and isocarboxazid. Lancet 346: 1298, 1995.

Knoll Pharmaceutical C: Sibutramine (Meridia) Product Information. 2002.

Koch-Weser J: Hemorrhagic reactions and drug interactions in 500 warfarin-treated patients. Clin Pharamcol Ther 14: 139, 1973.

Koe BK et al.: Marked depletion of brain serotonin by p-chlorophenylalanine. Fed Proc 25: 452, 1966.

Kostowski W et al.: Activity of diltiazem and nifedipine in some animal models of depression. Pol J Pharmacol Pharm 42: 121, 1990.

Kostowski W et al.: A study of the effects of clonidine on the EEG in rats treated with single and multiple doses of antidepressants. Psychopharmacology (Berl) 84: 85, 1984.

Krahenbuhl S et al.: Pharmacokinetic interaction between diltiazem and nortriptyline. Eur J Clin Pharmacol 49: 417, 1996.

Kranzler HR et al.: Placebo-controlled trial of fluoxetine as an adjunct to relapse prevention in alcoholics. Am J Psychiatry 152: 391, 1995.

Krisko I et al.: Severe hyperpyrexia due to tranylcypromine-amphetamine toxicity. Ann Intern Med 70: 559, 1969.

Kudoh A et al.: Antidepressant treatment for chronic depressed patients should not be discontinued prior to anesthesia. Can J Anaesth 49: 132, 2002.

Kuo FJ et al.: Extrapyramidal symptoms after addition of fluvoxamine to clozapine. J Clin Psychopharmacol 18: 483, 1998.

Kurtz DL et al.: The effect of sertraline on the pharmacokinetics of desipramine and imipramine. Clin Pharmacol Ther 62: 145, 1997.

Kusumoto M et al.: Effect of fluvoxamine on the pharmacokinetics of mexiletine in healthy Japanese men. Clin Pharmacol Ther 69: 104, 2001.

Laine K et al.: Inhibition of cytochrome P4502D6 activity with paroxetine normalizes the ultrarapid metabolizer phenotype as measured by nortriptyline pharmacokinetics and the debrisoquin test. Clin Pharmacol Ther 70: 327, 2001.

Lamberg TS et al.: The effect of fluvoxamine on the pharmacokinetics and pharmacodynamics of buspirone. Eur J Clin Pharmacol 54: 761, 1998.

Landauer AA et al.: Alcohol and amitriptyline effects on skills related to driving behavior. Science 163: 1467, 1969.

Lange-Asschenfeldt C et al.: Serotonin syndrome as a result of fluoxetine in a patient with tramadol abuse: plasma level-correlated symptomatology. J Clin Psychopharmacol 22: 440, 2002.

Lantz MS et al.: St. John's wort and antidepressant drug interactions in the elderly. J Geriatr Psychiatry Neurol 12: 7, 1999.

Lantz MS et al.: Serotonin syndrome following the administration of tramadol with paroxetine. Int J Geriat Psychiatry 13: 343, 1998.

Laplaud PM et al.: Antioxidant action of Vaccinium myrtillus extract on human low density lipoproteins in vitro: initial observations. Fundam Clin Pharmacol 11: 35, 1997.

Larochelle P et al.: Responses to tyramine and norepinephrine after imipramine and trazodone. Clin Pharmacol Ther 26: 24, 1979.

Larson AA et al.: Effect of fluoxetine hydrochloride (Lilly 110140), a specific inhibitor of serotonin uptake, on morphine analgesia and the development of tolerance. Life Sci 21: 1807, 1977.

Lazarus A: Rhabdomyolysis in a depressed patient following overdose with combined drug therapy and alcohol. J Clin Psychopharmacol 10:154, 1990.

Lee DO et al.: Serotonin syndrome in a child associated with erythromycin and sertraline. Pharmacotherapy 19: 894, 1999.

Lee RL et al.: Effect of tricyclic antidepressants on analgesic activity in laboratory animals. Postgrad Med J 56 Suppl 1: 19, 1980.

Leibovitz A et al.: Elevated serum digoxin level associated with co-administered fluoxetine. Arch Intern Med 158: 1152, 1998.

Leishman AW et al.: Antagonism of guanethidine by imipramine. Lancet 1: 112, 1963.

Lejoyeux M et al.: The serotonin syndrome. Am J Psychiatry 149: 1410, 1992.

Lejoyeux M et al.: Prospective evaluation of the serotonin syndrome in depressed inpatients treated with clomipramine. Acta Psychiatr Scand 88: 369, 1993.

Lemberger L et al.: Effect of fluoxetine on psychomotor performance, physiologic response, and kinetics of ethanol. Clin Pharmacol Ther 37: 658, 1985.

Leucht S et al.: Effect of adjunctive paroxetine on serum levels and side-effects of tricyclic antidepressants in depressive inpatients. Psychopharmacology (Berl) 147: 378, 2000.

Leung M et al.: Lack of an interaction between sumatriptan and selective serotonin reuptake inhibitors. Headache 35: 488, 1995.

Levy AB et al.: Myoclonus, hyperreflexia and diaphoresis in patients on phenelzine-tryptophan combination treatment. Can J Psychiatry 30: 434, 1985.

Liberzon I et al.: Bupropion and delirium. Am J Psychiatry 147: 1689, 1990.

Limke KK et al.: Fluvoxamine interaction with warfarin. Ann Pharmacother 36: 1890, 2002.

Linet LS: Treatment of a refractory depression with a combination of fluoxetine and d-amphetamine. Am J Psychiatry 146: 803, 1989.

Linnet K: Comparison of the kinetic interactions of the neuroleptics perphenazine and zuclopenthixol with tricyclic antidepressives. Ther Drug Monit 17: 308, 1995.

Linnoila M et al.: Effects of chronic zimelidine and ethanol on psychomotor performance. J Clin Psychopharmacol 5: 148, 1985.

Linnoila M et al.: Effects of fluvoxamine, alone and in combination with ethanol, on psychomotor and cognitive performance and on autonomic nervous system reactivity in healthy volunteers. J Clin Psychopharmacol 13: 175, 1993.

Liston HL et al.: Lack of citalopram effect on the pharmacokinetics of cyclosporine. Psychosomatics 42: 370, 2001.

Liu SJ et al.: Increased analgesia and alterations in distribution and metabolism of methadone by desipramine in the rat. J Pharmacol Exp Ther 195: 94, 1975.

Liu SJ et al.: Enhanced development of dispositional tolerance to methadone by desipramine given together with methadone. Life Sci 36: 745, 1985.

Loomis CW et al.: Drug interactions of amitriptyline and nortriptyline with warfarin in the rat. Res Commun Chem Pathol Pharmacol 30: 41, 1980.

Lu ML et al.: Fluvoxamine reduces the clozapine dosage needed in refractory schizophrenic patients. J Clin Psychiatry 61: 594, 2000.

Lu MR et al.: Ethanol intake of chickens treated with fenfluramine, fluoxetine, and dietary tryptophan. Alcohol Clin Exp Res 16: 852, 1992.

Lu MR et al.: Ethanol consumption following acute fenfluramine, fluoxetine, and dietary tryptophan. Pharmacol Biochem Behav 44: 931, 1993.

Lucena MI et al.: Interaction of fluoxetine and valproic acid. Am J Psychiatry 155: 575, 1998.

Lydiard RB et al.: Interactions between sertraline and tricyclic antidepressants. Am J Psychiatry 150: 1125, 1993.

Lyness WH et al.: Influence of dopaminergic and serotonergic neurons on intravenous ethanol self-administration in the rat. Pharmacol Biochem Behav 42: 187, 1992.

Maany I et al.: Increase in desipramine serum levels associated with methadone treatment. Am J Psychiatry 146: 1611, 1989.

Maany I et al.: Possible toxic interaction between disulfiram and amitriptyline. Arch Gen Psychiatry 39: 743, 1982.

MacCallum WA: Drug interactions in alcoholism treatment. Lancet 1: 313, 1969.

MacLeod DM: Chorea induced by tranquillizers. Lancet 41: 388, 1964.

Madani S et al.: Effect of terbinafine on the pharmacokinetics and pharmacodynamics of desipramine in healthy volunteers identified as cytochrome P450 2D6 (CYP2D6) extensive metabolizers. J Clin Pharmacol 42: 1211, 2002.

Madsen H et al.: Fluvoxamine inhibits the CYP2C9 catalyzed biotransformation of tolbutamide. Clin Pharmacol Ther 69: 41, 2001.

Maes M et al.: Effects of trazodone and fluoxetine in the treatment of major depression: therapeutic pharmacokinetic and pharmacodynamic interactions through formation of meta-chlorophenylpiperazine. J Clin Psychopharmacol 17: 358, 1997.

Mahlberg R et al.: Serotonin syndrome with tramadol and citalopram. Am J Psychiatry 161: 1129, 2004.

Malec D et al.: Effect of quipazine and fluoxetine on analgesic-induced catalepsy and antinociception in the rat. J Pharm Pharmacol 32: 71, 1980.

Mamiya K et al.: Phenytoin intoxication induced by fluvoxamine. Ther Drug Monit 23: 75, 2001.

Manos GH: Possible serotonin syndrome associated with buspirone added to fluoxetine. Ann Pharmacother 34: 871, 2000.

Marathe PH et al.: Metabolic kinetics of pseudoracemic propranolol in human liver microsomes. Enantioselectivity and quinidine inhibition. Drug Metab Dispos 22: 237, 1994.

Marchiando RJ et al.: Probable terfenadine-fluoxetine-associated cardiac toxicity. Ann Pharmacother 29: 937, 1995.

Margolese HC et al.: Serotonin syndrome from addition of low-dose trazodone to nefazodone. Am J Psychiatry 157: 1022, 2000.

Markel H et al.: LSD flashback syndrome exacerbated by selective serotonin reuptake inhibitor antidepressants in adolescents. J Pediatr 125:817, 1994.

Markovitz PJ et al.: Buspirone augmentation of fluoxetine in obsessive-compulsive disorder. Am J Psychiatry 147: 798, 1990.

Markowitz JS et al.: Rifampin-induced selective serotonin reuptake inhibitor withdrawal syndrome in a patient treated with sertraline. J Clin Psychopharmacol 20: 109, 2000.

Marley E et al.: Interactions of a non-selective monoamine oxidase inhibitor, phenelzine, with inhibitors of 5-hydroxytryptamine, dopamine or noradrenaline re-uptake. J Psychiatr Res 18: 173, 1984.

Martin DE et al.: Paroxetine does not affect the cardiac safety and pharmacokinetics of terfenadine in healthy adult men. J Clin Psychopharmacol 17: 451, 1997.

Martinelli V et al.: An interaction between carbamazepine and fluvoxamine. Br J Clin Pharmacol 36: 615, 1993.

Maskall DD et al.: Increased plasma concentration of imipramine following augmentation with fluvoxamine. Am J Psychiatry 150: 1566, 1993.

Mason BJ et al.: Possible serotonin syndrome associated with tramadol and sertraline coadministration. Ann Pharmacother 31: 175, 1997.

Mason BJ et al.: Desipramine treatment of alcoholism. Psychopharmacol Bull 27: 155, 1991.

Mathew NT et al.: Serotonin syndrome complicating migraine pharmacotherapy. Cephalalgia 16: 323, 1996.

McBride WJ et al.: Effects of Ro 15-4513, fluoxetine and desipramine on the intake of ethanol, water and food by the alcohol-preferring (P) and -nonpreferring (NP) lines of rats. Pharmacol Biochem Behav 30: 1045, 1988.

McCormick S et al.: Reversal of fluoxetine-induced anorgasmia by cyproheptadine in two patients. J Clin Psychiatry 51: 383, 1990.

McCue RE et al.: Venlafaxine- and trazodone-induced serotonin syndrome. Am J Psychiatry 158: 2088, 2001.

Meert TF: Effects of various serotonergic agents on alcohol intake and alcohol preference in Wistar rats selected at two different levels of alcohol preference. Alcohol Alcohol 28: 157, 1993.

Metz A et al.: Combination of fluoxetine with pemoline in the treatment of major depressive disorder. Int Clin Psychopharmacol 6: 93, 1991.

Meyer D et al.: Toxicity secondary to meperidine in patients on monoamine oxidase inhibitors: a case report and critical review. J Clin Psychopharmacol 1: 319, 1981.

Meyer JF et al.: Insidious and prolonged antagonism of guanethidine by amitriptyline. JAMA 213: 1487, 1970.

Miller DD et al.: Cimetidine-imipramine interaction: a case report. Am J Psychiatry 140: 351, 1983a.

Miller DD et al.: Cimetidine's effect on steady-state serum nortriptyline concentrations. Drug Intell Clin Pharm 17: 904, 1983b.

Miller FP et al.: Comparative effects of p-chloroamphetamine and p-chloro-N-methylamphetamine on rat brain norepinephrine, serotonin and 5-hydroxyindole-3-acetic acid. Biochem Pharmacol 19: 435, 1970.

Miller LG: Herbal medicinals: selected clinical considerations focusing on known or potential drug-herb interactions. Arch Intern Med 158: 2200, 1998.

Milner G et al.: The effects of doxepin, alone and together with alcohol, in relation to driving safety. Med J Aust 1: 837, 1978.

Mindham RH: Psychiatric symptoms in Parkinsonism. J Neurol Neurosurg Psychiatry 33: 188, 1970.

Mirchandani H et al.: Fatal malignant hyperthermia as a result of ingestion of tranylcypromine (Parnate) combined with white wine and cheese. J Forensic Sci 30: 217, 1985.

Mitchell JR et al.: Guanethidine and related agents. 3. Antagonism by drugs which inhibit the norepinephrine pump in man. J Clin Invest 49: 1596, 1970.

Mittino D et al.: Serotonin syndrome associated with tramadol-sertraline coadministration. Clin Neuropharmacol 27: 150, 2004.

Mochizucki D: Serotonin and noradrenaline reuptake inhibitors in animal models of pain. Hum Psychopharmacol 19 Suppl 1: S15, 2004.

Montastruc JL et al.: Pseudophaeochromocytoma in parkinsonian patient treated with fluoxetine plus selegiline. Lancet 341: 555, 1993.

Moody JP et al.: Pharmacokinetic aspects of protriptyline plasma levels. Eur J Clin Pharmacol 11: 51, 1977.

Morazzoni P et al.: Effects of V. myrtillus anthocyanosides on prostacyclin-like activity in rat arterial tissue. Fitoterapia 57: 11, 1986.

Morgan JP et al.: Imipramine-mediated interference with levodopa absorption from the gastrointestinal tract in man. Neurology 25: 1029, 1975.

Muller N et al.: Extremely long plasma half-life of amitriptyline in a woman with the cytochrome P450IID6 29/29-kilobase wild-type allele—a slowly reversible interaction with fluoxetine. Ther Drug Monit 13: 533, 1991.

Murphy DL et al.: Monoamine oxidase-inhibiting antidepressants. A clinical update. Psychiatr Clin North Am 7: 549, 1984.

Murphy JM et al.: Monoamine uptake inhibitors attenuate ethanol intake in alcohol-preferring (P) rats. Alcohol 2: 349, 1985.

Murphy JM et al.: Effects of fluoxetine on the intragastric self-administration of ethanol in the alcohol preferring P line of rats. Alcohol 5: 283, 1988.

Namaka M et al.: A treatment algorithm for neuropathic pain. Clin Ther 26: 951, 2004.

Naranjo CA et al.: Acute pharmacokinetic and pharmacodynamic interactions of zimelidine and ethanol. Clin Pharmacol Ther 35: 362, 1984b.

Naranjo CA et al.: Fluoxetine differentially alters alcohol intake and other consummatory behaviors in problem drinkers. Clin Pharmacol Ther 47: 490, 1990.

Naranjo CA et al.: Serotonin uptake inhibitors attenuate ethanol intake in problem drinkers. Recent Dev Alcohol 7: 255, 1989.

Naranjo CA et al.: Zimelidine-induced variations in alcohol intake by nonde-pressed heavy drinkers. Clin Pharmacol Ther 35: 374, 1984a.

Nelson JC et al.: A preliminary, open study of the combination of fluoxetine and desipramine for rapid treatment of major depression. Arch Gen Psychiatry 48: 303, 1991.

Nelson JC et al.: Combining norepinephrine and serotonin reuptake inhibition mechanisms for treatment of depression: a double-blind, randomized study. Biol Psychiatry 55: 296, 2004.

Newberry DL et al.: A fluconazole/amitriptyline drug interaction in three male adults. Clin Infect Dis 24: 270, 1997.

Niemi M et al.: Effects of fluconazole and fluvoxamine on the pharmacokinetics and pharmacodynamics of glimepiride. Clin Pharmacol Ther 69: 194, 2001.

Nierenberg AA: Treatment choice after one antidepressant fails: a survey of northeastern psychiatrists. J Clin Psychiatry 52: 383, 1991.

Nierenberg DW et al.: The central nervous system serotonin syndrome. Clin Pharmacol Ther 53: 84, 1993.

Nies A et al.: Monoamine oxidase inhibitors. In: Paykel ES (ed.), Handbook of Affective Disorders. New York: Guilford, 1982; p. 245.

Normann C et al.: Increased plasma concentration of maprotiline by coadministration of risperidone. J Clin Psychopharmacol 22: 92, 2002.

Novartis Pharmaceuticals Corp: Mellaril Product Information. 2000.

Nunes EV et al.: Imipramine treatment of alcoholism with comorbid depression. Am J Psychiatry 150: 963, 1993.

Ober KF et al.: Drug interactions with guanethidine. Clin Pharmacol Ther 14: 190, 1973.

Ochs HR et al.: Chronic treatment with fluvoxamine, clovoxamine, and placebo: interaction with digoxin and effects on sleep and alertness. J Clin Pharmacol 29: 91, 1989.

Oesterheld J et al.: Grapefruit juice and clomipramine: shifting metabolic ratios. J Clin Psychopharmacol 17: 62, 1997.

Ogura C et al.: Combined thyroid (triiodothyronine)-tricyclic antidepressant treatment in depressive states. Folia Psychiatr Neurol Jpn 28: 179, 1974.

Olesen OV et al.: Fluvoxamine-clozapine drug interaction: inhibition in vitro of five cytochrome P450 isoforms involved in clozapine metabolism. J Clin Psychopharmacol 20: 35, 2000.

O'Reardon JP et al.: Desipramine toxicity with terbinafine. Am J Psychiatry 159: 492, 2002.

Ossipov MH et al.: Augmentation of central and peripheral morphine analgesia by desipramine. Arch Int Pharmacodyn Ther 259: 222, 1982.

Ouellet D et al.: Effect of fluoxetine on pharmacokinetics of ritonavir. Antimicrob Agents Chemother 42: 3107, 1998.

Ozdemir V et al.: Paroxetine potentiates the central nervous system side effects of perphenazine: contribution of cytochrome P4502D6 inhibition in vivo. Clin Pharmacol Ther 62: 334, 1997.

Pataki CS et al.: Side effects of methylphenidate and desipramine alone and in combination in children. J Am Acad Child Adolesc Psychiatry 32: 1065, 1993.

Pathak SK: Gross oedema during treatment for depression. Br Med J 1: 1220, 1977.

Patman J et al.: The combined effect of alcohol and amitriptyline on skills similar to motor-car driving. Med J Aust 2: 946, 1969.

Paul KL et al.: Anticholinergic delirium possibly associated with protriptyline and fluoxetine. Ann Pharmacother 31: 1260, 1997.

Paykel ES. Hallucinosis on combined methyldopa and pargyline. Br Med J 5490: 803, 1966.

Pearson HJ. Interaction of fluoxetine with carbamazepine. J Clin Psychiatry 51: 126, 1990.

Perel JM et al.: Inhibition of imipramine metabolism by methylphenidate. Fed Proc 28: 148, 1969.

Perez V et al.: Randomised, double-blind, placebo-controlled trial of pindolol in combination with fluoxetine antidepressant treatment. Lancet 349: 1594, 1997.

Perucca E et al.: Inhibition of diazepam metabolism by fluvoxamine: a pharmacokinetic study in normal volunteers. Clin Pharmacol Ther 56: 471, 1994a.

Perucca E et al.: Clinical pharmacokinetics of fluvoxamine. Clin Pharmacokinet 27: 175, 1994b.

Perucca E et al.: Interaction between phenytoin and imipramine. Br J Clin Pharmacol 4: 485, 1977.

Pfizer Inc. Zoloft® (Sertraline HCl) Product Information. 2003.

Phillips SD et al.: Phenelzine and venlafaxine interaction. Am J Psychiatry 152: 1400, 1995.

Pick CG et al.: Potentiation of opioid analgesia by the antidepressant nefazodone. Eur J Pharmacol 211: 375, 1992.

Picker W et al.: Potential interaction of LSD and fluoxetine. Am J Psychiatry 149: 843, 1992.

Pihlsgard M et al.: Significant reduction of sertraline plasma levels by carbamazepine and phenytoin. Eur J Clin Pharmacol 57: 915, 2002.

Pinninti NR et al.: Interaction of sertraline with clozapine. J Clin Psychopharmacol 17:119, 1997.

Pinto YM et al.: QT lengthening and life-threatening arrhythmias associated with fexofenadine. Lancet 353: 980, 1999.

Poldinger W: Combined administration of desipramine and reserpine or tetrabenazine in depressive patients. Psychopharmacologia 4: 308, 1963.

Pollak PT et al.: Delirium probably induced by clarithromycin in a patient receiving fluoxetine. Ann Pharmacother 29: 486, 1995.

Pond SM et al.: Effects of tricyclic antidepressants on drug metabolism. Clin Pharmacol Ther 18: 191, 1975.

Pope HG, Jr. et al.: Testosterone gel supplementation for men with refractory depression: a randomized, placebo-controlled trial. Am J Psychiatry 160: 105, 2003.

Pope HG, Jr. et al.: Toxic reactions to the combination of monoamine oxidase inhibitors and tryptophan. Am J Psychiatry 142: 491, 1985.

Prange AJ, Jr. et al.: Hormonal alteration of imipramine response: a review. In: Sachar EJ (ed.), Hormones, Behavior, and Psychopathology. New York: Raven Press, 1976; p. 41.

Prange AJ, Jr. et al.: Enhancement of imipramine antidepressant activity by thyroid hormone. Am J Psychiatry 126: 457, 1969.

Preskorn SH: Should bupropion dosage be adjusted based upon therapeutic drug monitoring? Psychopharmacol Bull 27: 637, 1991.

Preskorn SH et al.: Pharmacokinetics of desipramine co-administered with sertraline or fluoxetine. J Clin Psychopharmacol 14: 90, 1994.

Preskorn SH et al.: Fatality associated with combined fluoxetine-amitriptyline therapy. JAMA 277: 1682, 1997.

Preskorn SH et al.: Serious adverse effects of combining fluoxetine and tricyclic antidepressants. Am J Psychiatry 147: 532, 1990.

Priskorn M et al.: Pharmacokinetic interaction study of citalopram and cimetidine in healthy subjects. Eur J Clin Pharmacol 52: 241, 1997.

Priskorn M et al.: Investigation of multiple dose citalopram on the pharmacokinetics and pharmacodynamics of racemic warfarin. Br J Clin Pharmacol 44: 199, 1997.

Rabkin J et al.: Adverse reactions to monoamine oxidase inhibitors. Part I. A comparative study. J Clin Psychopharmacol 4: 270, 1984.

Rabkin JG et al.: Adverse reactions to monoamine oxidase inhibitors. Part II. Treatment correlates and clinical management. J Clin Psychopharmacol 5: 2, 1985.

Randell J: Combining the antidepressant drugs. Br Med J 1: 521, 1965.

Raskin DE: Dangers of monoamine oxidase inhibitors. J Clin Psychopharmacol 4: 238, 1984.

Rauch PK et al.: Digoxin toxicity possibly precipitated by trazodone. Psychosomatics 25: 334, 1984.

Reeves RR et al.: Serotonin syndrome produced by paroxetine and low-dose trazodone. Psychosomatics 36: 159, 1995.

Reggev A et al.: Bradycardia induced by an interaction between phenelzine and beta blockers. Psychosomatics 30: 106, 1989.

Richelson E et al.: Antagonism by antidepressants of neurotransmitter receptors of normal human brain in vitro. J Pharmacol Exp Ther 230: 94, 1984.

Risch SC et al.: The effects of psychotropic drugs on the cardiovascular system. J Clin Psychiatry 43: 16, 1982.

Rivera-CalimLim L et al.: L-dopa treatment failure: explanation and correction. Br Med J 4: 93, 1970.

Robinson RF et al.: Syncope associated with concurrent amitriptyline and fluconazole therapy. Ann Pharmacother 34: 1406, 2000.

Rohrig TP et al.: Fluoxetine overdose: a case report. J Anal Toxicol 13: 305, 1989.

Rosebraugh CJ et al.: Visual hallucination and tremor induced by sertraline and oxycodone in a bone marrow transplant patient. J Clin Pharmacol 41: 224, 2001.

Roth A et al.: Delirium associated with the combination of a neuroleptic, an SSRI, and benztropine. J Clin Psychiatry 55: 492, 1994.

Rothschild BS: Fluoxetine-nortriptyline therapy of treatment-resistant major depression in a geriatric patient. J Geriatr Psychiatry Neurol 7: 137, 1994.

Rowe H et al.: The effect of fluoxetine on warfarin metabolism in the rat and man. Life Sci 23: 807, 1978.

Saiz-Ruiz J et al.: Delirium induced by association of propranolol and maprotiline. J Clin Psychopharmacol 8: 77, 1988.

Salonen JS et al.: Comparative studies on the cytochrome p450-associated metabolism and interaction potential of selegiline between human liver-derived in vitro systems. Drug Metab Dispos 31: 1093, 2003.

Salsali M et al.: Inhibitory effects of the monoamine oxidase inhibitor tranylcypromine on the cytochrome P450 enzymes CYP2C19, CYP2C9, and CYP2D6. Cell Mol Neurobiol 24: 63, 2004.

Sandoz M et al.: Biotransformation of amitriptyline in alcoholic depressive patients. Eur J Clin Pharmacol 24: 615, 1983.

Sargent W: Combining the antidepressant drugs (letter). Br Med J 1: 251, 1965.

Sargent W: Safety of combined antidepressant drugs. Br Med J 1: 555, 1971.

Sauget D et al.: [Possible serotonergic syndrome caused by combination of tramadol and sertraline in an elderly woman]. Therapie 57: 309, 2002.

Schenker S et al.: Fluoxetine disposition and elimination in cirrhosis. Clin Pharmacol Ther 44: 353, 1988.

Schlienger RG et al.: Seizures associated with therapeutic doses of venlafaxine and trimipramine. Ann Pharmacother 34: 1402, 2000.

Schmidt D et al.: [How is oxcarbazepine different from carbamazepine?]. Nervenarzt 75: 153, 2004.

Schuckit M et al.: Tricyclic antidepressants and monoamine oxidase inhibitors. Arch Gen Psychiatry 24: 509, 1971.

Seifritz E et al.: Increased trimipramine plasma levels during fluvoxamine comedication. Eur Neuropsychopharmacol 4: 15, 1994.

Self T et al.: Case report: interaction of rifampin and nortriptyline. Am J Med Sci 311: 80, 1996.

Seppala T et al.: Effect of tricyclic antidepressants and alcohol in psychomotor skills related to driving. Clin Pharmacol Ther 17: 515, 1975.

Sethna ER: A study of refractory cases of depressive illnesses and their response to combined antidepressant treatment. Br J Psychiatry 124: 265, 1974.

Shad MU et al.: The economic consequences of a drug interaction. J Clin Psychopharmacol 21: 119, 2001.

Shad MU et al.: A possible bupropion and imipramine interaction. J Clin Psychopharmacol 17: 118, 1997.

Shad MU et al.: Drug interaction in reverse: possible loss of phenytoin efficacy as a result of fluoxetine discontinuation. J Clin Psychopharmacol 19: 471, 1999.

Shader RI: Can patients on MAOIs safely drink white wine? J Clin Psychopharmacol 6: 254, 1986.

Shader RI et al.: MAOIs and drug interactions—a proposal for a clearinghouse. J Clin Psychopharmacol 5: A17, 1985a.

Shader RI et al.: Phenelzine and the dream machine—ramblings and reflections. J Clin Psychopharmacol 5: 65, 1985b.

Shader RI et al.: Fluoxetine inhibition of phenytoin metabolism. J Clin Psychopharmacol 14: 375, 1994.

Sherman KE et al.: Amitriptyline and asymptomatic hypoglycemia. Ann Intern Med 109: 683, 1988.

Shim JC et al.: Fluoxetine augmentation of haloperidol in chronic schizophrenia. J Clin Psychopharmacol 23: 520, 2003.

Shrivastava RK et al.: Hypoglycemia associated with imipramine. Biol Psychiatry 18: 1509, 1983.

Shulman KI et al.: Dietary restriction, tyramine, and the use of monoamine oxidase inhibitors. J Clin Psychopharmacol 9: 397, 1989.

Sides CA: Hypertension during anaesthesia with monoamine oxidase inhibitors. Anaesthesia 42: 633, 1987.

Silverman G et al.: Interaction of benzodiazepines with tricyclic antidepressants. Br Med J 4: 111, 1972.

Singleton JR et al.: Polyneuropathy with impaired glucose tolerance: implications for diagnosis and therapy. Curr Treat Options Neurol 7: 33, 2005.

Sjoqvist F et al.: The pH-dependent excretion of monomethylated tricyclic antidepressants. Clin Pharmacol Ther 10: 826, 1969.

Skjelbo E et al.: Inhibitors of imipramine metabolism by human liver microsomes. Br J Clin Pharmacol 34: 256, 1992.

Skop BP et al.: The serotonin syndrome associated with paroxetine, an over-the-counter cold remedy, and vascular disease. Am J Emerg Med 12: 642, 1994.

Slaughter RL et al.: Recent advances: the cytochrome P450 enzymes. Ann Pharmacother 29: 619, 1995.

Small NL et al.: Interaction between warfarin and trazodone. Ann Pharmacother 34: 734, 2000.

Smilkstein MJ et al.: A case of MAO inhibitor/MDMA interaction: agony after ecstasy. J Toxicol Clin Toxicol 25: 149, 1987.

Smookler S et al.: Hypertensive crisis resulting from an MAO inhibitor and an over-the-counter appetite suppressant. Ann Emerg Med 11: 482, 1982.

Solai LK et al.: Effect of sertraline on plasma nortriptyline levels in depressed elderly. J Clin Psychiatry 58: 440, 1997.

Sovner R et al.: A potential drug interaction between fluoxetine and valproic acid. J Clin Psychopharmacol 11: 389, 1991.

Sperber AD: Toxic interaction between fluvoxamine and sustained release theophylline in an 11-year-old boy. Drug Saf 6: 460, 1991.

Spigset O et al.: Serotonin syndrome caused by a moclobemide-clomipramine interaction. Br Med J 306: 248, 1993.

Spiller HA et al.: Prospective multicenter evaluation of tramadol exposure. J Toxicol Clin Toxicol 35: 361, 1997.

Spina E et al.: Decreased plasma concentrations of imipramine and desipramine following cholestyramine intake in depressed patients. Ther Drug Monit 16: 432, 1994.

Spina E et al.: The effect of carbamazepine on the 2-hydroxylation of desipramine. Psychopharmacology (Berl) 117: 413, 1995.

Spina E et al.: Effect of ketoconazole on the pharmacokinetics of imipramine and desipramine in healthy subjects. Br J Clin Pharmacol 43: 315, 1997.

Spina E et al.: Plasma concentrations of risperidone and 9-hydroxyrisperidone during combined treatment with paroxetine. Ther Drug Monit 23: 223, 2001.

Spina E et al.: Carbamazepine coadministration with fluoxetine or fluvoxamine. Ther Drug Monit 15: 247, 1993b.

Spina E et al.: Interaction between fluvoxamine and imipramine/desipramine in four patients. Ther Drug Monit 14: 194, 1992.

Spina E et al.: Fluvoxamine-induced alterations in plasma concentrations of imipramine and desipramine in depressed patients. Int J Clin Pharmacol Res 13: 167, 1993a.

Spina E et al.: Effect of fluvoxamine on the pharmacokinetics of imipramine and desipramine in healthy subjects. Ther Drug Monit 15: 243, 1993c.

Sprung J et al.: Treating intraoperative hypotension in a patient on long-term tricyclic antidepressants: a case of aborted aortic surgery. Anesthesiology 86: 990, 1997.

Staufenberg EF et al.: Malignant hyperpyrexia syndrome in combined treatment. Br J Psychiatry 154: 577, 1989.

Steiner E et al.: Inhibition of desipramine 2-hydroxylation by quinidine and quinine. Clin Pharmacol Ther 43: 577, 1988.

Steiner W et al.: Toxic reaction following the combined administration of fluoxetine and L-tryptophan: five case reports. Biol Psychiatry 21: 1067, 1986.

Sternbach H: Danger of MAOI therapy after fluoxetine withdrawal. Lancet 2: 850, 1988.

Sternbach H: The serotonin syndrome. Am J Psychiatry 148: 705, 1991a.

Sternbach H: Fluoxetine-associated potentiation of calcium-channel blockers. J Clin Psychopharmacol 11: 390, 1991b.

Stewart DE: High-fiber diet and serum tricyclic antidepressant levels. J Clin Psychopharmacol 12: 438, 1992.

Stiff JL et al.: Clonidine withdrawal complicated by amitriptyline therapy. Anesthesiology 59: 73, 1983.

Suchowersky O et al.: Interaction of fluoxetine and selegiline. Can J Psychiatry 35: 571, 1990.

Sullivan EA et al.: Diet and monoamine oxidase inhibitors: a re-examination. Can J Psychopharmacol 3: 249, 1983.

Sullivan EA et al.: Diet and monoamine oxidase inhibitors: a re-examination. Can J Psychiatry 29: 707, 1984.

Sutherland DL et al.: The influence of cimetidine versus ranitidine on doxepin pharmacokinetics. Eur J Clin Pharmacol 32: 159, 1987.

Sved AF et al.: Studies on the antihypertensive action of L-tryptophan. J Pharmacol Exp Ther 221: 329, 1982.

Svedmyr N: The influence of a tricyclic antidepressive agent (protriptyline) on some of the circulatory effects of noradrenaline and adrenaline in man. Life Sci 7: 77, 1968.

Swims MP: Potential terfenadine-fluoxetine interaction. Ann Pharmacother 27: 1404, 1993.

Szabo CP: Fluoxetine and sumatriptan: possibly a counterproductive combination. J Clin Psychiatry 56: 37, 1995.

Szymura-Oleksiak J et al.: Pharmacokinetic interaction between imipramine and carbamazepine in patients with major depression. Psychopharmacology (Berl) 154: 38, 2001.

Tackley RM et al.: Fatal disseminated intravascular coagulation following a monoamine oxidase inhibitor/tricyclic interaction. Anaesthesia 42: 760, 1987.

Taiwo YO et al.: Potentiation of morphine antinociception by monoamine reuptake inhibitors in the rat spinal cord. Pain 21: 329, 1985.

Tanquary J et al.: Paradoxical reaction to buspirone augmentation of fluoxetine. J Clin Psychopharmacol 10: 377, 1990.

Targum SD et al.: Thyroid hormone and the TRH stimulation test in refractory depression. J Clin Psychiatry 45: 345, 1984.

Teitelbaum ML et al.: Imipramine toxicity and terbinafine. Am J Psychiatry 158: 2086, 2001.

Tephly TR et al.: Inhibition of drug metabolism. V. Inhibition of drug metabolism by steroids. Mol Pharmacol 4: 10, 1968.

Teychenne PF et al.: Interactions of levodopa with inhibitors of monoamine oxidase and L-aromatic amino acid decarboxylase. Clin Pharmacol Ther 18: 273, 1975.

Thase ME et al.: Treatment of imipramine-resistant recurrent depression: I. An open clinical trial of adjunctive L-triiodothyronine. J Clin Psychiatry 50: 385, 1989.

Thomas JM et al.: Case report of a toxic reaction from a combination of tryptophan and phenelzine. Am J Psychiatry 141: 281, 1984.

Thomas M et al.: The dilemma of the prolonged QT interval in early drug studies. Br J Clin Pharmacol 41: 77, 1996.

Thomson AH et al.: Interaction between fluvoxamine and theophylline. Pharm J 249: 137, 1992.

Tollefson G et al.: Effect of propranolol on maprotiline clearance. Am J Psychiatry 141: 148, 1984.

Tollefson GD: Monoamine oxidase inhibitors: a review. J Clin Psychiatry 44: 280, 1983.

Toyama SC et al.: Is it safe to combine a selective serotonin reuptake inhibitor with selegiline? Ann Pharmacother 28: 405, 1994.

Troy SM et al.: The influence of cimetidine on the disposition kinetics of the antidepressant venlafaxine. J Clin Pharmacol 38: 467, 1998.

True BL et al.: Profound hypoglycemia with the addition of a tricyclic antidepressant to maintenance sulfonylurea therapy. Am J Psychiatry 144: 1220, 1987.

Tsutsui S et al.: Combined therapy of T3, and antidepressants in depression. J Int Med Res 7: 138, 1979.

van den Brekel AM et al.: Toxic effects of theophylline caused by fluvoxamine. Cmaj 151: 1289, 1994.

van der Kuy PH et al.: Nortriptyline intoxication induced by terbinafine. Br Med J 316: 441, 1998.

van der Kuy PH et al.: Pharmacokinetic interaction between nortriptyline and terbinafine. Ann Pharmacother 36: 1712, 2002.

van Harten J: Clinical pharmacokinetics of selective serotonin reuptake inhibitors. Clin Pharmacokinet 24: 203, 1993.

van Harten J et al.: Fluvoxamine does not interact with alcohol or potentiate alcohol-related impairment of cognitive function. Clin Pharmacol Ther 52: 427, 1992.

van Putten T et al.: Delirium associated with bupropion. J Clin Psychopharmacol 10: 234, 1990.

van Zwieten PA: Interaction between centrally acting hypotensive drugs and tricyclic antidepressants. Arch Int Pharmacodyn Ther 214: 12, 1975.

Vandel S et al.: Fluvoxamine and fluoxetine: interaction studies with amitriptyline, clomipramine and neuroleptics in phenotyped patients. Pharmacol Res 31: 347, 1995.

Vandel S et al.: Valpromide increases the plasma concentrations of amitriptyline and its metabolite nortriptyline in depressive patients. Ther Drug Monit 10: 386, 1988.

Vaughan DA: Interaction of fluoxetine with tricyclic antidepressants. Am J Psychiatry 145: 1478, 1988.

Vella JP et al.: Interactions between cyclosporine and newer antidepressant medications. Am J Kidney Dis 31: 320, 1998.

Venlafaxine + tramadol: serotonin syndrome. Prescrire Int 13: 57, 2004.

Vesell ES et al.: Impairment of drug metabolism in man by allopurinol and nortriptyline. N Engl J Med 283: 1484, 1970.

Vigran IM: Dangerous potentiation of meperidine hydrochloride by pargyline hydrochloride. JAMA 187: 953, 1964.

von Moltke LL et al.: Inhibition of desipramine hydroxylation in vitro by serotonin-reuptake-inhibitor antidepressants, and by quinidine and ketoconazole: a model system to predict drug interactions in vivo. J Pharmacol Exp Ther 268: 1278, 1994.

von Moltke LL et al.: Inhibition of terfenadine metabolism in vitro by azole antifungal agents and by selective serotonin reuptake inhibitor antidepressants:

relation to pharmacokinetic interactions in vivo. J Clin Psychopharmacol 16: 104, 1996.

von Moltke LL et al.: Midazolam hydroxylation by human liver microsomes in vitro: inhibition by fluoxetine, norfluoxetine, and by azole antifungal agents. J Clin Pharmacol 36: 783, 1996.

Vu TN: Current pharmacologic approaches to treating neuropathic pain. Curr Pain Headache Rep 8: 15, 2004.

Walker JI et al.: Patient compliance with MAO inhibitor therapy. J Clin Psychiatry 45: 78, 1984.

Walley T et al.: Interaction of metoprolol and fluoxetine. Lancet 341: 967, 1993.

Wang Z et al.: The effects of St. John's wort (Hypericum perforatum) on human cytochrome P450 activity. Clin Pharmacol Ther 70: 317, 2001.

Warrington SJ et al.: Evaluation of possible interactions between ethanol and trazodone or amitriptyline. Neuropsychobiology 15 Suppl 1: 31, 1986.

Waters CH: Fluoxetine and selegiline—lack of significant interaction. Can J Neurol Sci 21: 259, 1994.

Weigmann H et al.: Fluvoxamine but not sertraline inhibits the metabolism of olanzapine: evidence from a therapeutic drug monitoring service. Ther Drug Monit 23: 410, 2001.

Weiner AL et al.: Serotonin syndrome: case report and review of the literature. Conn Med 61: 717, 1997.

Weiner LA et al.: Serotonin syndrome secondary to phenelzine-venlafaxine interaction. Pharmacotherapy 18: 399, 1998.

Weintraub D: Nortriptyline toxicity secondary to interaction with bupropion sustained-release. Depress Anxiety 13: 50, 2001.

Weller RA et al.: Psychotropic drugs and alcohol: pharmacokinetic and pharmacodynamic interactions. Psychosomatics 25: 301, 1984.

Wetzel H et al.: Pharmacokinetic interactions of clozapine with selective serotonin reuptake inhibitors: differential effects of fluvoxamine and paroxetine in a prospective study. J Clin Psychopharmacol 18: 2, 1998.

Wharton RN et al.: A potential clinical use for methylphenidate with tricyclic antidepressants. Am J Psychiatry 127: 1619, 1971.

Wheatley D: Potentiation of amitriptyline by thyroid hormone. Arch Gen Psychiatry 26: 229, 1972.

White K et al.: Combined monoamine oxidase inhibitor-tricyclic antidepressant treatment: a pilot study. Am J Psychiatry 137: 1422, 1980.

White K et al.: Combined MAOI-tricyclic antidepressant treatment: a reply to Dr. Davidson. J Clin Psychopharmacol 2: 286, 1982.

Whybrow PC et al.: Thyroid function and the response to liothyronine in depression. Arch Gen Psychiatry 26: 242, 1972.

Wigen CL et al.: Serotonin syndrome and linezolid. Clin Infect Dis 34: 1651, 2002.

Williams LT et al.: Thyroid hormone regulation of beta-adrenergic receptor number. J Biol Chem 252: 2787, 1977.

Wilner KD et al.: The effects of sertraline on the pharmacodynamics of warfarin in healthy volunteers. Biol Psychiatry 29: 354, 1991.

Wilson IC et al.: Methyltestosterone with imipramine in men: conversion of depression to paranoid reaction. Am J Psychiatry 131: 21, 1974.

Wing YK et al.: Paroxetine treatment and the prolactin response to sumatriptan. Psychopharmacology (Berl) 124: 377, 1996.

Winston F: Combined antidepressant therapy. Br J Psychiatry 118: 301, 1971.

Wong KC et al.: Influence of imipramine and pargyline on the arrhythmo-genicity of epinephrine during halothane, enflurane or methoxyflurane anesthesia in dogs. Life Sci 27: 2675, 1980.

Wong SL et al.: Effects of divalproex sodium on amitriptyline and nortripty-line pharmacokinetics. Clin Pharmacol Ther 60: 48, 1996.

Woods DJ et al.: Interaction of phenytoin and fluoxetine. N Z Med J 107: 19, 1994.

Woolfrey S et al.: Fluoxetine-warfarin interaction. Br Med J 307: 241, 1993.

Woosley R et al.: Analysis of potential adverse drug reactions—a case of mis-taken identity. Am J Cardiol 74: 208, 1994.

Wright JM et al.: Isoniazid-induced carbamazepine toxicity and vice versa: a double drug interaction. N Engl J Med 307: 1325, 1982.

Yagiela JA et al.: Drug interactions and vasoconstrictors used in local anes-thetic solutions. Oral Surg Oral Med Oral Pathol 59: 565, 1985.

Yao C et al.: Fluvoxamine-theophylline interaction: gap between in vitro and in vivo inhibition constants toward cytochrome P4501A2. Clin Pharmacol Ther 70: 415, 2001.

Yaryura-Tobias JA et al.: Fluoxetine and bleeding in obsessive-compulsive dis-order. Am J Psychiatry 148: 949, 1991.

Young JP et al.: Controlled trial of trimipramine, monoamine oxidase inhibitors, and combined treatment in depressed outpatients. Br Med J 2: 1315, 1979.

Zabik JE et al.: Serotonin and ethanol aversion in the rat. In: Research Advances in New Psychopharmacological Treatment for Alcoholism. In: Excerpta Medica, Amsterdam: Elsevier, 1985; p. 87.

Zeidenberg P et al.: Clinical and metabolic studies with imipramine in man. Am J Psychiatry 127: 1321, 1971.

Zetin M: Combined use of trazodone and phenelzine in depression: case report. J Clin Psychiatry 45: 182, 1984.

Zetin M et al.: MAOI reaction with powdered protein dietary supplement. J Clin Psychiatry 48: 499, 1987.

Ziegler MG et al.: Sertraline does not alter the beta-adrenergic blocking activ-ity of atenolol in healthy male volunteers. J Clin Psychiatry 57 Suppl 1: 12, 1996.

Zornberg GL et al.: Severe adverse interaction between pethidine and selegi-line. Lancet 337: 246, 1991.

Antipsychotics

OLIVER FREUDENREICH
DONALD C. GOFF

Pharmacology of Antipsychotic Agents

Drug interactions with antipsychotic agents can occur with many diverse classes of medication, from all fields of medicine and psychiatry. Because patients with mental illnesses may have numerous medical and psychiatric problems, polypharmacy is the norm rather than the exception (Ghaemi 2002). Drug combinations are often utilized to broaden the range of therapeutic effects (Hyman and Fenton 2003) or to achieve a better response if remission is only partial (Freudenreich and Goff 2003). Generally, the therapeutic index (risk ratio) is large for antipsychotics with respect to lethal versus therapeutic doses, and therefore most interactions are not life threatening. They may, however, adversely affect clinical outcome if not recognized and managed appropriately. Exceptions to the relative safety of antipsychotics do exist; for example, certain interactions can result in lengthening of the QTc interval and increase the risk of lethal arrhythmias (see the cardiac section of this chapter). Some pharmacodynamic interactions are subtle but potentially serious in the long run, such as the combination of agents that promote obesity and its associated long-term morbidities.

Antipsychotics can be broadly grouped into typical (conventional or first generation) antipsychotics and atypical (second generation) antipsychotics (Lohr and Braff 2003). No one definition of "atypicality" is accepted, but at a minimum this designation requires a drug to have little or no extrapyramidal side effects at typical clinical doses. All antipsychotics share antagonism of dopamine D2 receptors, and for conventional antipsychotics, D2 receptor affinity correlates highly with clinical potency (Creese et al. 1976). Positron emission tomography (PET) studies using D2-selective radioligands indicated that maximal D2 receptor occupancy of approximately 80% to 85% occurs at daily haloperidol doses of 10 to 15 mg and plasma concentrations of about 15 to 20 ng/mL, and probably corresponds with maximal antipsychotic efficacy in many patients (Farde et al. 1992). Clozapine, the prototype of the atypical antipsychotics, does not follow the same dose–response relationship with regards to D2 receptor occupancy, because it produces optimal therapeutic effects at occupancy levels of only 40% to 60%, reached at daily doses of 300 to 500 mg (Farde et al. 1994). Many newer antipsychotics are modeled after clozapine in that they combine D2 antagonism with serotonin 5-HT2 antagonism (Kapur et al. 1998, Nyberg et al 1999) . This receptor combination is thought to add some protection against extrapyramidal side effects, at least within a limited dose range, and some additional efficacy for negative symptoms and depression (Simpson and Lindenmayer 1997). More recently, antipsychotics have been characterized by their "tightness of binding" to the dopamine receptor, which is based on the ease with which antipsychotics are displaced from the dopamine receptor relative to dopamine (Kapur and Seeman 2001, Seeman and Tallerico 1999). In this scheme, clozapine and quetiapine show "loose binding"; conventionals, such as haloperidol and chlorpromazine are tightly bound; and olanzapine and ziprasidone are somewhere in between. Aripiprazole, having partial D2 antagonism, represents a new principle in antipsychotic drug development that goes beyond pure D2 antagonism (Grunder et al. 2003).

Virtually all antipsychotics are rapidly absorbed after oral administration (peak plasma concentrations in 2 to 4 hours), are relatively lipophilic, and have correspondingly large apparent volumes of distribution (Vd = 8 to 30 L/kg). Because all antipsychotics are subject to considerable first-pass enterohepatic metabolism when administered orally, their bioavailability is increased substantially following parenteral administration. For example, the bioavailability of the oral form of haloperidol has been calculated to be 60% to 70% compared with intravenous injection, whereas intramuscularly injected haloperidol or its decanoate achieve virtually 100% relative bioavailability (Forsman and Ohman 1977, Verghese et al. 1991). The "depot" decanoate esters of fluphenazine and haloperidol are injected intramuscularly in an oil vehicle and then converted to the free active drug by esterases in muscle, blood, and other tissues (Marder et al. 1989a). The diffusion of the esterified drug from the oil depot is the rate-limiting factor in the absorption of these preparations (Dreyfuss et al. 1976a, Dreyfuss et al. 1976b). The intramuscular preparations of typical antipsychotics differ from oral preparations not only in avoiding first-pass metabolism, but they also form metabolites in different ratios (Marder et al. 1989b, Hubbard et al. 1993). The first available long-acting, injectable formulation of an atypical antipsychotic, risperidone microspheres (marketed in the United States under the brand name Risperdal Consta) represents a new method for sustained release. Polymer-based microspheres containing the active drug, risperidone, are suspended in a water-based diluent and injected into muscle; after a delay of approximately three weeks, the risperidone is gradually released over several weeks as the microspheres begin to dissolve, producing optimal therapeutic blood levels when administered every two weeks (Kane et al. 2003a, Kane et al. 2003b).

With the exception of molindone, antipsychotics are highly protein bound. The proportion of free drug typically is less than 10% of total plasma concentration and may closely approximate concentrations in the cerebrospinal fluid (CSF); in some studies the plasma-free fraction of conventional agents correlated reasonably well with therapeutic outcome (Garver 1989). In addition, some highly lipophilic antipsychotic agents (such as the butyrophenones) concentrate 10- to 20-fold in brain tissue, so that levels of antipsychotic agents in the proximity of relevant receptor sites may be much higher than levels found in plasma or CSF (Sunderland and Cohen 1987).

Antipsychotic drugs are extensively metabolized by the liver, primarily through enzyme-mediated microsomal oxidation and conjugation reactions. Drug–drug interactions mediated by the superfamily of cytochrome P450 (CYP) enzymes are fairly well characterized for antipsychotic drugs (Kudo and Ishizaki 1999, Prior and Baker 2003), and a knowledge of this system can be used to predict drug interactions. Less is known about drug–drug interactions involving the phase II glucuronidation enzyme system (Liston et al. 2001). This second superfamily of metabolizing enzymes, known as uridine glucuronosyl transferases (UGT), mediates phase II metabolism through the conjugation of a sugar, glucuronic acid, to drug metabolites. Some antipsychotics (e.g., haloperidol and olanzapine) have a P450-independent pathway of deactivation through immediate glucuronidation, providing an additional safety margin. The potential importance of this alternative metabolic path is suggested by a report of a patient with deficient UGT activity (Gilbert syndrome), who developed olanzapine toxicity from a 10 mg daily dose (Martin-Escudero et al. 2003). Additional P450-independent metabolic pathways are important for some antipsychotics. Ziprasidone, for example, is predominantly (by two-thirds) metabolized via reduction by a cytosolic enzyme, aldehyde oxidase (Caley and Cooper 2002, Beedham et al. 2003). Aldehyde oxidase has no clinically relevant inhibitor or inducer, and no important polymorphisms. These properties make ziprasidone fairly impervious to drug interactions.

Generally, all antipsychotics are at least to some extent metabolized by one or more of the CYP3A4, CYP2D6, or CYP1A2 hepatic microsomal enzymes. A discrepancy often exists between the estimated relevance of enzyme systems deduced from in vitro studies compared to in vivo studies. The relative importance of a particular hepatic enzyme can be concentration-dependent, with different enzymes becoming important as drug plasma levels rise. Further, if one pathway is inhibited or deficient, other systems often can take over and compensate; for example, drug metabolism will be accomplished via CYP3A4 in patients who are CYP2D6 deficient (Shin et al. 1999). CYP3A4 is an important enzyme system, because it oxidizes most atypical antipsychotics to some extent. Due to the location of CYP3A4 in the small bowel and liver, its inhibition or induction affects first-pass metabolism. Some interactions with CYP3A4 inhibitors also may involve the inhibition of P-glycoprotein (P-gp) but are not well described for antipsychotics at this time (von Moltke et al. 1998, Yasuda et al. 2002). Antipsychotics in general do not inhibit P450 drug metabolism with the exception of CYP2D6, which is inhibited by many antipsychotics (Shin et al. 1999) and by the haloperidol metabolite, reduced haloperidol (Shin et al. 2001). Reported nominal plasma elimination half-lives for many antipsychotics fall in the range of 10 to 30 hours. Quetiapine has a short half-life of approximately 6 hours, and aripiprazole has an unusually long half-life of 75 hours. Sensitive assays have revealed complex, multicompartmental half-lives for haloperidol, with near-terminal elimination half-life values of 1 week or more (Hubbard et al. 1987, Khot et al. 1993, Midha et al. 1989). Moreover, some clinical PET studies suggest that the washout of haloperidol from the human brain may be even slower than the rate of disappearance of the drug from plasma. Any attempt to correlate clinical changes in peripheral drug metabolism is further complicated by the dissociation between the interaction of a drug and its receptor (initiation) and resulting downstream changes in gene expression and gene regulation (adaptation) (Hyman and Nestler 1996).

Variability in metabolism comes mainly from metabolic inhibition, metabolic induction, and genetically determined differences in the activity of the metabolizing enzymes (genetic polymorphism). Great interindividual variability exists in the metabolism of conventional antipsychotics, so that mean plasma concentrations may not correlate closely with oral dose, and may vary by more than 10-fold among patients receiving the same dose (Dahl 1986). Dysken et al. (1981) found a 40-fold variation in steady-state plasma concentrations of fluphenazine during treatment with oral daily doses of 20 mg. The activity of the CYP2D6 isoenzyme, which is the primary metabolic pathway for most conventional antipsychotics and risperidone, is determined by a single polymorphism, producing three phenotypes: poor metabolizers, extensive (normal) metabolizers, or ultra-rapid metabolizers (Guzey et al. 2000). De Leon et al. (1998) genotyped CYP2D6 in predominantly white state hospital populations and found that 14% of patients were CYP2D6 deficient (poor metabolizers), 5% carried alleles associated with ultra-rapid CYP2D6 metabolism, and 81% were normal (extensive) metabolizers. Pollock et al. (1995) demonstrated the potential value of genetic phenotyping in a study of 45 elderly patients with dementia. The five patients who were prospectively identified as poor CYP2D6 metabolizers experienced more sedation and extrapyramidal symptoms (EPS) when treated with perphenazine. In a study of Japanese patients, haloperidol levels were significantly determined by a particular mutation of the CYP2D6 gene (Mihara et al. 1999). Similarly, the ratio of risperidone to 9-hydroxyrisperidone is dependent on the CYP2D6 genotype (Yasui-Furukori et al. 2003) and can be used to estimate CYP2D6 activity (Berecz et al. 2002). Bork et al. found that poor metabolizers of CYP2D6 tolerated risperidone more poorly than extensive metabolizers (Bork et al. 1999).

In contrast to the complex array of active metabolites produced by the phenothiazines, thioxanthenes, and other tricyclic antipsychotic agents (Hubbard et al. 1993, Chetty et al. 1994), only the reduced metabolite of haloperidol, hydroxyhaloperidol, yields antipsychotic activity (Kudo and Ishizaki 1999). Other metabolites exist as well, one of which, HP^+, a quaternary pyridinium metabolite, might confer neurotoxicity (Fang et al. 1995). Clozapine is metabolized almost entirely by the liver, producing a prominent, active N-desmethyl metabolite, norclozapine, and several relatively inactive and less prevalent metabolites such as clozapine N-oxide (Centorrino et al. 1994b, Jann et al. 1993). The norclozapine metabolite has been hypothesized to be responsible for hematologic toxicity (Gerson et al. 1994). Structurally similar to clozapine, olanzapine is extensively metabolized, but no metabolite is pharmacologically active (Fulton and Goa 1997). Major metabolites are 4-N-desmethylolanzapine and a phase II metabolite, 10-N-glucuronide. Although quetiapine has many metabolites, two of which are active, they constitute only a small percentage of the active moiety (DeVane and Nemeroff 2001). Risperidone has one equipotent metabolite: 9-hydroxyrisperidone (Huang et al. 1993). Ziprasidone is highly metabolized, predominantly by a P450-independent enzyme, aldehyde oxidase (Beedham et al. 2003); no metabolite contributes significant activity (Caley and Cooper 2002). Table 3.1 summarizes

(text continues on page 184)

TABLE 3.1. METABOLISM OF ANTIPSYCHOTIC DRUGS

Agent	Clinically Relevant Metabolites	CYP450 Metabolism	Alternative Metabolism	References
First-Generation Antipsychotics				
Chlorpromazine	7-OH-CPZ[1] others	3A4 (2D6-minor)	glucuronidation	(Chetty et al. 1994) (Yeung et al. 1993) (Creese et al. 1978)
Fluphenazine	7-OH-FLU	2D6		(Marder et al. 1989b)
Haloperidol	reduced HAL (20%) HP[+ (2)]	3A4 2D6	glucuronidation	(Kudo and Ishizaki 1999)
Perphenazine	none known	2D6		(Eggert Hansen 1976) (Dahl-Puustinen et al. 1989)
Thioridazine	mesoridazine sulforidazine	2D6		(von Bahr et al. 1991) (Niedzwiecki et al. 1989)
Second-Generation Antipsychotics				
Aripiprazole	none active	3A4 2D6		(Bristol-Myers Squibb 2002)

Drug	Active metabolite	Principal metabolizing enzymes	References
Clozapine	nor-CLZ[3]	**1A2** **3A4** **2C19** (2D6-minimal)	(Jann et al. 1993) (Linnet and Olesen 1997) (Olesen and Linnet 2001)
Olanzapine	none active	**1A2** (2D6, 2C19?-minimal)	(Callaghan et al. 1999)
Quetiapine	none relevant	**3A4** (2D6-minimal) **glucuronidation**	(DeVane and Nemeroff 2001)
Risperidone	9-OH-RSP[4]	**2D6** (3A4-minor)	(Huang et al. 1993) (Schotte et al. 1996) (Bork et al. 1999) (Fang et al. 1999)
Ziprasidone	none relevant	**3A4** (33%) **aldehyde oxidase** (66%)	(Caley and Cooper 2002) (Beedham et al. 2003)

CLZ, clozapine; *CPZ*, chlorpromazine; *FLU*, fluphenazine; *HAL*, haloperidol; *OH*, hydroxy; *RSP*, risperidone. Principal metabolizing enzymes are in **bold**.
References as indicated. Package inserts for the respective drugs were also consulted.

[1]7-Hydroxychlorpromazine is equipotent with chlorpromazine (Creese et al. 1978).

[2]HP⁺ is a quaternary pyridinium metabolite of haloperidol; HP⁺ is likely a neurotoxic metabolite (Fang et al. 1995).

[3]Norclozapine is also denoted N-desmethylclozapine; norclozapine is possibly responsible for clozapine's hematologic toxicity (Gerson et al. 1994).

[4]Active moiety is risperidone plus 9-hydroxyrisperidone; 9-hydroxyrisperidone is equipotent with risperidone (Schotte et al. 1996).

major metabolic pathways and clinically relevant active or toxic metabolites for some commonly used first-generation and available second-generation antipsychotics.

Alcohol

EVIDENCE OF INTERACTION

Alcohol alters both the disposition and action of many drugs, yet its potential interactions with antipsychotic medications have received little attention. Acutely, alcohol acts as a competitive inhibitor against drugs metabolized by enzymes of the hepatic cytochrome CYP2E family. Upon repeated administration, alcohol induces synthesis and thus increases activity of these enzymes (Shoaf and Linnoila 1991). When a patient is actively drinking, metabolism of certain drugs may be competitively inhibited, whereas during periods of abstinence, metabolism may be enhanced (Lieber 1990). In addition, alcohol can affect the rate and extent of absorption of other drugs (Mezey 1976), and chronic alcohol use may reduce levels of plasma proteins, resulting in a higher free fraction of some highly bound drugs (Lieber 1988). These effects may be further complicated by the strong comorbidity between alcoholism and heavy cigarette smoking, because tobacco smoke is a potent inducer of hepatic microsomal enzymes (also see Tobacco, in this chapter). The focal application of alcohol in rat brain increases the release of dopamine, suggesting a potential pharmacodynamic interaction between alcohol and dopaminergic systems (Wozniak et al. 1991).

Despite the high frequency with which alcohol is consumed by patients treated with antipsychotic medication, interactions between these two drugs rarely have been reported. Morselli et al. (1971) measured blood alcohol levels and dexterity in 16 normal subjects after the administration of alcohol, then repeated this procedure after the subjects had received chlorpromazine 200 mg/day or haloperidol 6 mg/day for 10 days. Blood levels of alcohol were significantly elevated in subjects receiving haloperidol but not in subjects receiving chlorpromazine. Although dexterity and alertness were impaired to the greatest degree by alcohol in subjects pretreated with haloperidol, it is unclear if this effect represents a drug interaction, because the effect of haloperidol alone on these measures was not determined. Lutz (Lutz 1976) observed that akathisia and dystonic reactions occurred in seven patients receiving stable, previously well-tolerated doses of antipsychotic medications when they started drinking alcohol. The EPS quickly subsided when patients ceased drinking alcohol or when an anticholinergic agent was added. Assessed retrospectively, Green et al. (2003) found a decrease in alcohol consumption by patients with schizophrenia who were receiving clozapine but not with risperidone. Olanzapine similarly had an ameliorating effect on alcohol consumption in a double-blind study (Hutchison et al. 2001). Summarizing the manufacturer's experience with olanzapine, orthostatic changes were observed when olanzapine and alcohol were co-administered (Callaghan et al. 1999).

MECHANISM

Haloperidol may increase blood alcohol levels by inhibiting hepatic enzymes. Sedation and incoordination are additive when antipsychotics are combined with alcohol and may be further intensified by pharmacokinetic interactions that may raise plasma concentrations of each drug. Potential pharmacodynamic interactions mediated by the effects of alcohol on dopaminergic systems have not been formally studied.

CLINICAL IMPLICATIONS

Patients taking antipsychotic agents should be advised that consuming alcohol can result in potentially dangerous sedation and incoordination and may increase the risk for extrapyramidal reactions such as dystonia and akathisia. Haloperidol also may interfere with the metabolism of alcohol, so that patients may become intoxicated after consuming alcohol at previously tolerated levels. Chronic alcohol use can be expected to complicate antipsychotic therapy and is associated with poorer outcome, although probably due to the complex effects of comorbidity rather than a simple pharmacological interaction. The sudden appearance of EPS in patients treated with a stable dose of antipsychotic medication might raise the question of acute alcohol use, although this possible interaction has not been established firmly. Interactions between atypical antipsychotics and alcohol have not been well studied, although some evidence suggests that clozapine and olanzapine may decrease alcohol use. A potentially heightened risk of seizures with alcohol withdrawal and clozapine must be considered, however.

Antibiotics, Antibacterial, and Antifungal Agents

EVIDENCE OF INTERACTION

The antifungals of the azole class, particularly ketoconazole and itraconazole are strong inhibitors of CYP3A4. Yasui et al. (1999a) studied the effect of a 1-week course of itraconazole on 13 patients with schizophrenia treated with haloperidol 12 or 24 mg daily. Both haloperidol and reduced haloperidol serum concentrations were significantly increased, and patients experienced more extrapyramidal side effects. A prospective, controlled trial found no effect of added itraconazole on clozapine and norclozapine levels (Raaska and Neuvonen 1998).

Most macrolide antibiotics are inhibitors of CYP3A4; the most potent are erythromycin and clarithromycin. Several cases have been reported of patients developing toxic clozapine levels and side effects when erythromycin was added (Cohen et al. 1996, Funderburg et al. 1994). However, no effect on metabolism of a single 12.5 mg dose of clozapine was detected when 12 healthy male subjects were pretreated with erythromycin 1,500 mg daily in a randomized crossover study (Hagg et al. 1999). It has been suggested that some bacterial infections increase clozapine levels via a cytokine-mediated suppression of CYP1A2 activity rather than a pharmacokinetic interaction (Raaska et al. 2000b, de Leon and Diaz 2003). Pharmacodynamic interactions might underlie reports of agranulocytosis occurring in clozapine-treated patients after receiving erythromycin (Usiskin et al. 2000) or trimethoprim/sulfamethoxazole (TMP/SMX) (Henderson and Borba 2001). It is also possible that the antibiotics alone caused bone marrow toxicity, and that the presence of clozapine was incidental. Clarithromycin can inhibit pimozide metabolism via an inhibition of CYP3A4 (Desta et al. 1999), which may result in potentially lethal prolongation of the QTc (Flockhart et al. 2000a).

Many quinolone antibiotics, including ciprofloxacin, are potent inhibitors of CYP1A2. In a randomized, crossover study, ciprofloxacin 250 mg two times a day for 7 days increased clozapine and nor-clozapine levels by 31% and 29%, respectively (Raaska and Neuvonen 2000), confirming an earlier observation of a pharmacokinetic interaction (Markowitz et al. 1997). Similarly, ciprofloxacin was reported to elevate olanzapine levels in a single case report (Markowitz and DeVane 1999).

CLINICAL SIGNIFICANCE

Antipsychotics with significant CYP3A4 metabolism can be inhibited by strong CYP3A4 inhibitors like itraconazole, with resultant extrapyramidal side effects, as shown with haloperidol; or prolonged QTc, as shown with pimozide. Pimozide prolongs the QTc interval in a dose-dependent fashion, which makes administering a drug that can raise pimozide levels particularly dangerous. Clinically important CYP3A4 inhibitors come from a group of widely used antibiotic medications from different classes and include itraconazole, ketoconazole, clarithromycin, erythromycin, or ritonavir. Antibiotics that increase the plasma levels of antipsychotics with effects on the QTc or antibiotics that are QTc-prolonging themselves (e.g., erythromycin, clarithromycin, gatifloxacin, levofloxacin, moxifloxacin; halofantrine, mefloquine) should not be added to ziprasidone, thioridazine, chlorpromazine, or pimozide. Reassuringly, ketoconazole did not substantially increase QTc when added to ziprasidone in a trial mandated by the Food and Drug Administration (FDA) prior to ziprasidone approval. Although case reports have suggested a pharmacokinetic interaction between clozapine and erythromycin, this was not supported by a controlled trial. Clozapine levels can be influenced by ciprofloxacin via CYP1A2 inhibition. Some antibiotics are bone marrow toxic (e.g., TMP/SMX), and combining them with clozapine is problematic. Cases of granulocytopenia and/or agranulocytosis are difficult to interpret if they occur, and the patient might lose access to clozapine.

Antituberculosis Agents

EVIDENCE OF INTERACTION

A stable clozapine patient was started on rifampin for a mycobacterial infection. The patient became symptomatic three weeks after the initiation of rifampin treatment, and clozapine levels were found to be substantially lowered (Joos et al. 1998). Takeda et al. (1986) described increased haloperidol levels in patients who where receiving isoniazid (INH), and decreased haloperidol levels in patients treated with rifampin. Kim et al. (1996) documented the effects of starting or stopping rifampin in 12 patients treated with haloperidol; adding rifampin was associated with decreased haloperidol levels to one-third of baseline and worsening clinical status; stopping rifampin was associated with more than a tripling of haloperidol levels.

MECHANISM

Rifamycins such as rifampin are "pan-inducers" of phase I and phase II metabolism (Gallicano et al. 1999), and they have therefore the potential to significantly lower antipsychotic levels. Isoniazid's effects on metabolism of other drugs are poorly understood. Isoniazid alone has been reported to cause psychosis de novo (Alao and Yolles 1998, Upadhyaya and Chaturvedi 1989).

CLINICAL SIGNIFICANCE

The treatment of tuberculosis and other mycobacterial infections (e.g., *Mycobacterium avium* complex infections) involves the use of enzyme-inducing agents that have the potential to lower antipsychotic drug-levels.

Antiviral Agents

EVIDENCE OF INTERACTION

Patients infected with HIV are usually treated with multi-drug regimens, resulting in an increased risk for drug interactions (Preston 1998). All protease inhibitors (PIs) and the non-nucleoside reverse transcriptase inhibitors (NNRTIs) (but not the nucleoside-analog reverse transcriptase inhibitors, which are primarily eliminated by the kidney) have the potential for P450-mediated drug interactions. In one single-dose study of normal volunteers, ritonavir decreased by half the area-under-curve (AUC) of olanzapine and doubled its renal excretion (Penzak et al. 2002). A 35-year-old man with AIDS developed an acute dystonic reaction 1 week after two PIs, ritonavir and indinavir, were added to risperidone (Kelly et al. 2002). The authors attributed this adverse event to a pharmacokinetic interaction resulting in elevated risperidone levels. A similar pharmacokinetic interaction with the same two PIs combined with risperidone may have resulted in a reversible coma in a second case (Jover et al. 2002). In a third case, neuroleptic malignant syndrome (NMS) was in part attributed to an interaction between the same three drugs (Lee et al. 2000).

MECHANISM

All protease inhibitors and non-nucleoside reverse transcriptase inhibitors are metabolized by the P450 system and have enzyme-inhibiting and/or inducing properties (Tseng and Foisy 1999). As a rule, all PIs and NNRTIs except nevirapine inhibit CYP3A4 to some extent, ritonavir being almost as potent as the prototypical CYP3A4 inhibitor, ketoconazole (von Moltke et al. 1998). Indinavir and efavirenz are other potent inhibitors of CYP3A4. Predictions of drug interactions with ritonavir and efavirenz can be difficult, however, because both can also induce CYP3A4 and other enzymes. The only currently available fusion inhibitor, enfuvirtide, does not seem to have P450 interactions.

CLINICAL SIGNIFICANCE

Multidrug regimens, which are the standard treatment for HIV, have not been formally studied for interactions with antipsychotics. Patients infected with HIV typically receive a cocktail of antiviral agents that includes several potent inhibitors and/or inducers of CYP3A4 and other P450 enzymes. In addition, patients with AIDS may be more sensitive to EPS (Hriso et al. 1991). To further complicate matters, antifungal drugs often are used prophylactically in the treatment of HIV. Therefore, antipsychotics with a narrow therapeutic index (such as pimozide) should be avoided and, when relevant, plasma levels monitored (such as clozapine), particularly if the cocktail contains ritonavir. Of note, ritonavir is often "hidden" in fixed combinations (such as the lopinavir-ritonavir combination (Cvetkovic and Goa 2003). Antipsychotics with significant phase II metabolism (e.g., olanzapine) are probably safer choices from a pharmacokinetic viewpoint, because even slight increases in drug levels might be poorly tolerated in AIDS patients. On the other hand, the addition of ritonavir to olanzapine might decrease the olanzapine plasma level. Therapeutic drug monitoring might help clarify confusing clinical pictures.

Anticholinergic Agents

EVIDENCE OF INTERACTION

Anticholinergic agents are widely prescribed with typical antipsychotics to prevent or treat extrapyramidal symptoms, but they are usually unnecessary with atypicals. Prolonged treatment using anticholinergic agents may be necessary in patients who suffer from persistent parkinsonism and are unable to switch to an atypical agent, although some patients may experience partial attenuation of bradykinesia over time (World Health Organization 1990). The rapid withdrawal of an anticholinergic antiparkinsonism agent may precipitate a worsening of EPS (Goff et al. 1991a), presumably by transiently elevating central cholinergic activity (Tandon et al. 1989). Although gradual discontinuation may avoid this reaction, it may not prevent the emergence of parkinsonism and, in some cases, a worsening of psychiatric symptoms (Manos et al. 1981). The continued use of anticholinergic agents beyond early prophylaxis for dystonia may have important negative consequences, particularly in the elderly. Several studies have demonstrated substantial impairment of memory and cognitive functioning at typical clinical doses of these agents (Baker et al. 1983, McEvoy and Freter 1989, Minzenberg et al. 2004, Strauss et al. 1990, Tune et al. 1982). Cognitive impairment may be sufficiently severe as to interfere with efforts at rehabilitation. Newer antipsychotics appear to have a better profile with regards to cognitive impairment, although clozapine has substantial muscarinic anticholinergic activity.

The impact of anticholinergic agents on plasma concentrations and efficacy of typical antipsychotic agents has been the subject of disagreement. Some early studies indicated that trihexyphenidyl lowered plasma concentrations of chlorpromazine by as much as 45% (Rivera-Calimlim et al. 1973, Rivera-Calimlim et al. 1976, Gautier et al. 1977). However, better-designed trials did not confirm this observation (Simpson et al. 1980) and found no evidence of appreciable pharmacokinetic interactions between benztropine and haloperidol (Goff et al. 1991a), biperiden and haloperidol or thioridazine (Linnoila et al. 1980), biperiden and perphenazine (Hansen et al. 1979), or with other comparable drug combinations (Hitri et al. 1987, Otani et al. 1990). Simpson et al. (1980) added trihexyphenidyl or a placebo to chlorpromazine in middle-aged patients with chronic schizophrenia and found no effect on chlorpromazine levels, whereas Rockland et al. (1990) reported a 41% mean elevation of chlorpromazine levels in young adults.

Whether anticholinergic agents may affect antipsychotic efficacy through pharmacodynamic interactions also has been debated (Ziemba et al. 1978). Singh et al. (Singh and Kay 1975a, Singh and Kay 1975b, Singh and Smith 1973) reported that the addition of benztropine to haloperidol or chlorpromazine produced clinical worsening, consisting of increased hostility, belligerence, suspiciousness, and uncooperativeness. These results are difficult to interpret, however, because the specific clinical features that were affected were not consistent between or within trials. Two uncontrolled trials by other investigators also reported clinical worsening associated with the addition of an anticholinergic agent (Johnstone et al. 1988, Tandon et al. 1990). In a well-designed placebo-controlled trial, Johnstone et al. (Johnstone et al. 1983) added the anticholinergic agent procyclidine to the thioxanthene antipsychotic, flupentixol, and found an increase in ratings of psychosis, flat affect, and depression in the group receiving the anticholinergic agent. Conversely, the majority of trials did not find adverse effects on any clinical ratings when anticholinergic agents were added to an antipsychotic agent (Goff et al. 1991a, Simpson et al. 1980, Otani et al. 1990, Chien et al. 1979, Gardos et al. 1984, Gerlach et al. 1977, Hanlon et al. 1966, Johnson 1975).

Finally, combining an anticholinergic agent with a low-potency antipsychotic agent may produce additive anticholinergic adverse effects. Cases have been reported of fatal paralytic ileus and hyperpyrexia associated with combined treatment using a phenothiazine and an anticholinergic agent, although the same adverse reactions also have been reported with phenothiazines alone (Evans et al. 1979, Giordano et al. 1975, Mann and Boger 1978, Zelman and Guillan 1970). Two placebo-controlled trials detected only minimal peripheral anticholinergic side effects associated with the addition of benztropine mesylate (4 mg daily) to typical clinical doses of haloperidol (Goff et al. 1991a, Winslow et al. 1986), suggesting that additive toxicity is more probable when the antipsychotic itself is appreciably anticholinergic (such as clozapine, thioridazine, or mesoridazine).

MECHANISM OF INTERACTION

Anticholinergic antiparkinsonian agents act by blocking central muscarinic acetylcholine receptors in the basal ganglia; presumably, toxic effects arise from similar actions at central cognitive centers or in peripheral parasympathetically innervated tissues. Because low-potency antipsychotic agents also antagonize these receptors, anticholinergic side effects may be additive when such drugs are combined. Some antipsychotics have complex effects on muscarinic receptors, acting as agonists on some and as antagonists on other (e.g., olanzapine). Although it has been suggested that anticholinergic agents may reduce gastric motility and alter the absorption of antipsychotic agents, controlled trials have not demonstrated such an interaction consistently. In addition, cholinergic receptors are known to modulate dopaminergic activity, and an inverse relationship may exist between cholinergic and dopaminergic activity levels. Anticholinergic drugs can compromise temperature regulation by impairing heat dissipation; this may produce hyperthermia, including heat stroke, especially when combined with antipsychotics that perturb hypothalamic temperature control.

CLINICAL IMPLICATIONS

Because anticholinergics are old medicines, their metabolism has not been well characterized. It seems, however, that pharmacokinetic interactions between anticholinergic and antipsychotic agents, if they occur, appear to be inconsistent and generally of small magnitude. More important is the potential for cognitive impairment caused by additive anticholinergic activity, particularly in elderly patients given a low-potency antipsychotic drug. Probably underestimated are the effects of anticholinergics on complex attention and memory in all patients with schizophrenia, not just the elderly (Minzenberg et al. 2004). When an anticholinergic agent is combined with a low-potency antipsychotic agent, additional serious adverse events may result, such as delirium, paralytic ileus, or hyperthermia.

Antidepressants, Monoamine Oxidase Inhibitors

EVIDENCE OF INTERACTION

The combination of phenothiazine antipsychotics with MAOIs was reported to potentiate hypotension and EPS as well as the anticholinergic side effects of phenothiazines (Sjoqvist 1965). In a patient treated with the MAOI, pargyline, for 2 months, a fever of 106° F developed, with coma and death following the addition of the phenothiazine antipsychotic methotrimeprazine (Barsa and Saunders 1964). It should be emphasized that this fatality may have represented NMS rather than an interaction between the MAOI and antipsychotic. No systematic evidence has implicated MAOIs as a risk factor for NMS, however, and MAOIs have been well tolerated in combination with conventional antipsychotics in two controlled trials (Bucci 1987, Goff et al. 1993).

MECHANISM

MAOIs may interact pharmacokinetically and pharmacodynamically to potentiate the side effects of antipsychotics, but such interactions have not been studied systematically.

CLINICAL SIGNIFICANCE

Antipsychotics, in particular phenothiazines, when combined with MAOIs, have been reported to cause hypotension and anticholinergic side effects, although this has not been established. The combination of tranylcypromine and trifluoperazine is available in some countries as a single pill, suggesting that the combination is deemed safe in clinical practice.

Antidepressants, Heterocyclics

EVIDENCE OF INTERACTION

Several studies have indicated that tricyclic antidepressants and typical antipsychotic agents may interact by inhibiting the hepatic metabolism of both agents. Brosen and Gram (Brosen and Gram 1989, Gram et al. 1974, Gram and Overo 1972) reported that the urinary excretion of nortriptyline and imipramine decreased by as much as 50% following the addition of haloperidol, chlorpromazine, or perphenazine; plasma concentrations of nortriptyline increased by 10% to 30%. In additional studies (Overo et al. 1977), this group determined that the clearance of tricyclic antidepressants was reduced in some patients by 50% following the addition of antipsychotic agents, primarily as a result of inhibiting hepatic ring-hydroxylation of the tricyclic. However, Kragh-Sorensen et al. (1977) found no effect of perphenazine on nortriptyline metabolism. Vandel et al. (1979) observed that the addition of phenothiazine to amitriptyline produced significant elevations of nortriptyline levels but not of amitriptyline plasma levels. Nelson and Jatlow (1980) compared plasma concentrations of desipramine in 15 depressed patients receiving 2.5 mg/kg of desipramine daily versus 15 delusionally depressed patients receiving an antipsychotic agent with the same weight-adjusted dose of desipramine. Patients receiving the combination had a mean desipramine concentration twice that of patients given desipramine alone (225 versus 110 ng/mL). Toxic reactions, including urinary retention, generalized seizures, and delirium, developed in several patients receiving desipramine plus the antipsychotic. This group replicated this finding in 82 depressed inpatients treated with desipramine, 35 of whom were concurrently receiving a phenothiazine or butyrophenone antipsychotic added to their antidepressant (Bock et al. 1983). Desipramine concentrations were twice as high in patients treated with an antipsychotic drug (233 versus 166 ng/mL) and the ratios of plasma concentrations of the hydroxy-metabolite to desipramine were significantly decreased (0.29 versus 0.49). Similarly, Siris et al. (1982a) warned of potentially dangerous elevations of tricyclic antidepressant plasma concentrations in patients treated with fluphenazine decanoate. These authors reported a mean imipramine plus desipramine plasma concentration of 850 ng/mL in four patients treated with imipramine 300 mg/day added to fluphenazine decanoate.

Tricyclic antidepressants may, in turn, elevate the plasma concentrations of antipsychotic agents. Mean plasma concentrations of chlorpromazine (300 mg daily) increased by approximately 50% in seven patients with schizophrenia 1 week after nortriptyline was added at a daily dose of 150 mg, and this increase was associated with increases in agitation sufficient to cause a premature termination of the study (Loga et al. 1981). Plasma concentrations of nortriptyline were not measured. El-Yousef and Manier (el-Yousef and Manier 1974) studied the effect of desipramine (75 to 300 mg daily) added for 3 weeks to the phenothiazine, butaperazine, in a crossover study of eight male patients with schizophrenia. Butaperazine plasma concentrations were significantly elevated by the co-administration of desipramine, but only at daily doses of 150 mg or more of the antidepressant.

Antidepressants and antipsychotics are often used in combination to treat psychotic depression (Kocsis et al. 1990, Spiker et al. 1985). Kramer et al. (1989) reported that the addition of desipramine or amitriptyline in recently admitted depressed schizophrenia patients treated for 5 weeks with haloperidol failed to improve measures of depression and impaired the response of some psychotic symptoms, compared with addition of placebo to haloperidol. In stable, depressed outpatients, by contrast, Siris et al. (1982b, 1987) reported that the addition of imipramine (200 mg daily) to an antipsychotic improved depression, and, in one study, negative symptoms (Siris et al. 1991). Other investigators have found inconsistent results using the combination of an antidepressant with an antipsychotic for schizophrenia, with one study finding improvement of depressive symptoms but worsening of psychosis (Prusoff et al. 1979), and two others reporting no improvement in depressive symptoms (Becker 1983, Waehrens and Gerlach 1980). Chouinard (1975) studied the combination of amitriptyline and perphenazine in patients with schizophrenia not selected for depression and found no benefit over that of the phenothiazine alone. Plasky (1991) concluded that tricyclic antidepressants may exert a destabilizing effect when administered with antipsychotic agents during acute psychotic episodes, whereas the combination may be beneficial when administered to stable patients with schizophrenia who experience residual depressive symptoms or anhedonia.

Antidepressants, SSRIs and Other Newer Classes

EVIDENCE OF INTERACTION

Several studies and many cases have reported the emergence of EPS associated with the addition of selective serotonin reuptake inhibitors (SSRIs) to antipsychotic agents. A review of EPS associated with SSRIs found that antipsychotics were co-prescribed in 11 of 71 identified cases (Leo 1996).

Citalopram and Escitalopram

Taylor et al. (1998) reported five patients for whom citalopram 20 mg was started for depression after at least 2 weeks of clozapine treatment. In four patients, clozapine levels declined slightly; in one patient levels increased slightly. Citalopram 40 mg daily had no effect on phenothiazine or haloperidol levels, in a double-blind, placebo-controlled augmentation trial in 80 stable schizophrenia patients (Salokangas et al. 1996). No reports document escitalopram in combination with antipsychotics.

Fluoxetine

Four weeks of treatment with fluoxetine 20 mg daily added to stable risperidone 4 to 6 mg daily in nine patients resulted in an increase in blood levels of the active moiety (risperidone plus 9-hydroxyrisperidone) by 75% (Spina et al. 2002). Two patients developed parkinsonian symptoms. In an open study of 11 patients who received the same medication combination, at the same doses, fluoxetine increased the AUC of the active moiety by 40% in extensive metabolizers, but not significantly in poor metabolizers (Bondolfi et al. 2002). An increase of haloperidol levels by 30%, but no increase in EPS, was found in an open trial of 13 patients with schizophrenia on low-dose haloperidol (3 to 6 mg) after fluoxetine 20 mg was added (Avenoso et al. 1997).

Negative symptomatology was improved. In a placebo-controlled trial, the addition of fluoxetine 20 mg daily to stable doses of fluphenazine and haloperidol decanoate increased serum concentrations of fluphenazine by an average of 65% and haloperidol by 20%, although EPS was not increased (Goff et al. 1995). Another double-blind, placebo-controlled trial of fluoxetine added to conventional antipsychotics also found the combination to be well-tolerated and effective for depressive and negative symptoms (Spina et al. 1994). Centorrino et al. (1994) found that serum concentrations of clozapine and two of its major metabolites (norclozapine and clozapine-N-oxide) were increased up to twofold in patients taking fluoxetine, compared with a matched control group in a cross-sectional naturalistic study. These findings were confirmed in a prospective trial of fluoxetine 20 mg added to stable clozapine therapy, in which plasma concentrations of clozapine and its major metabolites increased by 36% (norclozapine) and 58% (clozapine) (Spina et al. 1998). In a pharmacokinetic study of 13 patients on quetiapine (600 mg daily dose), the addition of fluoxetine (60 mg daily dose) was tolerated without additional side effect burden and no significant change in quetiapine levels (Potkin et al. 2002a). The combination of fluoxetine with pimozide was associated with bradycardia in a single case report (Ahmed et al. 1993). A study in rats found more than 10-fold elevations of thioridazine and its metabolites in blood after fluoxetine was given to the animals (Daniel et al. 1999).

Fluvoxamine

Jerling et al. (1994) found that the addition of fluvoxamine increased clozapine levels 5- to 10-fold, which they attributed to an inhibition of CYP1A2 activity. Subsequent trials in larger samples confirmed the substantial elevation of clozapine levels by fluvoxamine (Fabrazzo 2000). Extrapyramidal symptoms, thought to be the result of pharmacodynamic interactions, also have been reported using the fluvoxamine–clozapine combination (Kuo et al. 1998). Similar to clozapine, olanzapine plasma levels were shown to increase by 12% to 112% in eight patients who received 100 mg fluvoxamine added to olanzapine 10 to 20 mg daily (Hiemke et al. 2002). N-desmethylolanzapine levels remained unchanged, and the combination was well tolerated.

Paroxetine

Ozdemir et al. (1997) added paroxetine to perphenazine in eight healthy subjects and found a 2- to 13-fold elevation in perphenazine peak plasma concentrations, resulting in sedation, EPS, and memory problems. The addition of paroxetine 20 mg for 4 weeks to a stable dose of risperidone (4 to 8 mg/day) in 10 patients increased serum concentrations of the active moiety (sum of risperidone and 9-hydroxyrisperidone) by 45% (Spina et al. 2001a); one patient developed parkinsonism. Paroxetine co-administration was found to increase clozapine levels by 31% and norclozapine levels by 20% in an uncontrolled, prospective trial in nine schizophrenia patients (Spina et al. 2000a), and this combination showed similarly increased clozapine levels in an uncontrolled cross-sectional study (Centorrino et al. 1996).

Sertraline

In a double-blind, 8-week, placebo-controlled trial of sertraline 50 mg/day added to ongoing haloperidol treatment, Lee et al. (1998) found no benefit in the clinical symptoms in 36 patients; haloperidol and reduced haloperidol levels were unaffected by this low dose of sertraline. Similarly, sertraline 50 to 100 mg daily added to clozapine for 3 weeks was well-tolerated and had no effect on plasma clozapine and norclozapine levels (Spina et al. 2000a).

Bupropion

Bupropion in doses from 150 to 300 mg daily has been added to antipsychotics to aid in smoking cessation for clinically stable patients with schizophrenia (Evins et al. 2001, George et al. 2002); the combination was well-tolerated according to one case report (Evins and Tisdale 1999) and the aforementioned trials. One of the trials reported beneficial effects on negative symptoms, without worsening of positive symptoms, while rates of smoking cessation significantly increased (George et al. 2002). No formal study of drug–drug interactions between bupropion and antipsychotics is available.

Mirtazapine

A double-blind, placebo-controlled trial showed a reduction in negative symptoms when mirtazapine was added to 5 mg daily of haloperidol for schizophrenia without significant side effects (Berk et al. 2001).

Nefazodone

Nefazodone is a strong inhibitor of CYP3A4. When given together with haloperidol in a study of healthy volunteers, nefazodone significantly increased the AUC of haloperidol (Barbhaiya et al. 1996). Co-administration of clozapine with nefazodone in six patients modestly increased clozapine and norclozapine levels by 4% and 19%, respectively (Taylor et al. 1999). In contrast to these small increases from the combination, Khan and Preskorn (2001) reported a single case in which the addition of 300 mg nefazodone to clozapine led to an almost doubling of clozapine and norclozapine levels.

Venlafaxine

A single-dose study of 1 mg risperidone in healthy subjects showed weak inhibition of risperidone metabolism by steady-state venlafaxine (Amchin et al. 1999).

Several case reports describe the development of a serotonin syndrome when antipsychotics with potent serotonin antagonism were given together with serotonergic antidepressants. In one case, olanzapine 10 mg/day was added to mirtazapine 45 mg/day and tramadol 150 mg/day, resulting in a serotonin syndrome 1 week later (Duggal and Fetchko 2002). The clinical picture dramatically improved within 12 hours of the discontinuation of all medications. A second case of serotonin syndrome developed within 2 hours in a patient who was restarted on 40 mg of paroxetine and 6 mg of risperidone after having been off medication for 1 week (Hamilton and Malone 2000). In a third case, serotonin syndrome developed on the combination of olanzapine, lithium, and citalopram (Haslett and Kumar 2002).

MECHANISM

Dose-related side effects, such as EPS with typical agents and somnolence with certain atypical agents, theoretically can result from co-administration with SSRIs, because SSRIs are potent inhibitors of key metabolic pathways, including CYP2D6 (inhibited by fluoxetine, norfluoxetine, sertraline, and paroxetine), CYP1A2 (inhibited by fluvoxamine), and CYP3A4 (inhibited by fluvoxamine and nefazodone) (Ereshefsky et al. 1995, Nemeroff et al. 1996, Sproule et al. 1997). Citalopram and venlafaxine would be expected to be relatively free of pharmacokinetic interactions. Haloperidol and phenothiazines may elevate the plasma concentrations of tricyclic antidepressants moderately, apparently by inhibiting hepatic CYP2D6 metabolism by aromatic ring-hydroxylation (Brosen and Gram 1989).

Moreover, a pharmacodynamic interaction is also likely with SSRIs. Fluoxetine administered alone is reported to produce a syndrome indistinguishable from neuroleptic-induced akathisia (Lipinkski et al. 1989). Pretreatment with serotonin reuptake blockers potentiates neuroleptic-induced catalepsy in rats (Balsara et al. 1979), and dystonia and parkinsonism in monkeys (Korsgaard et al. 1985). In rats, Zhang et al. (2000) observed the synergistic effects of olanzapine and fluoxetine on norepinephrine and dopamine release in prefrontal cortex.

Serotonin syndrome is thought to result from the excessive stimulation of 5-HT1a receptors. The addition of an antipsychotic with a strong blockade of 5-HT2 receptors to an SSRI potentially may over-activate 5-HT1a receptors via an indirect mechanism. Although the original criteria for serotonin syndrome did not allow for a diagnosis if antipsychotics were added or the dose increased (Sternbach 1991), several cases could be interpreted as the result of serotonergic over-stimulation because NMS was ruled out.

CLINICAL IMPLICATIONS

The combination of an antipsychotic agent with an antidepressant is an effective treatment for delusional depression and possibly for refractory depression in psychotic patients. If tricyclics are combined with antipsychotics, plasma concentrations should be monitored, as well as clinical signs of toxicity. SSRIs have the potential to interact with antipsychotics both pharmacodynamically and pharmacokinetically. In susceptible individuals, adding an SSRI to ongoing antipsychotic treatment might result in the emergence of EPS, as a result of serotoninergic inhibitory effects on dopaminergic pathways. Side effects can also emerge as a result of increased levels of the antipsychotic, if an SSRI that inhibits metabolizing enzymes is added (such as paroxetine impairing risperidone or perphenazine elimination, or fluvoxamine inhibiting clozapine metabolism). Care must be taken with clozapine, pimozide, and thioridazine because of their relatively narrow therapeutic indexes. At a minimum, close clinical observation is indicated when SSRIs are added to ongoing antipsychotic therapy. In selected cases, antipsychotic plasma levels are helpful to monitor pharmacokinetic interactions. Bupropion is often added to ongoing antipsychotic treatment for smoking cessation. The safety of this combination, especially with respect to seizure threshold when added to antipsychotics like chlorpromazine or clozapine, is inadequately studied. It is possible that certain antidepressants are partially effective against the negative symptoms of schizophrenia when combined with antipsychotics (Goff and Evins 1998).

A pharmacodynamic interaction leading to serotonin syndrome is possible if atypical antipsychotics that have strong 5-HT2 blocking effects are combined with antidepressants that increase serotonergic tone. This appears to be more likely if additional serotonergic medications are co-administered. It is not known how common this interaction is, but atypicals are frequently co-prescribed with SSRIs, for example, in treating depression and obsessive compulsive disorder (OCD), without adverse consequences. One particular combination, olanzapine plus fluoxetine, is approved by the FDA as a combination drug for bipolar depression.

Antiepileptic Drugs

EVIDENCE OF INTERACTION

For the purpose of predicting drug interactions, antiepilepsy drugs (AEDs) can broadly be divided into whether they induce metabolic enzymes or not: phenytoin, phenobarbital, and carbamazepine are classified as enzyme inducers; valproate, gabapentin, levetiracetam, lamotrigine, oxcarbazepine, and tiagabine are generally not considered inducers (Riva et al. 1996).

Hesslinger et al. (1999) compared clinical outcomes in a controlled 4-week trial in which patients were randomized to receive haloperidol alone, haloperidol with carbamazepine, or haloperidol with valproate. Although the addition of valproate had no effect on haloperidol levels or clinical symptoms after 4 weeks, the addition of carbamazepine significantly lowered haloperidol levels and impeded symptomatic improvement. Worsening of psychosis and an average decrease of haloperidol concentrations by 60% were also observed in a trial of seven patients in which carbamazepine was added to haloperidol (Arana et al. 1986). Of note was a marked worsening of psychosis after the addition of carbamazepine in those patients who were receiving 10 mg or less of haloperidol; haloperidol became nondetectable in these patients. Carbamazepine was discontinued in five patients treated with haloperidol or fluphenazine, and all patients subsequently displayed improvement in clinical status, although most developed EPS within 30 days (Jann et al. 1989). Antipsychotic plasma levels increased two- to fourfold. A doubling of clozapine levels was reported in two cases after carbamazepine was stopped (Raitasuo et al. 1993), and in four cases, clozapine, chlorpromazine, and haloperidol levels doubled when carbamazepine was switched to oxcarbazepine (Raitasuo et al. 1994). Clozapine levels were reported to be lowered by 50% following the addition of carbamazepine (Jerling et al. 1994), and risperidone and 9-hydroxyrisperidone levels similarly decreased by up to half (Ono et al. 2002). A significant induction of olanzapine metabolism by carbamazepine was also suggested by the finding in a sample of 194 patients that the mean ratio of olanzapine serum concentrations to olanzapine doses was 70 % lower in patients coprescribed carbamazepine compared to patients treated with olanzapine alone (Skogh et al. 2002). Data from healthy volunteers also have shown a decrease in ziprasidone serum concentrations with carbamazepine co-administration (Miceli et al. 2000).

Increasingly, valproate is added to hasten the response to typical and atypical antipsychotics in acute exacerbations of schizophrenia

(Wassef et al. 2002, Casey et al. 2003). In one prospective controlled study, valproate had negligible effect on risperidone metabolism (Spina et al. 2000b). The addition of valproate to clozapine has been associated with small elevations of clozapine levels in a case-controlled (Centorrino et al. 1994a) and a prospective study (Facciola et al. 1999), but also was reported to decrease clozapine levels in another study (Conca et al. 2000). Chlorpromazine, but not haloperidol, was noted to decrease valproate clearance (Ishizaki et al. 1984).

Phenytoin is a potent inducer of several important enzyme systems, including CYP3A and the UGT system (Riva et al. 1996). In a study of 10 patients with chronic psychotic disorders, Wong et al. (2001) added phenytoin 100 mg three times a day to a stable dose of quetiapine. The clearance of quetiapine increased more than fivefold. Chlorpromazine, haloperidol, and mesoridazine serum concentrations were noted to be decreased when co-administered with phenytoin (Linnoila et al. 1980, Haidukewych and Rodin 1985). Miller reported two cases in which clozapine plasma levels were decreased by 65% to 85% under co-medication with phenytoin (Miller 1991).

Barbiturates, as pan-inducers, significantly lower the plasma concentrations of chlorpromazine and haloperidol when co-administered with these agents (Linnoila et al. 1980, Forrest et al. 1970). The combination of phenobarbital and thioridazine resulted in decreased concentrations of both phenobarbital and mesoridazine (a prominent active metabolite of thioridazine) (Linnoila et al. 1980).

MECHANISM

Carbamazepine is the prototype and most widely studied of an enzyme-inducing anticonvulsant. It increases its own metabolism as well as the phase I and phase II metabolism of other drugs. Its epoxide metabolite confers neurotoxicity. Other "pan-inducers" are phenytoin and barbiturates, such as phenobarbital. As would be expected, antipsychotic drug levels can be reduced significantly if the antipsychotic metabolism depends on the induced enzymes. This is well documented for haloperidol, risperidone, and olanzapine. In addition, a patient's CYP2D6 genotype is important for risperidone, because CYP2D6-deficient patients might rely more on CYP3A4 metabolism (Spina et al. 2001b). In the case of olanzapine, accelerated glucuronidation could be an important mechanism (Linnet and Olesen 2002) in addition to the induction of CYP1A2 (Lucas et al. 1998). In the case of ziprasidone, CYP3A4 induction can lower ziprasidone levels (Miceli et al. 2000). Some antipsychotics might interfere with the epoxide metabolism, leading to toxicity from increased epoxide levels. Lamotrigine is metabolized through phase II glucuronidation and appears relatively free of drug interactions. Valproate seems to interact minimally with antipsychotics, whereas chlorpromazine can inhibit valproate clearance.

CLINICAL IMPLICATIONS

Clinicians should monitor for the emergence of psychotic symptoms and be prepared to increase the dose of antipsychotic after the addition of carbamazepine, phenytoin, or a barbiturate. Because the induction of hepatic metabolism may require several weeks, clinical deterioration can be gradual or delayed. A clinically relevant lowering of haloperidol levels following the addition of carbamazepine is well documented in controlled trials. This is particularly important if low (neuroleptic-threshold) doses of haloperidol are used (McEvoy et al. 1991). Clinicians can anticipate drug interactions by increasing the antipsychotic dose by 30% to 50% when adding an enzyme-inducing anticonvulsant. The reverse, an increase in plasma levels, is expected if carbamazepine is discontinued; clinicians should monitor for EPS or other signs of antipsychotic toxicity, and decrease the antipsychotic dose. Whereas oxcarbazepine, the 10-keto analog of carbamazepine, does not produce the epoxide form, it can induce hepatic enzymes as well. Valproate does not enhance the clearance of antipsychotics, and it may even increase drug levels slightly. Generally, valproate, topiramate, gabapentin, and lamotrigine can be added safely to antipsychotics, including clozapine (Navarro et al. 2001).

Antipsychotics

EVIDENCE OF INTERACTION

Combining antipsychotics is common practice despite insufficient evidence for increased efficacy and little data on risk (Freudenreich and Goff 2003). Some empirical support exists for adding a tightly bound D2 blocker like risperidone to clozapine. Although individual cases have been reported of increased clozapine levels when risperidone was co-prescribed (Tyson et al. 1995), this was not confirmed in prospective augmentation studies of 18 patients (Raaska et al. 2002a) and 12 patients (Henderson and Goff 1996). Potkin et al. (2002b) openly but randomly added risperidone (6 mg daily), haloperidol (15 mg daily), or thioridazine (400 mg daily) to quetiapine treatment (600 mg daily) and found that only thioridazine significantly increased the clearance of quetiapine. Side effects were increased in the combined treatments compared with antipsychotic monotherapy. Prolactin can be elevated if clozapine is augmented by haloperidol or risperidone (Kapur et al. 2001, Henderson et al. 2001).

MECHANISM

Many conceivable pharmacodynamic and pharmacokinetic interactions are possible if antipsychotics are co-prescribed, but this has not been well-studied empirically.

CLINICAL IMPLICATIONS

If antipsychotics are combined, monitor for side effects, preferably starting before the combination is used. The atypicality of a compound may be lost if it is combined with a conventional agent. Combinations that have overlapping side effects, such as anticholinergic effects or QTc prolongation, are best avoided.

Anxiolytics

EVIDENCE OF INTERACTION

Benzodiazepines

The combination of benzodiazepines with antipsychotic agents has been studied in the treatment of mania or agitation in a variety of acute psychotic states, and in the treatment of chronically symptomatic schizophrenic patients. Diazepam augmentation has been shown to be as effective as increasing the antipsychotic dose in staving off relapse (Carpenter et al. 1999). Douyon et al. (1989) added alprazolam to stable doses of typical antipsychotics in nine patients with schizophrenia and found a mean increase of 23% in plasma concentrations of haloperidol and fluphenazine. Several investigators have reported significant improvement of both positive and negative symptoms of schizophrenia on the addition of benzodiazepines to antipsychotic agents (Pato et al. 1989, Wolkowitz et al. 1988). However, the benefits of benzodiazepine supplementation are most likely during acute exacerbations of illness, are found in only about 30% to 50% of chronically ill patients, and may diminish over time (Wolkowitz and Pickar 1991).

Side effects reported with the addition of benzodiazepines to clozapine have included sedation, sialorrhea, ataxia, and, in rare cases, fainting, loss of consciousness, and respiratory arrest (Tupala et al. 1999, Klimke and Klieser 1994, Cobb et al. 1991, Friedman et al. 1991). The etiologic role of benzodiazepines in producing these reactions remains uncertain; if such an interaction does occur, it is evidently rare (Wokowitz and Pickar 1991). The competitive inhibition of the glucuronidation pathway by benzodiazepines might have caused elevated clozapine levels in some of these cases (Liston et al. 2001).

Buspirone

In an open trial, the addition of buspirone at a mean daily dose of 24 mg to typical antipsychotics in 20 patients with schizophrenia was associated with improvements in depression, tension, and parkinsonian symptoms (Goff et al. 1991b). Another open trial reported improved psychosis, negative symptoms, and anxiety in 13 patients with schizophrenia who received a (high) mean dose of 100 mg buspirone in addition to stable doses of haloperidol 10 to 20 mg (Sirota et al. 2001). Huang et al. (1996) added buspirone 10 mg three times a day to stable haloperidol doses (10 to 40 mg daily) and found no effect on haloperidol and reduced haloperidol levels, consistent with the lack of effect of buspirone on the CYP3A4-mediated oxidation of haloperidol to reduced haloperidol (Kalgutkar et al. 2003).

MECHANISM

Alprazolam may lower antipsychotic plasma concentrations slightly, although the mechanism is not known. The enhancement of antipsychotic effects on agitation and possibly on psychotic and negative symptoms of schizophrenia may simply be the result of benzodiazepine-induced sedation, or may represent a pharmacodynamic interaction between γ-aminobutyric acid (GABA) and dopaminergic systems. Buspirone's effect on psychopathology and EPS in schizophrenia are possibly mediated via buspirone's partial 5-HT1a agonism.

CLINICAL SIGNIFICANCE

Benzodiazepines (e.g., lorazepam, alprazolam, diazepam, and clonazepam) are effective when combined with moderate doses of high-potency conventional antipsychotic agents in the treatment of acute psychotic or manic agitation. Atypical parenteral antipsychotics (ziprasidone or olanzapine) might be similarly effective. During the early stages of treatment, adjuvant benzodiazepine use may allow lower doses of conventional antipsychotic agents, and thus reduce the risk of EPS. Benzodiazepines and buspirone may improve psychotic and negative symptoms when combined with antipsychotics in some chronic patients with schizophrenia, although this effect is variable, typically minor, and, in the case of benzodiazepines, may not be sustained. Combinations of buspirone with clozapine, ziprasidone, or aripiprazole are not recommended, because all share similar degrees of partial serotonin 1a-receptor agonism and might therefore constitute "irrational" pharmacotherapy (Newman-Tancredi et al. 2003).

Cardiovascular Drugs, Antihypertensives

EVIDENCE OF INTERACTION

A variety of agents control hypertension through several differing mechanisms, and each type may interact differently with antipsychotic agents. Propranolol and pindolol can increase the circulating levels of chlorpromazine and thioridazine when co-administered at typical doses (Greendyke and Gulya 1988, Greendyke and Kanter 1987, Peet et al. 1980, Silver et al. 1986, Vestal et al. 1979), whereas haloperidol concentrations are not affected by these agents (Greendyke and Gulya 1988, Greendyke and Kanter 1987). In turn, chlorpromazine and thioridazine, but not haloperidol, can increase the plasma concentrations of propranolol and pindolol (Greendyke and Gulya 1988, Greendyke and Kanter 1987, Peet et al. 1980, Silver et al. 1986, Vestal 1979). The full clinical implications of combining antipsychotics and β-blockers remain unclear, although such combinations are generally well tolerated (Yorkston et al. 1977). Vestal et al. (1979) described a case of orthostatic syncope after chlorpromazine 50 mg daily was added to propranolol. More ominously, Alexander et al. (1984) reported three episodes of severe hypotension and cardiopulmonary arrest in a 48-year-old woman with schizophrenia treated with haloperidol 10 mg and propranolol 40 mg daily; she tolerated both haloperidol and propranolol when separately combined with other psychotropic drugs. Thioridazine and chlorpromazine frequently cause postural hypotension when administered alone (Goff and Shader 2003). Although it has not been studied systematically, the addition of a β-blocker might further compromise cardiovascular function by adding β-adrenergic blockade to the anti–α-adrenergic actions of chlorpromazine and thioridazine, and perhaps other low-potency antipsychotics (particularly clozapine). Whereas generally considered safer with regards to orthostatic hypotension, newer antipsychotics are not exempt (Goff and Shader 2003, Markowitz et al. 2002).

Other antihypertensives also have been reported to produce hypotension when combined with low-potency conventional antipsychotics. White (White 1986) described a patient in whom orthostatic hypotension and syncope developed when the angiotensin-converting enzyme (ACE) inhibitor captopril (12.5 mg) was added to chlorpromazine; the patient later tolerated each drug separately, but again became hypotensive when rechallenged with the combination. Similarly, Fruncillo (1985) reported two cases of severe hypotension when clonidine was added to chlorpromazine as well as other medications. Delirium occurred in a 39-year-old patient treated with fluphenazine decanoate following the addition of clonidine; this reaction cleared after a discontinuation of clonidine and recurred when the patient was rechallenged (Allen and Flemenbaum 1979).

The catecholamine synthesis inhibitor, α-methyldopa, also has been reported to produce hypotension and delirium when added to antipsychotic agents. Chouinard et al. (1973a, 1973b) evaluated methyldopa as a possible adjuvant to antipsychotic therapy. In their first study, methyldopa was gradually increased to 1,000 mg in combination with chlorpromazine 400 mg daily. In the second study, methyldopa 500 mg was combined with haloperidol 10 mg daily. Both regimens produced substantial orthostatic hypotension, with dizziness as well as impressive clinical responses, but their interpretation is limited by the absence of a control group. In addition, three cases of cognitive or behavioral deterioration were associated with the combination of methyldopa and haloperidol. One, a 74-year-old man, tolerated 100 mg of thioridazine combined with 500 mg of methyldopa daily, but became irritable, aggressive, and assaultive when the antipsychotic was changed to haloperidol 4 mg daily (Nadel and Wallach 1979). Two other patients became confused when haloperidol was added at doses of 6 or 8 mg daily to 500 mg of methyldopa, but improved after the discontinuation of haloperidol (Thornton 1976).

Finally, several studies have evaluated the effect of antipsychotic agents on blood pressure when co-administered with the peripheral antisympathetic agent guanethidine. Janowsky et al. (1972) stabilized otherwise medication-free patients on guanethidine (60 to 150 mg daily) alone for 7 days before adding chlorpromazine, haloperidol, or thiothixene. After a delay of several days, the antipsychotic agents significantly reversed the antihypertensive effect of guanethidine and, in some patients, increased blood pressure; this effect was most apparent using chlorpromazine (100 to 400 mg daily). The blockade of the antihypertensive effect of guanethidine by chlorpromazine was also observed by Fann et al. (1971). Unlike chlorpromazine, molindone does not block the neural uptake of guanethidine in rats (Gilder et al. 1976) and, when administered at doses of 30 to 120 mg daily, molindone did not interfere with the antihypertensive effect of guanethidine in seven hypertensive patients (Gilder et al. 1976).

Cardiovascular Drugs, Antiarrhythmics

EVIDENCE OF INTERACTION

Many antipsychotic agents have direct myocardial depressant effects that are reflected in prolongation of the QT interval and nonspecific T-changes on the electrocardiogram (ECG) (Risch et al. 1981, Glassman and Bigger 2001). Thioridazine exhibits a particularly strong myocardial depressant effect and may prolong atrial and ventricular conduction and refractory periods (Descotes et al. 1979, Yoon and Han 1979). It was noted that thioridazine at clinical doses has calcium-channel–blocking properties comparable to clinically available calcium channel blockers (Gould et al. 1984). Chlorpromazine also depresses myocardial function and can increase QT duration at daily doses as low as 150 mg. Of great concern have been early reports of sudden death associated with antipsychotic doses of thioridazine (Giles and Modlin 1968), and higher rates of sudden cardiac deaths in patients treated with conventional antipsychotics (Ray et al. 2001). The cardiac safety of thioridazine, particularly at higher doses, has been called into further question by a cohort study using administrative data in which elevated rates of cardiac arrests and ventricular arrhythmias were found in patients treated with thioridazine, when compared with other antipsychotics (Hennessy et al. 2002), and by a case-controlled study in which the odds ratio for sudden death was 5.3 for thioridazine-treated patients compared with untreated patients (Reilly et al. 2002). Higher thioridazine levels can be reached inadvertently, as reported by Silver et al. (1986), who found thioridazine plasma levels more than doubled after high-dose propranolol was added to the antipsychotic to treat aggression.

Pimozide can produce clinically significant cardiac depressant effects as a result of its calcium-channel–blocking action (Opler and Feinberg 1991). These effects are concentration-dependent and observed at recommended doses of the drug. ECG conduction intervals should be monitored when pimozide is initiated, particularly in children and the elderly, and this drug should not be combined with other calcium channel blockers (e.g., nifedipine, diltiazem, and verapamil). Because pimozide is strongly metabolized by CYP3A4, special care should be taken to avoid potential pharmacokinetic interactions leading to high plasma levels of pimozide. Torsade de pointes, a life-threatening ventricular arrhythmia associated with QT prolongation, can occur if CYP3A4 inhibitors are co-administered with pimozide (Dresser et al. 2000).

Pimozide, thioridazine, chlorpromazine, and ziprasidone appear to be especially likely to produce QT prolongation (Risch et al. 1981, Glassman and Bigger 2001, Ban and St. Jean 1964, Drolet et al. 2001, Haddad and Anderson 2002). Effects on cardiac conduction may be additive, so these agents should not be combined or added to similarly acting drugs (such as quinidine-like antiarrhythmics) without close monitoring of the ECG. Thioridazine produced the largest QTc interval change in a prospective study of 183 patients assigned to haloperidol, thioridazine, ziprasidone, quetiapine, olanzapine, or risperidone

(Harrigan et al. 2004); ziprasidone was intermediate between thioridazine and the other antipsychotics studied. QTc prolongation by ziprasidone was not strongly concentration-dependent; a 31% elevation of ziprasidone blood levels following the addition of ketoconazole did not appreciably increase QT interval duration.

Extremely high doses of intravenous haloperidol (up to 1,000 mg in 24 hours) have been administered safely to patients with cardiac disease in combination with antiarrhythmic agents, although rare cases of QT interval prolongation and torsade de pointes have been reported at these doses (Metzger and Friedman 1993, Di Salvo and O'Gara 1995, Perrault et al. 2000, Hunt and Stern 1995, O'Brien et al. 1999, Sharma et al. 1998), and also somewhat unpredictably during oral, low-dose treatment (Jackson et al. 1997). Because droperidol can lengthen the QTc interval, its cardiac safety has been questioned despite a good clinical record (Shale et al. 2003).

Cardiovascular Drugs, Pressors

EVIDENCE OF INTERACTION

Because low-potency and some high-potency antipsychotics block α- but not β-adrenergic receptors, the administration of epinephrine may cause severe hypotension as a result of unopposed β-agonist activity at visceral beds (Ginsbug and Duff 1956).

MECHANISM

The β-blockers propranolol and pindolol elevate the circulating levels of some phenothiazines, presumably by impairing hepatic metabolism. Antipsychotic agents, particularly thioridazine and chlorpromazine, also can interact with cardiovascular agents as a result of their α-adrenergic blockade, as well as mild quinidine-like direct depression of cardiac conduction. Several antipsychotics (molindone is an exception) also block the uptake of guanethidine into postganglionic sympathetic neurons, and thereby reduce its antihypertensive efficacy. Pimozide and thioridazine have calcium-channel–blocking properties that can depress cardiac conduction and produce severe additive cardiac or hypotensive effects when combined with other calcium channel blockers. The combination of low-potency antipsychotic agents with β-adrenergic agonist pressors can result in hypotension, as a result peripheral β-adrenergic agonist activity, unopposed by α-receptor–mediated vasoconstriction which is blocked. One of the main molecular mechanisms by which many medications, including some antipsychotics, lengthen the QTc interval appears to be the blockade of a potassium channel encoded by the gene HERG (Human Ether-a-go-go-Related Gene)

(Witchel et al. 2003). Other mechanisms, such as calcium channel blockade (in the case of pimozide and thioridazine), likely contribute to the potential cardiotoxicity of a drug.

CLINICAL SIGNIFICANCE

High-potency antipsychotic agents such as haloperidol or fluphenazine, and newer antipsychotics such as aripiprazole and olanzapine, produce substantially less hypotension and cardiac depression than do thioridazine or chlorpromazine, and so are preferable for patients with cardiovascular disease and the elderly. Unlike certain phenothiazines, haloperidol plasma levels are not elevated by the co-administration of propranolol or pindolol. Drugs that impair cardiac conduction (including tricyclic antidepressants) should not be added to QTc-prolonging antipsychotics (thioridazine and its metabolite, mesoridazine; pimozide; chlorpromazine; droperidol; or ziprasidone), unless the ECG is monitored, especially in elderly or cardiac patients. Drugs that are relatively contraindicated to be given concomitantly with QTc-prolonging antipsychotics are drugs that (a) themselves have the potential for QTc prolongation, such as cardiac drugs like sotalol, quinidine, or other class Ia and class III antiarrhythmics; antibiotics such as erythromycin, clarithromycin, sparfloxacin, gatifloxacin, and moxifloxacin (Iannini 2002); antimalaria agents such as halofantrine or mefloquine (Nosten et al. 1993); and some antipsychotics; or (b) increase the antipsychotic plasma levels via pharmacokinetic interactions. ECG monitoring also is recommended when patients are started on pimozide or when the dose is increased. Because of their potentially serious effects on cardiac conduction, thioridazine, mesoridazine, and pimozide are not antipsychotics of first choice, and other antipsychotics usually can be substituted. Finally, pressors, such as epinephrine, should not be combined with low-potency agents because severe hypotension can result from excessive and unopposed β-adrenergic activity.

Coffee or Tea

EVIDENCE OF INTERACTION

Early studies raised concern that coffee or tea may decrease the bioavailability of antipsychotic agents. Kulhanek et al. (1979) mixed tea or coffee with elixirs (alcohol solutions) of fluphenazine and haloperidol in vitro and observed the formation of insoluble precipitates. When fluphenazine was given to rats orally in a solution of coffee or tea, the degree and duration of catalepsy was decreased when compared with the administration of fluphenazine alone (Kulhanek and Linde 1981). Zaslove et al. (1991) reported that the substitution of caffeinated beverages with decaffeinated beverages on an inpatient psychiatric ward resulted in a decrease in assaults and property destruction. Subsequent clinical trials have not confirmed an interaction, however. Koczapski et al. (1991) compared the plasma levels of chlorpromazine, haloperidol, fluphenazine, and trifluoperazine, measured by radioreceptor assay, in 16 patients given these drugs with coffee or tea versus fruit juice, and found no difference. Similarly, Bowen et al. (1981) substituted fruit juice for coffee and tea in 16 patients with mental retardation and psychosis. No change in antipsychotic drug levels or behavior was noted. Wallace et al. (1981) found no effect of coffee or tea on the plasma concentrations of fluphenazine in 12 normal volunteers. Although consistent effects of the consumption of caffeinated beverages have not been demonstrated in patients treated with antipsychotic drugs, the acute administration of a high dose of caffeine (10 mg/kg) increased arousal and measures of psychosis in patients with schizophrenia receiving oral fluphenazine (Lucas et al. 1990).

MECHANISM

The psychostimulant effects of caffeine are mediated through its antagonism of adenosine A(2A) receptors. Adenosine and dopamine signaling pathways converge on an intracellular phosphoprotein, DARRP-32, suggesting the possibility of a pharmacodynamic rather than pharmacokinetic interaction between antipsychotics and caffeine in some patients, although this is not well understood (Lindskog et al. 2002).

CLINICAL SIGNIFICANCE

Clinical evidence inadequately suggests a significant pharmacokinetic interaction between caffeinated beverages and antipsychotic agents. However, patients with schizophrenia often consume copious amounts of coffee (e.g., in excess of six cups or 600 mg of caffeine), which leads to caffeinism. Such high levels of caffeine alone cause anxiety and can exacerbate psychopathology, with a concomitant increased need for antipsychotics to counteract unpleasant caffeine effects. Caffeinism can be confused with akathisia or psychotic exacerbation. Caffeine withdrawal states may present with headache, lassitude, and nausea.

Disulfiram

EVIDENCE OF INTERACTION

Hansen and Larsen (1982) reported a case in which the addition of disulfiram to perphenazine resulted in decreased plasma concentrations of perphenazine, increased concentrations of the inactive sulfoxide metabolite, and a deterioration in the patient's psychiatric condition.

MECHANISM

The interaction is presumed to be pharmacokinetic, through an increase in the first-pass metabolism of the antipsychotic. Because disulfiram inhibits only CYP2E1, but not enzymes thought to be relevant for the metabolism of antipsychotics, the mechanism remains unexplained.

CLINICAL SIGNIFICANCE

In one reported case, this interaction was of a magnitude sufficient to result in clinical deterioration. Disulfiram has not been studied systematically in relation to other antipsychotic agents, but clinicians should be aware of this potential interaction, presumed to be pharmacokinetic in nature. Brenner et al. (1994) report on the successful use of clozapine plus disulfiram. The patient remained clinically stable, but no pharmacokinetic data were obtained that could clarify the impact of disulfiram on antipsychotic drug levels, in this case clozapine.

Donepezil

EVIDENCE OF INTERACTION

Two case reports have linked parkinsonian side effects to the addition of donepezil to risperidone in elderly patients with Alzheimer's disease (Magnuson et al. 1998, Liu et al. 2002). In a formal study in which 24 healthy volunteers received donepezil 5 mg and risperidone 1 mg daily, no pharmacokinetic interaction was observed (Zhao et al. 2003).

MECHANISM OF ACTION

In neither case report were the plasma levels of risperidone obtained. Both authors attributed the development of EPS to a change in the dopamine–acetylcholine balance in the striatum, resulting in increased susceptibility to the antidopaminergic blockade by risperidone. It is not clear if EPS was in fact the result of the combined treatment.

CLINICAL SIGNIFICANCE

Combining cholinesterase inhibitors with dopamine-blocking agents might increase the risk for parkinsonism through a pharmacodynamic interaction. This might be particularly relevant in patient populations who are already at risk for EPS, such as elderly patients with dementia, who have very little nigrostriatal dopaminergic reserve. No formal studies in populations at risk have been performed.

Gastrointestinal Agents: Antacids and Food

EVIDENCE OF INTERACTION

Antacids may impair the absorption of antipsychotic agents. Forrest et al. (1970) administered a suspension of aluminum and magnesium hydroxide for 2 to 7 days to 10 patients who had been receiving chlorpromazine at daily doses of 400 to 1,200 mg for at least 12 weeks. The antacids decreased the urinary excretion of chlorpromazine by 10% to 45%. Fann et al. (1973) measured plasma concentrations before and 2 hours after the administration of a liquid suspension of chlorpromazine to 67 patients who had been medication-free for 7 days. Two days later, this procedure was repeated, but with the additional administration of 30 ml of a gel of magnesium trisilicate with aluminum hydroxide immediately before, plus 10 minutes after, the administration of chlorpromazine. Plasma chlorpromazine concentrations were lower in all six patients when the antipsychotic was co-administered with the antacid. Although this study demonstrated impaired absorption, it is not possible to determine whether the antacid decreased or merely delayed absorption. A case of clinical worsening was associated with the administration of aluminum hydroxide gel to a patient with schizophrenia previously stabilized on haloperidol (Goldstein 1982). A formal study of Maalox co-administration with ziprasidone in healthy volunteers revealed no appreciable interaction (Wilner et al. 2000).

MECHANISM

It is assumed that chlorpromazine, and possibly other antipsychotic drugs, become bound to the gel-type antacids, thus reducing or delaying drug absorption (Forrest et al. 1970). The alteration of urinary pH level as a result of antacid therapy also might affect the urinary excretion of chlorpromazine metabolites, although such an effect is probably minor.

CLINICAL IMPLICATIONS

The intestinal absorption of chlorpromazine is impaired when administered with gel-type antacids composed of magnesium or aluminum hydroxide. This potential interaction has not generally been studied systematically, although a case report by Goldstein et al. (1982) suggests that it may occur with haloperidol as well. On the other hand, ziprasidone absorption does not seem to be affected by the co-administration of Maalox. The clinical significance of such an interaction is difficult to estimate, because it depends in part on plasma concentrations achieved prior to the addition of the antacid, and on the temporal relation between the administration of the two drugs. Patients treated with a relatively low dose of antipsychotic medication given within 2 hours of a gel antacid may experience clinically significant loss of antipsychotic efficacy. This problem is best avoided by administering the drugs separately—for example, the antipsychotic at bedtime, at least 4 hours after the last daily dose of antacid, or by use of parenteral (depot) forms of antipsychotic.

Gastrointestinal Agents: Antidiarrheal Agents

EVIDENCE OF INTERACTION

Sorby and Liu (1966) demonstrated a decreased rate and extent of urinary excretion of the phenothiazine promazine following the administration of an antidiarrheal mix of attapulgite and pectin in repeated studies in a single normal subject.

MECHANISM

Attapulgite is a clay mineral adsorbent. It appears to decrease the rate and extent of promazine absorption from the gastrointestinal tract.

CLINICAL IMPLICATIONS

Although this finding is preliminary and has only been studied in a single-dose design with promazine, it may apply to other antipsychotics as well. It is unclear if this pharmacokinetic interaction is likely to produce a clinically significant lowering of drug plasma concentrations. Because attapulgite is contained in many over-the-counter antidiarrheal preparations, clinicians should monitor for such an interaction when a patient reports taking an adsorbent antidiarrheal compound.

Gastrointestinal Agents: H₂-Blockers

EVIDENCE OF INTERACTION

Histamine H_2 antagonists affect hepatic metabolic enzymes to varying degrees. Cimetidine is a nonspecific inhibitor of P450 enzymes and of glucuronidation. Howes et al. (1983) reported that the addition of cimetidine 1,200 mg daily orally for 7 days to eight patients receiving stable doses of chlorpromazine reduced plasma concentrations of chlorpromazine by 33%. This contrasts with a report of two cases of chlorpromazine-treated patients who became sedated when cimetidine was added (Byrne and O'Shea 1989). Szymanski (1991) reported a possible interaction between cimetidine and clozapine, characterized by severe dizziness, diaphoresis, emesis, and weakness. The patient subsequently tolerated ranitidine 300 mg daily. The addition of cimetidine (400 mg three times a day) led to a slight increase in quetiapine levels due to reduced clearance in seven patients (Strakowski et al. 2002), whereas ziprasidone was not affected by cimetidine (Wilner et al. 2000). Famotidine added to ongoing antipsychotic treatment might lead to improved psychopathology in patients with schizophrenia, as initially reported in one case report (40 mg daily dose) (Kaminsky et al. 1990) and several open trials (Rosse et al. 1996, Oyewumi et al. 1994). No placebo-controlled trials have been performed.

MECHANISM

Changes in the metabolite ratios in urine indicate that the hepatic metabolism of chlorpromazine is inhibited by cimetidine, consistent with other drug interactions of this agent. However, the significant reduction in plasma concentration of chlorpromazine indicates that decreased absorption is the more important mechanism responsible for this interaction. Cimetidine probably elevates plasma concentrations of clozapine by inhibiting hepatic microsomal enzymes, most importantly via 1A2 (Taylor 1997), but also conceivably by inhibiting glucuronidation (Liston et al. 2001).

CLINICAL IMPLICATIONS

Gastro-intestinal reflux disease (GERD) is a common ailment, and several classes of medications are used to treat GERD; all can interfere with antipsychotics (Flockhart et al. 2000b). Cimetidine can produce a substantial decrease in plasma concentrations of chlorpromazine, which may have adverse clinical effects in patients treated with relatively low doses of the antipsychotic agent. It is not known whether other antipsychotic agents are similarly affected, but levels of clozapine may increase. Cimetidine is a non-specific P450 inhibitor and an inhibitor of glucuronidation and, as such, can potentially inhibit the metabolism of many psychotropics; the case report by Szymanski (1991) of an interaction with clozapine is consistent with such an effect. Clinicians should be prepared to either increased or decreased antipsychotic levels when cimetidine is added. Other H_2 blockers might be considered instead of cimetidine for patients on clozapine.

Gastrointestinal Agents: Proton Pump Inhibitors

EVIDENCE OF INTERACTION

In two clozapine-treated patients, a reduction of clozapine levels by more than 40% was reported after omeprazole was added (Frick et al. 2003).

MECHANISM

Omeprazole can induce CYP1A2, one of the enzymes responsible for clozapine metabolism (Meyer 1996). Lansoprazole, but not pantoprazole, can similarly induce CYP1A2.

CLINICAL IMPLICATIONS

Omeprazole may lower clozapine levels. The combination of a proton pump inhibitor with clozapine is used frequently because of the possibility of gastrointestinal discomfort in patients treated with clozapine, and interactions should be anticipated. Pantoprazole might be considered as a first choice to avoid interactions. The degree to which reduced gastric acidity from proton pump inhibitors affects the absorption of antipsychotics is unknown.

Grapefruit Juice

EVIDENCE OF INTERACTION

Twelve patients with schizophrenia who were receiving haloperidol (12 mg daily) were given grapefruit juice for 7 days (Yasui et al. 1999b). No changes in haloperidol or reduced haloperidol serum concentrations were noted, nor were changes in side effects and psychopathology observed. Lane et al. (2001) studied 15 patients treated with stable clozapine doses; 2 weeks of grapefruit juice (250 mg two times a day) had no effect on clozapine and its metabolites or measures of drug efficacy and side effects.

MECHANISM

Grapefruit juice contains substances that can substantially inhibit the intestinal (but not the hepatic) CYP3A4 enzyme as well as P-gp. The effect is not merely a matter of timing, because the inhibition of the enzyme is prolonged rather than transient.

CLINICAL SIGNIFICANCE

If large quantities of grapefruit are consumed, first-pass metabolism may be altered. Reassuringly, studies by Lane (2001) and Yasui (1999b) did not find an effect on clozapine or haloperidol clearance when grapefruit juice was repeatedly given.

Herbal Preparations

EVIDENCE OF INTERACTION

Two patients with schizophrenia developed severe EPS after a period of heavy betel nut (*Areca catechu*) consumption (Deahl 1989). Both patients additionally received depot neuroleptics, and the anticholinergic agent procyclidine. Betel nut combined with flupentixol or fluphenazine was also reported to result in extrapyramidal symptoms (Fugh-Berman 2000). These reports contrast with a cross-sectional study of patients with schizophrenia in Palau, Micronesia, comparing 40 chewers of betel nut with 30 nonchewers (Sullivan et al. 2000). Whereas betel nut chewers had milder psychiatric symptomatology, they did not experience more EPS. In a case series of four patients, kava (*Piper methysticum*) was thought to be responsible for EPS (Schelosky et al. 1995).

MECHANISM

The betel nut contains a pro-cholinergic alkaloid, arecoline, that can directly antagonize anticholinergic medications or possibly shift the dopamine–acetylcholine balance toward a propensity for EPS. The root extracts of the kava plant might possess antidopaminergic properties, as suggested experimentally in mice. Other interactions (such as between ginseng and haloperidol, or between primrose oil (rich in the essential fatty acid, linoleic acid) and phenothiazines (Wong et al. 1998)) are poorly characterized and not understood.

CLINICAL SIGNIFICANCE

Herbal remedies are widely used (Eisenberg et al. 1998) and not always reported or inquired about. Because of possible worsening of EPS or loss of antipsychotic efficacy, betel nut and kava are probably best avoided in patients treated with antipsychotics. While not yet reported for antipsychotics, St. John's wort is a potent inducer of CYP3A4 and has the potential to substantially lower 3A4 substrates (Markowitz et al. 2003), resulting in loss of efficacy. At a minimum, herbal co-medication should be inquired about (Cupp 1999), because herbal medications can produce serious psychiatric and neurological adverse effects (Ernst 2003).

Lithium

EVIDENCE OF INTERACTION

In one study, the co-administration of lithium carbonate was associated with 40% lower peak plasma concentrations of chlorpromazine (Rivera-Calimlim et al. 1978). In rats given lithium and chlorpromazine orally, the concentrations of chlorpromazine in plasma and brain were significantly lower and the percent of chlorpromazine remaining in the stomach was significantly higher than in matched controls given chlorpromazine alone (Rivera-Calimlim 1976). These findings have not been replicated, and their clinical significance is not established. Of greater concern is the question of a potential neuro-toxic reaction to the combination of lithium and conventional antipsychotic agents. Cohen and Cohen (1974) first reported four cases of an irreversible neurologic reaction to the combination of lithium with haloperidol. In this and subsequent reports, a toxic interaction between lithium and antipsychotic agents was suspected and described as being similar to NMS. It consisted of confusion, impaired consciousness, rigidity, tremor, akathisia, akinesia, dyskinesia, dystonia, and, less commonly, cerebellar signs and hyperthermia (Cohen and Cohen 1974, Prakash 1982). Prakash et al. (1982) reviewed 39 reported cases and noted that 67% involved haloperidol, whereas the other third were associated with thioridazine, perphenazine, flupentixol, or thiothixene. It remains unclear whether this rare phenomenon is specific to an interaction of lithium with haloperidol, particularly since a similar syndrome has been reported with thioridazine and lithium (Spring 1979), and even with clozapine and lithium (Pope 1986). Haloperidol may have been implicated because it was used very commonly in combination with lithium. Prakash et al. also noted that in 10% of cases the neurological deficits, including dementia, persisted after the discontinuation of the psychotropics. The early case reports emphasized high lithium levels as a risk factor, whereas a study of 22 manic patients determined that the six patients in whom neurotoxicity developed with the combination were receiving relatively high doses of haloperidol but did not have high serum levels of lithium (Miller and Menninger 1987).

Despite the considerable attention that this putative drug interaction has received, whether a drug interaction is in fact responsible for this neurotoxic syndrome continues to be debated. Two groups retrospectively studied a total of 494 patients treated with lithium and an antipsychotic drug and did not identify a single case of this neurotoxic reaction (Miller and Menninger 1987, Goldney and Spence 1986). Similar neurotoxicity can occur as an adverse reaction to lithium or the antipsychotic agents alone, rather than as a true drug interaction. For example, lithium toxicity can manifest as confusion and ataxia, as well as cogwheel rigidity and irreversible nonspecific cerebellar neurotoxicity in the absence of an antipsychotic agent (Asnis et al. 1979, Kane et al. 1978, Schou 1984). In addition, some cases of neurotoxicity attributed to a lithium-neuroleptic syndrome may actually represent NMS. The co-administration of lithium has not been established firmly as a risk factor for NMS, although recent evidence supports this possibility (Rosebush and Stewart 1989). Interestingly, two cases were reported of bipolar patients who had relapses of NMS when rechallenged with lithium alone (Susman and Addonizio 1987). Finally, several reports have suggested that lithium co-administration may increase the frequency and severity of reversible EPS in patients treated with conventional neuroleptics (Addonizio 1985, Sachdev 1986). However, Goldney and Spence (1986) found no increase in EPS in 69 manic patients treated with a combination of lithium and a neuroleptic agent, compared with 60 manic patients treated with a neuroleptic alone. More recently, Goldman (1996) used the FDA spontaneous reporting database and the published literature to conclude that indeed a spectrum of pathology exists in lithium–antipsychotic combinations.

Among the atypical agents, few reports exist on combinations with lithium. In one case, a patient became disoriented when 5 mg olanzapine was added to longstanding lithium treatment (Swartz 1996). Chen and Cardasis (1996) described the development of a delirium in a lithium-treated elderly woman when 6 mg daily risperidone replaced 5 mg daily thiothixene. A reversible neurologic syndrome was associated with the combination of risperidone and lithium (Swanson et al. 1995), and with the combination of clozapine and lithium (Blake et al. 1992). Small et al. (2003) examined the safety and tolerability of added lithium to clozapine therapy in a randomized trial of 20 patients with schizophrenia and schizoaffective disorder. No clinical effect was discernible in the 10 patients with schizophrenia, but two of them developed neurotoxic reactions. By contrast, the patients with schizoaffective disorder showed improved psychopathology and no adverse effects.

MECHANISM

Although lithium may elevate the plasma concentrations of chlorpromazine by undetermined pharmacokinetic mechanisms, such an effect is poorly established. Rare central neurotoxic reactions, if they occur, are more likely the result of synergistic pharmacodynamic interactions. Both antipsychotics and lithium can produce extrapyramidal and neurotoxic symptoms when administered alone, so that additive toxicity remains possible. Whether co-administration may increase the risk for NMS remains an important question.

CLINICAL SIGNIFICANCE

Reports of a potentially irreversible, though rare, neurotoxic syndrome associated with the combined use of lithium and antipsychotic agents are of great concern, but it is unclear whether this effect represents a drug interaction or neurotoxicity that can be produced by either drug administered alone. Given the high morbidity of this rare syndrome, clinicians should monitor patients with particular care when administering lithium with an antipsychotic agent, and avoid high serum levels of lithium as well as high antipsychotic doses. The evidence of a greater risk of neurotoxicity associated with haloperidol or risperidone than with other antipsychotic agents remains unconvincing, and does not merit a specific avoidance of the combined use of haloperidol or risperidone and lithium, in our opinion.

In contrast to concerns about combining lithium with clozapine, lithium can be used to increase the white blood cell count in patients who have a low baseline count but who are considered for clozapine treatment. This maneuver allows treatment with clozapine in situations that would otherwise exclude patients from a potentially effective treatment (Adityanjee 1995, Blier et al. 1998, Silverstone 1998, Boshes et al. 2001).

Modafinil

EVIDENCE OF INTERACTION

Narendran et al. (2002) described a worsening of psychosis in a previously stable 61-year-old patient with schizophrenia in whom a high dose of modafinil (200 mg four times daily) was added for clozapine-induced sedation. No blood levels were reported. A second report described the development of dizziness and an unsteady gait after 100 mg of modafinil was added for clozapine-induced sedation (Dequardo 2002); clozapine blood levels increased by 64% (856 to 1400 ng/mL) following addition of modafinil.

MECHANISM

No pharmacodynamic mechanism has been identified to explain a putative worsening of psychosis using the clozapine–modafinil combination. Because modafinil inhibits CYPC19, and clozapine is at least partially metabolized through this enzyme, a pharmacokinetic interaction involving CYP2C19 is possible, but other enzymes might be involved as well, because the metabolisms of both clozapine and modafinil are complex.

CLINICAL SIGNIFICANCE

Modafinil has been used clinically to treat antipsychotic-induced sedation (Makela et al. 2003). Both reported cases of antipsychotic–modafinil interaction involved clozapine. Therapeutic drug monitoring should be considered if modafinil is added for clozapine-induced sedation, because clozapine levels might rise sufficiently to produce clinically significant side effects. The safety of the combination has not been established.

Stimulants

EVIDENCE OF INTERACTION

Antipsychotics can counteract many of the signs of stimulant toxicity. In addition, a few studies have explored the use of stimulants to control the side effects of antipsychotics, such as sedation and weight gain. Both haloperidol and chlorpromazine block amphetamine toxicity in dogs administered lethal doses of amphetamine (10 mg/kg intravenously) (Catraras et al. 1975). In rats, the metabolism of amphetamine is slowed by chlorpromazine but not by haloperidol: Lemberger et al. 1970. Because chlorpromazine may impair the metabolism of amphetamine and may exacerbate amphetamine-induced cardiovascular instability, chlorpromazine is not recommended for the treatment of amphetamine toxicity. A high-potency agent like haloperidol is less likely to produce adverse interactions but is not free of them. Several case reports suggested the possibility of an increased risk for dystonic reactions and neuroleptic malignant syndrome when haloperidol was given to cocaine-abusing patients. In a subsequent prospective study, van Harten et al. (1998) confirmed cocaine as a major risk factor for neuroleptic-induced acute dystonia by comparing nine cocaine users (five with schizophrenia) to 20 nonusers (15 with schizophrenia). Farren et al. (2000) pretreated eight cocaine-dependent patients with up to 50 mg clozapine, followed 2 hours later by intranasal cocaine. Clozapine treatment increased cocaine levels in a dose-dependent manner, and one patient had a near-syncope, consistent with an earlier report (Hameedi et al. 1996).

Chronic amphetamine abuse appears to produce sensitization, so that progressively smaller doses may produce the same level of response over time. Early studies suggested that psychotic symptoms develop in many normal subjects if they are given a sufficiently large amount of amphetamine; this psychotogenic effect is at least partially blocked by antipsychotics. However, stimulant abuse may have long-lasting effects on dopamine systems, and this can interfere with antipsychotic efficacy. Bowers et al. (1990) reported that a past history of stimulant abuse was associated with significantly poorer response to antipsychotic treatment and with lower baseline plasma concentration of the main metabolite of dopamine, homovanillic acid (HVA).

The stimulants also have been evaluated as a possible adjuvant treatment to control antipsychotic side effects. Burke and Sebastian (1993) reported that methylphenidate (5 to 30 mg daily) decreased clozapine-induced sedation in 2 patients without interfering with antipsychotic effect or adding other side effects. In contrast, Miller (1996) reported a case in which the effects of methylphenidate seemed to wear off a couple weeks after dose adjustment, and pre-existent tardive myoclonus worsened with each increase in methylphenidate dose. (Also see the Modafinil section in this chapter.)

MECHANISM

Although only studied in rats, chlorpromazine may elevate amphetamine plasma concentrations by impairing hepatic metabolism. Other interactions between these two classes of drugs are most likely pharmacodynamic in nature, because the stimulants increase the release of dopaminergic and norepinephrine. In addition, stimulant abuse may cause enduring changes in dopamine receptor levels and intracellular signaling pathways that are manifest clinically as behavioral sensitization to stimulant administration and possibly as diminished therapeutic response to antipsychotic agents and increased risk for motor side effects.

CLINICAL IMPLICATIONS

Because of the risk of cardiovascular complications, as well as a possible interference with hepatic metabolism of amphetamine, it is best to treat amphetamine intoxication with moderate doses of a high-potency antipsychotic.

Although a low dose of methylphenidate may improve clozapine-induced sedation, the routine use of stimulants with antipsychotic agents is not recommended because of the risk of exacerbating psychosis. The safety of prescribing clozapine in patients who use cocaine has not been established. Finally, clinicians should be aware that stimulant abuse can significantly impair antipsychotic efficacy, and past stimulant abuse may predict subsequent poor response. This is particularly relevant in the treatment of schizophrenic patients, because this population prefers stimulants, along with alcohol and cigarettes, as substances of abuse.

Tobacco

EVIDENCE OF INTERACTION

Surveys of patients with schizophrenia have reported rates of cigarette smoking between 60% and 90%, more than double the rate for the general population. Factors contributing to high smoking rates include institutionalization, impaired judgment, poor impulse control, and partial correction of attentional deficits in schizophrenia (Adler et al.

1992, Adler et al. 1998). These finding have led to a "self-medication" model for cigarette smoking in schizophrenia.

Smoking also might reflect an attempt by patients to lower their antipsychotic plasma drug level by taking advantage of a pharmacokinetic interaction between tobacco and antipsychotics. Patients with schizophrenia who smoke were found to receive conventional antipsychotic doses up to twice as high as patients who do not smoke (Goff et al. 1992). Cigarette smoking increases the clearance of haloperidol and fluphenazine by 44% to 67% and of fluphenazine decanoate by 133% (Ereshefsky et al. 1985, Jann et al. 1986). Haring et al. (1990) reported that cigarette smoking lowered steady-state plasma concentrations of clozapine in men by 32% but not in women. Using data form 9894 samples collected for the purpose of therapeutic drug monitoring, Rostami-Hodjegan et al. (2004) estimated that smoking lowers clozapine levels by about 50%, in both males and females, a percentage very similar to an estimate by Meyer (2001), deduced from six patients who quit smoking and for whom clozapine plasma levels were measured before and after quitting. Stimmel and Falloon (1983) described a patient with schizophrenia in whom EPS developed in association with an elevation of serum chlorpromazine levels when he stopped smoking cigarettes. The neurological side effects returned to baseline when this patient resumed smoking. Data from two naturalistic patient samples in whom olanzapine levels were determined for therapeutic drug monitoring showed that smokers received higher oral olanzapine doses, and that nonsmokers achieved a higher olanzapine concentration-to-dose ratio (Skogh et al. 2002, Gex-Fabry et al. 2003). In an experimental study, the olanzapine concentration-to-dose ratio was closely correlated to CYP1A2 activity (Carrillo et al. 2003).

Cigarette smoking also may affect antipsychotic efficacy and EPS through pharmacodynamic actions on brain cholinergic and dopaminergic systems. Smokers in the general populations may be at lower risk for idiopathic Parkinson's disease than nonsmokers. Nicotine improves attention, memory, and mood, and transiently may improve deficits in processing auditory stimuli that are reported to be characteristic of schizophrenia (Adler et al. 1998). Withdrawal from nicotine may produce adverse effects in some patients. Greeman and McClellan (1991) observed that attempts to ban smoking on an inpatient unit resulted in the exacerbation of symptoms in patients with schizophrenia.

MECHANISM

As a strong inducer of hepatic microsomal enzymes, particularly but not limited to CYP1A2, cigarette smoke can substantially lower plasma concentrations of typical antipsychotics and of those atypical antipsychotics with significant CYP1A2 metabolism [clozapine and olanzapine (Gex-Fabry et al. 2003)]. For typical antipsychotics, the mechanism must involve mechanisms other than CYP1A2 induction, because CYP1A2 is not thought to be a significant pathway; the induction of glucuronidation by polycyclic aromatic carbons in cigarette smoke is one possibility (Liston et al. 2001). In addition, nicotine may have activating effects on brain dopamine systems, resulting in pharmacodynamic interactions with antipsychotic agents. Cigarette smoking may reduce EPS, improve mood, and improve the attentional and neuropsychological impairments characteristic of schizophrenia. These beneficial effects may reinforce cigarette smoking, and lead patients to "self-medicate" with this agent.

CLINICAL IMPLICATIONS

Admission to "smoke-free" inpatient units may substantially alter a patient's metabolism of antipsychotic medications, in addition to worsening EPS and possibly exacerbating some clinical symptoms of the illness. From a pharmacokinetic point of view, this is most likely relevant only if the admission lasts more than just a few days. Rising plasma levels following forced smoking cessation can be particularly relevant in clozapine-treated patients (Zullino et al. 2002). Similarly, clozapine dose titrations in smoke-free settings will underestimate the dose needed once patients are discharged and resume smoking. The use of transdermal nicotine patches may reduce patients' discomfort but does not prevent the changes in antipsychotic metabolism, because constituents in tobacco smoke other than nicotine induce hepatic microsomal enzymes. Nicotine patches should be used with caution in unsupervised settings, because schizophrenia patients may continue to smoke heavily and thereby expose themselves to toxic nicotine levels. (Also see the section Bupropion in this chapter.)

REFERENCES

Addonizio G: Rapid induction of extrapyramidal side effects with combined use of lithium and neuroleptics. J Clin Psychopharmacol 5(5): 296–298, 1985.

Adityanjee: Modification of clozapine-induced leukopenia and neutropenia with lithium carbonate [letter]. Am J Psychiatry 152(4): 648–649, 1995.

Adler LE et al.: Normalization by nicotine of deficient auditory sensory gating in the relatives of schizophrenics. Biol Psychiatry 32: 607–616, 1992.

Adler LE et al.: Schizophrenia, sensory gating, and nicotinic receptors. Schizophr Bull 24(2): 189–202, 1998.

Ahmed I et al.: Possible interaction between fluoxetine and pimozide causing sinus bradycardia. Can J Psychiatry 38(1): 62–63, 1993.

Alao AO, Yolles JC: Isoniazid-induced psychosis. Ann Pharmacother 32(9): 889–891, 1998.

Alexander HE, Jr. et al.: Hypotension and cardiopulmonary arrest associated with concurrent haloperidol and propranolol therapy. JAMA 252(1): 87–88, 1984.

Allen RM, Flemenbaum A: Delirium associated with combined fluphenazine-clonidine therapy. J Clin Psychiatry 40(5): 236–237, 1979.

Amchin J et al.: Effect of venlafaxine on the pharmacokinetics of risperidone. J Clin Pharmacol 39(3): 297–309, 1999.

Arana GW et al.: Does carbamazepine-induced reduction of plasma haloperidol levels worsen psychotic symptoms? Am J Psychiatry 143(5): 650–651, 1986.

Asnis GM et al.: Cogwheel rigidity during chronic lithium therapy. Am J Psychiatry 136(9): 1225–1226, 1979.

Avenoso A et al.: Interaction between fluoxetine and haloperidol: pharmacokinetic and clinical implications. Pharmacol Res 35(4): 335–339, 1997.

Baker LA et al.: The withdrawal of benztropine mesylate in chronic schizophrenic patients. Br J Psychiatry 143: 584–590, 1983.

Balsara JJ et al.: Effect of drugs influencing central serotonergic mechanisms on haloperidol-induced catalepsy. Psychopharmacology (Berl) 62(1): 67–69, 1979.

Ban TA, St. Jean A: The effects of phenothiazines on the electrocardiogram. Can Med Assoc J 91: 537–540, 1964.

Barbhaiya RH et al.: Investigation of pharmacokinetic and pharmacodynamic interactions after co-administration of nefazodone and haloperidol. J Clin Psychopharmacol 16(1): 26–34, 1996.

Barsa JA, Saunders JC: A comparative study of tranylcypromine and pargyline. Psychopharmacologia 6(4): 295–298, 1964.

Becker RE: Implications of the efficacy of thiothixene and a chlorpromazine-imipramine combination for depression in schizophrenia. Am J Psychiatry 140(2): 208–211, 1983.

Beedham C et al.: Ziprasidone metabolism, aldehyde oxidase, and clinical implications. J Clin Psychopharmacol 23(3): 229–232, 2003.

Berecz R et al.: Relationship between risperidone and 9-hydroxy-risperidone plasma concentrations and CYP2D6 enzyme activity in psychiatric patients. Pharmacopsychiatry 35(6): 231–234, 2002.

Berk M et al.: Efficacy of mirtazapine add on therapy to haloperidol in the treatment of the negative symptoms of schizophrenia: a double-blind randomized placebo-controlled study. Int Clin Psychopharmacol 16(2): 87–92, 2001.

Blake LM et al.: Reversible neurologic symptoms with clozapine and lithium. J Clin Psychopharmacol 12(4): 297–299, 1992.

Blier P et al.: Lithium and clozapine-induced neutropenia/agranulocytosis. Int Clin Psychopharmacol 13(3): 137–140, 1998.

Bock JL et al.: Desipramine hydroxylation: variability and effect of antipsychotic drugs. Clin Pharmacol Ther 33(3): 322–328, 1983.

Bondolfi G et al.: The effect of fluoxetine on the pharmacokinetics and safety of risperidone in psychiatric patients. Pharmacopsychiatry 35(2): 50–56, 2002.

Bork JA et al.: A pilot study on risperidone metabolism: the role of cytochromes P450 2D6 and 3A. J Clin Psychiatry 60(7): 469–476, 1999.

Boshes RA et al.: Initiation of clozapine therapy in a patient with preexisting leukopenia: a discussion of the rationale of current treatment options. Ann Clin Psychiatry 13(4): 233–237, 2001.

Bowen S et al.: Effect of coffee and tea on blood levels and efficacy of antipsychotic drugs. Lancet 1: 1217–1218, 1981.

Bowers Jr. MB et al.: Psychotogenic drug use and neuroleptic response. Schizophr Bull 16(1): 81–85, 1990.

Brenner LM et al.: Short-term use of disulfiram with clozapine. J Clin Psychopharmacol 14(3): 213–215, 1994.

Bristol-Myers Squibb Company: Product Information: Abilify (Aripiprazole) tablets. Princeton, NJ, 2002.

Brosen K, Gram LF: Clinical significance of the sparteine/debrisoquine oxidation polymorphism. Eur J Clin Pharmacol 36(6): 537–547, 1989.

Bucci L: The negative symptoms of schizophrenia and the monoamine oxidase inhibitors. Psychopharmacology (Berl) 91(1): 104–108, 1987.

Burke M, Sebastian CS: Treatment of clozapine sedation [letter]. Am J Psychiatry 150(12): 1900–1901, 1993.

Byrne A, O'Shea B: Adverse interaction between cimetidine and chlorpromazine in two cases of chronic schizophrenia. Br J Psychiatry 155: 413–415, 1989.

Caley CF, Cooper CK: Ziprasidone: the fifth atypical antipsychotic. Ann Pharmacother 36(5): 839–851, 2002.

Callaghan JT et al.: Olanzapine. Pharmacokinetic and pharmacodynamic profile. Clin Pharmacokinet 37(3): 177–193, 1999.

Carpenter WT, Jr. et al.: Diazepam treatment of early signs of exacerbation in schizophrenia. Am J Psychiatry 156(2): 299–303, 1999.

Carrillo JA et al.: Role of the smoking-induced cytochrome P450 (CYP)1A2 and polymorphic CYP2D6 in steady-state concentration of olanzapine. J Clin Psychopharmacol 23(2): 119–127, 2003.

Casey DE et al.: Effect of divalproex combined with olanzapine or risperidone in patients with an acute exacerbation of schizophrenia. Neuropsychopharmacology 28(1): 182–192, 2003.

Centorrino F et al.: Serum concentrations of clozapine and its major metabolites: effects of cotreatment with fluoxetine or valproate. Am J Psychiatry 151(1): 123–125, 1994a.

Centorrino F et al.: Serum levels of clozapine and norclozapine in patients treated with selective serotonin reuptake inhibitors. Am J Psychiatry 153(6): 820–822, 1996.

Centorrino F et al.: Clozapine and metabolites: concentrations in serum and clinical findings during treatment of chronically psychotic patients. J Clin Psychopharmacol 14(2): 119–125, 1994b.

Chen B, Cardasis W: Delirium induced by lithium and risperidone combination. Am J Psychiatry 153(9): 1233–1234, 1996.

Chetty M et al.: Important metabolites to measure in pharmacodynamic studies of chlorpromazine. Ther Drug Monit 16(1): 30–36, 1994.

Chien CP et al.: Prophylactic usage of antiparkinsonian drugs for akinesia [proceedings]. Psychopharmacol Bull 15(2): 75–78, 1979.

Chouinard G et al.: Amitriptyline-perphenazine interaction in ambulatory schizophrenic patients. A controlled study of drug interaction. Arch Gen Psychiatry 32(10): 1295–1307, 1975.

Chouinard G et al.: Potentiation of haloperidol by methyldopa in the treatment of schizophrenic patients. Curr Ther Res Clin Exp 15(7): 473–483, 1973a.

Chouinard G et al.: Alpha methyldopa-chlorpromazine interaction in schizophrenic patients. Curr Ther Res Clin Exp 15(2): 60–72, 1973b.

Cobb CD et al.: Possible interaction between clozapine and lorazepam [letter]. Am J Psychiatry 148(11): 1606–1607, 1991.

Cohen LG et al.: Erythromycin-induced clozapine toxic reaction. Arch Intern Med 156(6): 675–677, 1996.

Cohen WJ, Cohen NH: Lithium carbonate, haloperidol, and irreversible brain damage. JAMA 230(9): 1283–1287, 1974.

Conca A et al.: A case of pharmacokinetic interference in comedication of clozapine and valproic acid. Pharmacopsychiatry 33(6): 234–235, 2000.

Creese I et al.: 3H-Haloperidol binding to dopamine receptors in rat corpus striatum: influence of chlorpromazine metabolites and derivatives. Eur J Pharmacol 47(3): 291–296, 1978.

Creese I et al.: Dopamine receptor binding predicts clinical and pharmacological potencies of antischizophrenic drugs. Science 192: 481–483, 1976.

Cupp MJ: Herbal remedies: adverse effects and drug interactions. Am Fam Physician 59(5): 1239–1245, 1999.

Cvetkovic RS, Goa KL: Lopinavir/ritonavir: a review of its use in the management of HIV infection. Drugs 63(8): 769–802, 2003.

Dahl SG: Plasma level monitoring of antipsychotic drugs. Clinical utility. Clin Pharmacokinet 11(1): 36–61, 1986.

Dahl-Puustinen ML et al.: Disposition of perphenazine is related to polymorphic debrisoquin hydroxylation in human beings. Clin Pharmacol Ther 46(1): 78–81, 1989.

Daniel WA et al.: The influence of selective serotonin reuptake inhibitors (SSRIs) on the pharmacokinetics of thioridazine and its metabolites: in vivo and in vitro studies. Exp Toxicol Pathol 51(4–5): 309–314, 1999.

de Leon J et al.: Pilot study of the cytochrome P450-2D6 genotype in a psychiatric state hospital. Am J Psychiatry 155(9): 1278–1280, 1998.

de Leon J, Diaz FJ: Serious respiratory infections can increase clozapine levels and contribute to side effects: a case report. Prog Neuropsychopharmacol Biol Psychiatry 27(6): 1059–1063, 2003.

Deahl M: Betel nut-induced extrapyramidal syndrome: an unusual drug interaction. Mov Disord 4(4): 330–332, 1989.

Dequardo JR: Modafinil-associated clozapine toxicity [letter]. Am J Psychiatry 159(7): 1243–1244, 2002.

Descotes J et al.: Study of thioridazine cardiotoxic effects by means of His bundle activity recording. Acta Pharmacol Toxicol (Copenh) 44(5): 370–376, 1979.

Desta Z et al.: Effect of clarithromycin on the pharmacokinetics and pharmacodynamics of pimozide in healthy poor and extensive metabolizers of cytochrome P450 2D6 (CYP2D6). Clin Pharmacol Ther 65(1): 10–20, 1999.

DeVane CL, Nemeroff CB: Clinical pharmacokinetics of quetiapine. An atypical antipsychotic. Clin Pharmacokinet 40(7): 509–522, 2001.

Di Salvo TG, O'Gara PT: Torsade de pointes caused by high-dose intravenous haloperidol in cardiac patients. Clin Cardiol 18(5): 285–290, 1995.

Douyon R et al.: Neuroleptic augmentation with alprazolam: clinical effects and pharmacokinetic correlates. Am J Psychiatry 146(2): 231–234, 1989.

Dresser GK et al.: Pharmacokinetic-pharmacodynamic consequences and clinical relevance of cytochrome P450 3A4 inhibition. Clin Pharmacokinet 38(1): 41–57, 2000.

Dreyfuss J et al.: Fluphenazine enanthate and fluphenazine decanoate: intramuscular injection and esterification as requirements for slow-release characteristics in dogs. J Pharm Sci 65(9): 1310–1315, 1976a.

Dreyfuss J et al.: Release and elimination of 14C-fluphenazine enanthate and decanoate esters administered in sesame oil to dogs. J Pharm Sci 65(4): 502–507, 1976b.

Drolet B et al.: Pimozide (Orap) prolongs cardiac repolarization by blocking the rapid component of the delayed rectifier potassium current in native cardiac myocytes. J Cardiovasc Pharmacol Ther 6(3): 255–260, 2001.

Duggal HS, Fetchko J: Serotonin syndrome and atypical antipsychotics. Am J Psychiatry 159(4): 672–673, 2002.

Dysken MW et al.: Fluphenazine pharmacokinetics and therapeutic response. Psychopharmacology (Berl) 73(3): 205–210, 1981.

Eggert Hansen C et al.: Clinical pharmacokinetic studies of perphenazine. Br J Clin Pharmacol 3(5): 915–923, 1976.

Eisenberg DM et al.: Trends in alternative medicine use in the United States, 1990–1997: results of a follow-up national survey. JAMA 280(18): 1569–1575, 1998.

el-Yousef MK, Manier DH: Letter: Tricyclic antidepressants and phenothiazines. JAMA 229(11): 1419, 1974.

Ereshefsky L et al.: Antidepressant drug interactions and the cytochrome P450 system. The role of cytochrome P450 2D6. Clin Pharmacokinet 29 Suppl 1: 10–8 discussion 18–19, 1995.

Ereshefsky L et al.: Effects of smoking on fluphenazine clearance in psychiatric inpatients. Biol Psychiatry 20(3): 329–332, 1985.

Ernst E: Serious psychiatric and neurological adverse effects of herbal medicines—a systematic review. Acta Psychiatr Scand 108(2): 83–91, 2003.

Evans DL et al.: Intestinal dilatation associated with phenothiazine therapy: a case report and literature review. Am J Psychiatry 136(7): 970–972, 1979.

Evins AE et al.: A pilot trial of bupropion added to cognitive behavioral therapy for smoking cessation in schizophrenia. Nicotine Tob Res 3(4): 397–403, 2001.

Evins AE, Tisdale T: Bupropion and smoking cessation [letter]. Am J Psychiatry 156(5): 798–799, 1999.

Fabrazzo M et al.: Fluvoxamine increases plasma and urinary levels of clozapine and its major metabolites in a time- and dose-dependent manner. J Clin Psychopharmacol 20(6): 708–710, 2000.

Facciola G et al.: Small effects of valproic acid on the plasma concentrations of clozapine and its major metabolites in patients with schizophrenic or affective disorders. Ther Drug Monit 21(3): 341–345, 1999.

Fang J et al.: Comparison of cytotoxicity of a quaternary pyridinium metabolite of haloperidol (HP+) with neurotoxin N-methyl-4-phenylpyridinium (MPP+) towards cultured dopaminergic neuroblastoma cells. Psychopharmacology (Berl) 121(3): 373–378, 1995.

Fang J et al.: Metabolism of risperidone to 9-hydroxyrisperidone by human cytochromes P450 2D6 and 3A4. Naunyn Schmiedebergs Arch Pharmacol 359(2): 147–151, 1999.

Fann WE et al.: Chlorpromazine: effects of antacids on its gastrointestinal absorption. J Clin Pharmacol 13(10): 388–390, 1973.

Fann WE et al.: Chlorpromazine reversal of the antihypertensive action of guanethidine. Lancet 2(7721): 436–437, 1971.

Farde L et al.: D1-, D2-. and 5-HT2-receptor occupancy in clozapine-treated patients. J Clin Psychiatry 55 (9, suppl B): 67–69, 1994.

Farde L et al.: Positron emission tomographic analysis of central D1 and D2 dopamine receptor occupancy in patients treated with classical neuroleptics and clozapine. Relation to extrapyramidal side effects. Arch Gen Psychiatry 49: 538–544, 1992.

Farren CK et al.: Significant interaction between clozapine and cocaine in cocaine addicts. Drug Alcohol Depend 59(2): 153–163, 2000.

Flockhart DA et al.: Studies on the mechanism of a fatal clarithromycin-pimozide interaction in a patient with Tourette syndrome. J Clin Psychopharmacol 20(3): 317–324, 2000a.

Flockhart DA et al.: Selection of drugs to treat gastro-intestinal reflux disease: the role of drug interactions. Clin Pharmacokinet 39(4): 295–309, 2000b.

Forrest FM et al.: Modification of chlorpromazine metabolism by some other drugs frequently administered to psychiatric patients. Biol Psychiatry 2(1): 53–58, 1970.

Forsman A, Ohman R: Studies on serum protein binding of haloperidol. Curr Ther Res Clin Exp 21(2): 245–255, 1977.

Freudenreich O, Goff DC: Antipsychotic combination therapy in schizophrenia. A review of efficacy and risks of current combinations. Acta Psychiatr Scand 106(5): 323–330, 2003.

Frick A et al.: Omeprazole reduces clozapine plasma concentrations—a case report. Pharmacopsychiatry 36(3): 121–123, 2003.

Friedman LJ et al.: Clozapine—a novel antipsychotic agent [letter]. N Engl J Med 325(7): 518–519, 1991.

Fruncillo RJ et al.: Severe hypotension associated with concurrent clonidine and antipsychotic medication [letter]. Am J Psychiatry 142(2): 274, 1985.

Fugh-Berman A: Herb-drug interactions. Lancet 355(9198)((9198)): 134–138, 2000.

Fulton B, Goa KL: Olanzapine. A review of its pharmacological properties and therapeutic efficacy in the management of schizophrenia and related psychoses. Drugs 53(2): 281–298, 1997.

Funderburg LG et al.: Seizure following addition of erythromycin to clozapine treatment [letter]. Am J Psychiatry 151(12): 1840–1841, 1994.

Gallicano KD et al.: Induction of zidovudine glucuronidation and amination pathways by rifampicin in HIV-infected patients. Br J Clin Pharmacol 48(2): 168–179, 1999.

Gardos G et al.: Anticholinergic challenge and neuroleptic withdrawal. Changes in dyskinesia and symptom measures. Arch Gen Psychiatry 41(11): 1030–1035, 1984.

Garver DL: Neuroleptic drug levels and antipsychotic effects: a difficult correlation potential advantage of free (or derivative) versus total plasma levels. J Clin Psychopharmacol 9(4): 277–281, 1989.

Gautier J et al.: Influence of the antiparkinsonian drugs on the plasma level of neuroleptics. Biol Psychiatry 12(3): 389–399, 1977.

George TP et al.: A placebo controlled trial of bupropion for smoking cessation in schizophrenia. Biol Psychiatry 52(1): 53–61, 2002.

Gerlach J et al.: Antiparkinsonian agents and long-term neuroleptic treatment. Effect of G 31.406, orphenadrine, and placebo on parkinsonism, schizophrenic symptoms, depression and anxiety. Acta Psychiatr Scand 55(4): 251–260, 1977.

Gerson SL et al.: N-desmethylclozapine: a clozapine metabolite that suppresses haemopoiesis. Br J Haematol 86(3): 555–561, 1994.

Gex-Fabry M et al.: Therapeutic drug monitoring of olanzapine: the combined effect of age, gender, smoking, and comedication. Ther Drug Monit 25(1): 46–53, 2003.

Ghaemi SN (ed.): *Polypharmacy in Psychiatry*, New York, Marcel Dekker, Inc., 2002.

Gilder DA et al.: A comparison of the abilities of chlorpromazine and molindone to interact adversely with guanethidine. J Pharmacol Exp Ther 198(2): 255–263, 1976.

Giles TD, Modlin RK: Death associated with ventricular arrhythmia and thioridazine hydrochloride. JAMA 205(2): 108–110, 1968.

Ginsburg J, Duff RS: Effect of chlorpromazine on adrenaline vasoconstriction in man. Br J Pharmacol 11: 180, 1956.

Giordano J et al.: Fatal paralytic ileus complicating phenothiazine therapy. South Med J 68(3): 351–353, 1975.

Glassman AH, Bigger JT, Jr.: Antipsychotic drugs: prolonged QTc interval, torsade de pointes, and sudden death. Am J Psychiatry 158(11): 1774–1782, 2001.

Goff DC et al.: A placebo-controlled trial of fluoxetine added to neuroleptic in patients with schizophrenia. Psychopharmacology (Berl) 117(4): 417–423, 1995.

Goff DC et al.: A placebo-controlled trial of selegiline (L-deprenyl) in the treatment of tardive dyskinesia. Biol Psychiatry 33(10): 700–706, 1993.

Goff DC et al.: Cigarette smoking in schizophrenia: relationship to psychopathology and medication side effects. Am J Psychiatry 149(9): 1189–1194, 1992.

Goff DC et al.: The effect of benztropine on haloperidol-induced dystonia, clinical efficacy and pharmacokinetics: a prospective, double-blind trial. J Clin Psychopharmacol 11(2): 106–112, 1991a.

Goff DC et al.: An open trial of buspirone added to neuroleptics in schizophrenic patients. J Clin Psychopharmacol 11(3): 193–197, 1991b.

Goff DC, Evins AE: Negative symptoms in schizophrenia: neurobiological models and treatment response. Harv Rev Psychiatry 6(2): 59–77, 1998.

Goff DC, Shader RI: Non-neurological side-effects of antipsychotic drugs. In Hirsch SR Weinberger DR (eds.), *Schizophrenia*, Oxford, Blackwell Publishing, 2003 , pp. 573–588.

Goldman SA: Lithium and neuroleptics in combination: the spectrum of neurotoxicity [corrected]. Psychopharmacol Bull 32(3): 299–309, 1996.

Goldney RD, Spence ND: Safety of the combination of lithium and neuroleptic drugs. Am J Psychiatry 143(7): 882–884, 1986.

Goldstein BJ: Interaction of antacids with psychotropics. Hosp Community Psychiatry 33(2): 96, 1982.

Gould RJ et al.: Calcium channel blockade: possible explanation for thioridazine's peripheral side effects. Am J Psychiatry 141(3): 352–357, 1984.

Gram LF et al.: Influence of neuroleptics and benzodiazepines on metabolism of tricyclic antidepressants in man. Am J Psychiatry 131(8): 863–866, 1974.

Gram LF, Overo KF: Drug interaction: inhibitory effect of neuroleptics on metabolism of tricyclic antidepressants in man. Br Med J 1(798): 463–465, 1972.

Greeman M, McClellan TA: Negative effects of a smoking ban on an inpatient psychiatric service. Hosp Community Psychiatry 42(4): 408–412, 1991.

Green AI et al.: Alcohol and cannabis use in schizophrenia: effects of clozapine versus risperidone. Schizophr Res 60(1): 81–85, 2003.

Greendyke RM, Gulya A: Effect of pindolol administration on serum levels of thioridazine, haloperidol, phenytoin, and phenobarbital. J Clin Psychiatry 49(3): 105–107, 1988.

Greendyke RM, Kanter DR: Plasma propranolol levels and their effect on plasma thioridazine and haloperidol concentrations. J Clin Psychopharmacol 7(3): 178–182, 1987.

Grunder G et al.: Mechanism of new antipsychotic mechanisms: occupancy is not just antagonism. Arch Gen Psychiatry 60(10): 974–977, 2003.

Guzey C et al.: Risperidone metabolism and the impact of being a cytochrome P450 2D6 ultrarapid metabolizer (letter). J Clin Psychiatry 61(8): 600–601, 2000.

Haddad PM, Anderson IM: Antipsychotic-related QTc prolongation, torsade de pointes and sudden death. Drugs 62(11): 1649–1671, 2002.

Hagg S et al.: Absence of interaction between erythromycin and a single dose of clozapine. Eur J Clin Pharmacol 55(3): 221–226, 1999.

Haidukewych D, Rodin EA: Effect of phenothiazines on serum antiepileptic drug concentrations in psychiatric patients with seizure disorder. Ther Drug Monit 7(4): 401–404, 1985.

Hameedi FA et al.: Near syncope associated with concomitant clozapine and cocaine use [letter]. J Clin Psychiatry 67(8): 371–372, 1996.

Hamilton S, Malone K: Serotonin syndrome during treatment with paroxetine and risperidone [letter]. J Clin Psychopharmacol 20(1): 103–105, 2000.

Hanlon TE et al.: Perphenazine-benztropine mesylate treatment of newly admitted psychiatric patients. Psychopharmacologia 9(4): 328–339, 1966.

Hansen LB et al.: Plasma levels of perphenazine and its major metabolites during simultaneous treatment with anticholinergic drugs. Br J Clin Pharmacol 7(1): 75–80, 1979.

Hansen LB, Larsen NE: Metabolic interaction between perphenazine and disulfiram. Lancet 2(8313): 1472, 1982.

Haring C et al.: Influence of patient-related variables on clozapine plasma levels. Am J Psychiatry 147(11): 1471–1475, 1990.

Harrigan EP et al.: A randomized evaluation of the effects of six antipsychotic agents on QTc, in the absence and presence of metabolic inhibition. J Clin Psychopharmacol 24(1): 62–69, 2004.

Haslett CD, Kumar S: Can olanzapine be implicated in causing serotonin syndrome? Psychiatry Clin Neurosci 56(5): 533–535, 2002.

Henderson DC et al.: Risperidone added to clozapine: impact on serum prolactin levels. J Clin Psychiatry 62(8): 605–608, 2001.

Henderson DC, Borba CP: Trimethoprim-sulfamethoxazole and clozapine [letter]. Psychiatr Serv 52(1): 111–112, 2001.

Henderson DC, Goff DC: Risperidone as an adjunct to clozapine therapy in chronic schizophrenics. J Clin Psychiatry 57(9): 395–397, 1996.

Hennessy S et al.: Cardiac arrest and ventricular arrhythmia in patients taking antipsychotic drugs: cohort study using administrative data. Br Med J 325(7372): 1070, 2002.

Hesslinger B et al.: Effects of carbamazepine and valproate on haloperidol plasma levels and on psychopathologic outcome in schizophrenic patients. J Clin Psychopharmacol 19(4): 310–315, 1999.

Hiemke C et al.: Fluvoxamine augmentation of olanzapine in chronic schizophrenia: pharmacokinetic interactions and clinical effects. J Clin Psychopharmacol 22(5): 502–506, 2002.

Hitri A et al.: Drug levels and antiparkinsonian drugs in neuroleptic-treated schizophrenic patients. Clin Neuropharmacol 10(3): 261–271, 1987.

Howes CA et al.: Reduced steady-state plasma concentrations of chlorpromazine and indomethacin in patients receiving cimetidine. Eur J Clin Pharmacol 24(1): 99–102, 1983.

Hriso E et al.: Extrapyramidal symptoms due to dopamine-blocking agents in patients with AIDS encephalopathy. Am J Psychiatry 148(11): 1558–1561, 1991.

Huang HF et al.: Lack of pharmacokinetic interaction between buspirone and haloperidol in patients with schizophrenia. J Clin Pharmacol 36(10): 963–969, 1996.

Huang ML et al.: Pharmacokinetics of the novel antipsychotic agent risperidone and the prolactin response in healthy subjects. Clin Pharmacol Ther 54(3): 257–268, 1993.

Hubbard JW et al.: Metabolism of phenothiazine and butyrophenone antipsychotic drugs. A review of some recent research findings and clinical implications. Br J Psychiatry Suppl 22: 19–24, 1993.

Hubbard JW et al.: Prolonged pharmacologic activity of neuroleptic drugs. Arch Gen Psychiatry 44(1): 99–100, 1987.

Hunt N, Stern TA: The association between intravenous haloperidol and torsade de pointes. Three cases and a literature review. Psychosomatics 36(6): 541–549, 1995.

Hutchison KE et al.: Olanzapine reduces urge to drink after drinking cues and a priming dose of alcohol. Psychopharmacology (Berl) 155(1): 27–34, 2001.

Hyman SE, Fenton WS: Medicine. What are the right targets for psychopharmacology? Science 299(5605): 350–351, 2003.

Hyman SE, Nestler EJ: Initiation and adaptation: a paradigm for understanding psychotropic drug action. Am J Psychiatry 153(2): 151–162, 1996.

Iannini PB: Cardiotoxicity of macrolides, ketolides and fluoroquinolones that prolong the QTc interval. Expert Opin Drug Saf 1(2): 121–128, 2002.

Ishizaki T et al.: The effects of neuroleptics (haloperidol and chlorpromazine) on the pharmacokinetics of valproic acid in schizophrenic patients. J Clin Psychopharmacol 4(5): 254–261, 1984.

Jackson T et al.: Torsade de pointes and low-dose oral haloperidol. Arch Intern Med 157(17): 2013–2015, 1997.

Jann MW et al.: Clinical implications of increased antipsychotic plasma concentrations upon anticonvulsant cessation. Psychiatry Res 28(2): 153–159, 1989.

Jann MW et al.: Effects of smoking on haloperidol and reduced haloperidol plasma concentrations and haloperidol clearance. Psychopharmacology 90(4): 468–470, 1986.

Jann MW et al.: Pharmacokinetics and pharmacodynamics of clozapine. Clin Pharmacokinet 24(2): 161–176, 1993.

Jerling M et al.: Fluvoxamine inhibition and carbamazepine induction of the metabolism of clozapine: evidence from a therapeutic drug monitoring service. Ther Drug Monit 16(4): 368–374, 1994.

Johnson DA: Observations on the dose regime of fluphenazine decanoate in maintenance therapy of schizophrenia. Br J Psychiatry 126: 457–461, 1975.

Johnstone EC et al.: Adverse effects of anticholinergic medication on positive schizophrenic symptoms. Psychol Med 13(3): 513–527, 1983.

Johnstone EC et al.: The Northwick Park "functional" psychosis study: diagnosis and treatment response. Lancet 2(8603): 119–125, 1988.

Joos AA et al.: Pharmacokinetic interaction of clozapine and rifampicin in a forensic patient with an atypical mycobacterial infection [letter]. J Clin Psychopharmacol 18(1): 83–85, 1998.

Jover F et al.: Reversible coma caused by risperidone-ritonavir interaction. Clin Neuropharmacol 25(5): 251–253, 2002.

Kalgutkar AS et al.: Assessment of the contributions of CYP3A4 and CYP3A5 in the metabolism of the antipsychotic agent haloperidol to its potentially neurotoxic pyridinium metabolite and effect of antidepressants on the bioactivation pathway. Drug Metab Dispos 31(3): 243–249, 2003.

Kaminsky R et al.: Effect of famotidine on deficit symptoms of schizophrenia. Lancet 335(8701): 1351–1352, 1990.

Kane J et al.: Extrapyramidal side effects with lithium treatment. Am J Psychiatry 135(7): 851–853, 1978.

Kane JM et al.: Long-acting injectable risperidone: efficacy and safety of the first long-acting atypical antipsychotic. Am J Psychiatry 160(6): 1125–1132, 2003b.

Kane JM et al.: Strategies for improving compliance in treatment of schizophrenia by using a long-acting formulation of an antipsychotic: clinical studies. J Clin Psychiatry 64 Suppl 16(6): 34–40, 2003a.

Kapur S et al.: 5-HT2 and D2 receptor occupancy of olanzapine in schizophrenia: a PET investigation. Am J Psychiatry 155(7): 921–928, 1998.

Kapur S et al.: Increased dopamine D2 receptor occupancy and elevated prolactin level associated with addition of haloperidol to clozapine. Am J Psychiatry 158(2): 311–314, 2001.

Kapur S, Seeman P: Does fast dissociation from the dopamine D2 receptor explain the action of atypical antipsychotics?: A new hypothesis. Am J Psychiatry 158(3): 360–369, 2001.

Kelly DV et al.: Extrapyramidal symptoms with ritonavir/indinavir plus risperidone. Ann Pharmacother 36(5): 827–830, 2002.

Khan AY, Preskorn SH: Increase in plasma levels of clozapine and norclozapine after administration of nefazodone [letter]. J Clin Psychiatry 62(5): 375–376, 2001.

Khot V et al.: The assessment and clinical implications of haloperidol acute-dose, steady-state, and withdrawal pharmacokinetics. J Clin Psychopharmacol 13(2): 120–127, 1993.

Kim YH et al.: Effect of rifampin on the plasma concentration and the clinical effect of haloperidol concomitantly administered to schizophrenic patients. J Clin Psychopharmacol 16(3): 247–252, 1996.

Klimke A, Klieser E: Sudden death after intravenous application of lorazepam in a patient treated with clozapine [letter]. Am J Psychiatry 151(5): 780, 1994.

Kocsis JH et al.: Response to treatment with antidepressants of patients with severe or moderate nonpsychotic depression and of patients with psychotic depression. Am J Psychiatry 147(5): 621–624, 1990.

Koczapski A et al.: Effects of caffeine on behavior of schizophrenic inpatients. Schiophr Bull 1989 15(2): 339–344, 1991.

Korsgaard S et al.: Behavioral aspects of serotonin-dopamine interaction in the monkey. Eur J Pharmacol 118(3): 245–252, 1985.

Kragh-Sorensen P et al.: Effect of simultaneous treatment with low doses of perphenazine on plasma and urine concentrations of nortriptyline and 10-hydroxynortriptyline. Eur J Clin Pharmacol 11(6): 479–483, 1977.

Kramer MS et al.: Antidepressants in "depressed" schizophrenic inpatients. A controlled trial. Arch Gen Psychiatry 46(10): 922–928, 1989.

Kudo S, Ishizaki T: Pharmacokinetics of haloperidol: an update. Clin Pharmacokinet 37(6): 435–456, 1999.

Kulhanek F et al.: Precipitation of antipsychotic drugs in interaction with coffee or tea. Lancet 2: 1130, 1979.

Kulhanek F, Linde OK: Coffee and tea influence pharmacokinetics of antipsychotic drugs. Lancet 2: 359–360, 1981.

Kuo FJ et al.: Extrapyramidal symptoms after addition of fluvoxamine to clozapine [letter]. J Clin Psychopharmacol 18(6): 483–484, 1998.

Lane HY et al.: Repeated ingestion of grapefruit juice does not alter clozapine's steady-state plasma levels, effectiveness, and tolerability. J Clin Psychiatry 62(10): 812–817, 2001.

Lee MS et al.: A double-blind study of adjunctive sertraline in haloperidol-stabilized patients with chronic schizophrenia. J Clin Psychopharmacol 18(5): 399–403, 1998.

Lee SI et al.: Neuroleptic malignant syndrome associated with use of risperidone, ritonavir, and indinavir: a case report [letter]. Psychosomatics 41(5): 453–454, 2000.

Leo RJ: Movement disorders associated with the serotonin selective reuptake inhibitors. J Clin Psychiatry 57(10): 449–454, 1996.

Lieber CS: Biochemical and molecular basis of alcohol-induced injury to liver and other tissues. N Engl J Med 319(25): 1639–1650, 1988.

Lieber CS: Interaction of alcohol with other drugs and nutrients. Implication for the therapy of alcoholic liver disease. Drugs 40 Suppl 3: 23–44, 1990.

Lindskog M et al.: Involvement of DARRP-32 phosphorylation in the stimulant action of caffeine. Nature 418(6899): 774–778, 2002.

Linnet K, Olesen OV: Free and glucuronidated olanzapine serum concentrations in psychiatric patients: influence of carbamazepine comedication. Ther Drug Monit 24(4): 512–517, 2002.

Linnet K, Olesen OV: Metabolism of clozapine by cDNA-expressed human cytochrome P450 enzymes. Drug Metab Dispos 25(12): 1379–1382, 1997.

Linnoila M et al.: Effect of anticonvulsants on plasma haloperidol and thioridazine levels. Am J Psychiatry 137(7): 819–821, 1980.

Lipinski JF, Jr. et al.: Fluoxetine-induced akathisia: clinical and theoretical implications. J Clin Psychiatry 50(9): 339–342, 1989.

Liston HL et al.: Drug glucuronidation in clinical psychopharmacology. J Clin Psychopharmacol 21(5): 500–515, 2001.

Liu H-C et al.: Extrapyramidal side effects due to drug combination of risperidone and donepezil [letter]. Psychiatry Clin Neurosci 56: 479, 2002.

Loga S et al.: Interaction of chlorpromazine and nortriptyline in patients with schizophrenia. Clin Pharmacokinet 6(6): 454–462, 1981.

Lohr JB, Braff DL: The value of referring to recently introduced antipsychotics as "second generation". Am J Psychiatry 160(8): 1371–1372, 2003.

Lucas PB et al.: Effects of the acute administration of caffeine in patients with schizophrenia. Biol Psychiatry 28(1): 35–40, 1990.

Lucas RA et al.: A pharmacokinetic interaction between carbamazepine and olanzapine: observations on possible mechanism. Eur J Clin Pharmacol 54(8): 639–643, 1998.

Lutz EG: Neuroleptic-induced akathisia and dystonia triggered by alcohol. JAMA 236(21): 2422–2423, 1976.

Magnuson TM et al.: Extrapyramidal side effects in a patient treated with risperidone plus donepezil [letter]. Am J Psychiatry 155(10): 1458–1459, 1998.

Makela EH et al.: Three case reports of modafinil use in treating sedation induced by antipsychotic medications [letter]. J Clin Psychiatry 64(4): 485–486, 2003.

Mann SC, Boger WP: Psychotropic drugs, summer heat and humidity, and hyperpyrexia: a danger restated. Am J Psychiatry 135(9): 1097–1100, 1978.

Manos N et al.: The need for continuous use of antiparkinsonian medication with chronic schizophrenic patients receiving long-term neuroleptic therapy. Am J Psychiatry 138(2): 184–188, 1981.

Marder SR et al.: Pharmacokinetics of long-acting injectable neuroleptic drugs: clinical implications. Psychopharmacology (Berl) 98(4): 433–439, 1989a.

Marder SR et al.: Plasma levels of parent drug and metabolites in patients receiving oral and depot fluphenazine. Psychopharmacol Bull 25(3): 479–482, 1989b.

Markowitz JS et al.: Effect of St. John's wort on drug metabolism by induction of cytochrome P450 3A4 enzyme. JAMA 290(11): 1500–1504, 2003.

Markowitz JS et al.: Hypotension and bradycardia in a healthy volunteer following a single 5 mg dose of olanzapine. J Clin Pharmacol 42(1): 104–106, 2002.

Markowitz JS et al.: Fluoroquinolone inhibition of clozapine metabolism [letter]. Am J Psychiatry 154(6): 881, 1997.

Markowitz JS, DeVane CL: Suspected ciprofloxacin inhibition of olanzapine resulting in increased plasma concentration [letter]. J Clin Psychopharmacol 19(3): 289–291, 1999.

Martin-Escudero JC et al.: Olanzapine toxicity in unconjugated hyperbilirubinaemia (Gilbert's syndrome) [letter]. Br J Psychiatry 182: 267, 2003.

McEvoy JP et al.: Optimal dose of neuroleptic in acute schizophrenia. A controlled study of the neuroleptic threshold and higher haloperidol dose. Arch Gen Psychiatry 48(8): 739–745, 1991.

McEvoy JP, Freter S: The dose-response relationship for memory impairment by anticholinergic drugs. Compr Psychiatry 30(2): 135–138, 1989.

Metzger E, Friedman R: Prolongation of the corrected QT and torsade de pointes cardiac arrhythmia associated with intravenous haloperidol in the medically ill. J Clin Psychopharmacol 13(2): 128–132, 1993.

Meyer JM: Individual changes in clozapine levels after smoking cessation: results and a predictive model. J Clin Psychopharmacol 21(6): 569–574, 2001.

Meyer UA: Metabolic interactions of the proton-pump inhibitors lansoprazole, omeprazole and pantoprazole with other drugs. Eur J Gastroenterol Hepatol 8 Suppl 1: S21–25, 1996.

Mezey E: Ethanol metabolism and ethanol-drug interactions. Biochem Pharmacol 25(8): 869–875, 1976.

Miceli JJ et al.: The effect of carbamazepine on the steady-state pharmacokinetics of ziprasidone in healthy volunteers. Br J Clin Pharmacol 49 Suppl 1: 65S–70S, 2000.

Midha KK et al.: Intersubject variation in the pharmacokinetics of haloperidol and reduced haloperidol. J Clin Psychopharmacol 9(2): 98–104, 1989.

Mihara K et al.: Effects of the CYP2D6 #10 allele on the steady-state plasma concentrations of haloperidol and reduced haloperidol in Japanese patients with schizophrenia. Clin Pharmacol Ther 65(3): 291–294, 1999.

Miller DD: Effect of phenytoin on plasma clozapine concentrations in two patients. J Clin Psychiatry 52(1): 23–25, 1991.

Miller F, Menninger J: Lithium-neuroleptic neurotoxicity is dose dependent. J Clin Psychopharmacol 7(2): 89–91, 1987.

Miller SC: Methylphenidate for clozapine sedation [letter]. Am J Psychiatry 153(9): 1231–1232, 1996.

Minzenberg MJ et al.: Association of anticholinergic load with impairment of complex attention and memory in schizophrenia. Am J Psychiatry 161(1): 116–124, 2004.

Morselli PL et al.: Further observations on the interaction between ethanol and psychotropic drugs. Arzneimittelforschung 2: 20–23, 1971.

Nadel I, Wallach M: Drug interaction between haloperidol and methyldopa [letter]. Br J Psychiatry 135: 484, 1979.

Narendran R et al.: Is psychosis exacerbated by modafinil [letter]? Arch Gen Psychiatry 59(3): 292–293, 2002.

Navarro V et al.: Topiramate for clozapine-induced seizures [letter]. Am J Psychiatry 158: 968–969, 2001.

Nelson JC, Jatlow PI: Neuroleptic effect on desipramine steady-state plasma concentrations. Am J Psychiatry 137(10): 1232–1234, 1980.

Nemeroff CB et al.: Newer antidepressants and the cytochrome P450 system. Am J Psychiatry 153(3): 311–320, 1996.

Newman-Tancredi A et al.: Comparison of hippocampal G protein activation by 5-HT(1A) receptor agonists and the atypical antipsychotics clozapine and S16924. Naunyn Schmiedebergs Arch Pharmacol 368(3): 188–199, 2003.

Niedzwiecki DM et al.: Comparative antidopaminergic properties of thioridazine, mesoridazine and sulforidazine on the corpus striatum. J Pharmacol Exp Ther 250(1): 117–125, 1989.

Nosten F et al.: Cardiac effects of antimalaria treatment with halofantrine. Lancet 341(8852): 1054–1056, 1993.

Nyberg S et al.: Suggested minimal effective dose of risperidone based on PET-measured D2 and 5-HT2A receptor occupancy in schizophrenic patients. Am J Psychiatry 156(6): 869–875, 1999.

O'Brien JM et al.: Haloperidol-induced torsade de pointes. Ann Pharmacother 33(10): 1046–1050, 1999.

Olesen OV, Linnet K: Contributions of five human cytochrome P450 isoforms to the N-demethylation of clozapine in vitro at low and high concentrations. J Clin Pharmacol 41(8): 823–832, 2001.

Ono S et al.: Significant pharmacokinetic interaction between risperidone and carbamazepine: its relationship with CYP2D6 genotypes. Psychopharmacology (Berl) 162(1): 50–54, 2002.

Opler LA, Feinberg SS: The role of pimozide in clinical psychiatry: a review. J Clin Psychiatry 52(5): 221–233, 1991.

Otani K et al.: Biperiden and piroheptine do not affect the serum level of zotepine, a new antipsychotic drug. Br J Psychiatry 157: 128–130, 1990.

Overo KF et al.: Interaction of perphenazine with the kinetics of nortriptyline. Acta Pharmacol Toxicol (Copenh) 40(1): 97–105, 1977.

Oyewumi LK et al.: Famotidine as an adjunct treatment of resistant schizophrenia. J Psychiatry Neurosci 19(2): 145–150, 1994.

Ozdemir V et al.: Paroxetine potentiates the central nervous system side effects of perphenazine: contribution of cytochrome P4502D6 inhibition in vivo. Clin Pharmacol Ther 62(3): 334–347, 1997.

Pato CN et al.: Benzodiazepine augmentation of neuroleptic treatment in patients with schizophrenia. Psychopharmacol Bull 25(2): 263–266, 1989.

Peet M et al.: Pharmacokinetic interaction between propranolol and chlorpromazine in schizophrenic patients. Lancet 2(8201): 978, 1980.

Penzak SR et al.: Influence of ritonavir on olanzapine pharmacokinetics in healthy volunteers. J Clin Psychopharmacol 22(4): 366–370, 2002.

Perrault LP et al.: Torsade de pointes secondary to intravenous haloperidol after coronary bypass grafting surgery. Can J Anaesth 47(3): 251–254, 2000.

Plasky P: Antidepressant usage in schizophrenia. Schizophr Bull 17(4): 649–657, 1991.

Pollock BG et al.: Prospective cytochrome P450 phenotyping for neuroleptic treatment in dementia. Psychopharmacol Bull 31(2): 327–331, 1995.

Pope HG, Jr. et al.: Apparent neuroleptic malignant syndrome with clozapine and lithium. J Nerv Ment Dis 174(8): 493–495, 1986.

Potkin SG et al.: Effect of fluoxetine and imipramine on the pharmacokinetics and tolerability of the antipsychotic quetiapine. J Clin Psychopharmacol 22(2): 174–182, 2002a.

Potkin SG et al.: The safety and pharmacokinetics of quetiapine when coadministered with haloperidol, risperidone, or thioridazine. J Clin Psychopharmacol 22(2): 121–130, 2002b.

Prakash R et al.: Neurotoxicity with combined administration of lithium and a neuroleptic. Compr Psychiatry 23(6): 567–571, 1982.

Prakash R: Lithium-haloperidol combination and brain damage [letter]. Lancet 1(8287): 1468–1469, 1982.

Preston SL et al.: Drug interactions in HIV-positive patients initiated on protease inhibitor therapy. Aids 12(2): 228–230, 1998.

Prior TI, Baker GB: Interactions between the cytochrome P450 system and the second-generation antipsychotics. J Psychiatry Neurosci 28(2): 99–112, 2003.

Prusoff BA et al.: Treatment of secondary depression in schizophrenia. A double-blind, placebo-controlled trial of amitriptyline added to perphenazine. Arch Gen Psychiatry 36(5): 569–575, 1979.

Raaska K et al.: Therapeutic drug monitoring data: risperidone does not increase serum clozapine concentration. Eur J Clin Pharmacol 58(9): 587–591, 2002a.

Raaska K et al.: Bacterial pneumonia can increase serum concentration of clozapine. Eur J Clin Pharmacol 58(5): 321–322, 2002b.

Raaska K, Neuvonen PJ: Ciprofloxacin increases serum clozapine and N-desmethylclozapine: a study in patients with schizophrenia. Eur J Clin Pharmacol 56(8): 585–589, 2000.

Raaska K, Neuvonen PJ: Serum concentrations of clozapine and N-desmethyl-clozapine are unaffected by the potent CYP3A4 inhibitor itraconazole. Eur J Clin Pharmacol 54(2): 167–170, 1998.

Raitasuo V et al.: Carbamazepine and plasma levels of clozapine [letter]. Am J Psychiatry 150(1): 169, 1993.

Raitasuo V et al.: Effect of switching carbamazepine to oxcarbazepine on the plasma levels of neuroleptics. A case report. Psychopharmacology (Berl) 116(1): 115–116, 1994.

Ray WA et al.: Antipsychotics and the risk of sudden cardiac death. Arch Gen Psychiatry 58(12): 1161–1167, 2001.

Reilly JG, ,et al.: Thioridazine and sudden unexplained death in psychiatric in-patients. Br J Psychiatry 180: 515–522, 2002.

Risch SC et al.: Interfaces of psychopharmacology and cardiology—Part two. J Clin Psychiatry 42(2): 47–59, 1981.

Riva R et al.: Pharmacokinetic interactions between antiepileptic drugs. Clinical considerations. Clin Pharmacokinet 31(6): 470–493, 1996.

Rivera-Calimlim L: Effect of lithium on gastric emptying and absorption of oral chlorpromazine. Psychopharmacol Commun 2(3): 263–272, 1976.

Rivera-Calimlim L et al.: Clinical response and plasma levels: effect of dose, dosage schedules, and drug interactions on plasma chlorpromazine levels. Am J Psychiatry 133(6): 646–652, 1976.

Rivera-Calimlim L et al.: Effect of lithium on plasma chlorpromazine levels. Clin Pharmacol Ther 23(4): 451–455, 1978.

Rivera-Calimlim et al.: Effects of mode of management on plasma chlorpromazine in psychiatric patients. Clin Pharmacol Ther 14(6): 978–986, 1973.

Rockland L et al.: Effects of trihexyphenidyl on plasma chlorpromazine in young schizophrenics. Can J Psychiatry 35(7): 604–607, 1990.

Rosebush P, Stewart T: A prospective analysis of 24 episodes of neuroleptic malignant syndrome. Am J Psychiatry 146(6): 717–725, 1989.

Rosse RB et al.: An open-label study of the therapeutic efficacy of high-dose famotidine adjuvant pharmacotherapy in schizophrenia: preliminary evidence for treatment efficacy. Clin Neuropharmacol 19(4): 341–348, 1996.

Rostami-Hodjegan A et al.: Influence of dose, cigarette smoking, age, sex, and metabolic activity on plasma clozapine concentrations: a predictive model and nomograms to aid clozapine dose adjustment and to assess compliance in individual patients. J Clin Psychopharmacol 24(1): 70–78, 2004.

Sachdev PS: Lithium potentiation of neuroleptic-related extrapyramidal side effects [letter]. Am J Psychiatry 143(7): 942, 1986.

Salokangas RK et al.: Citalopram as an adjuvant in chronic schizophrenia: a double-blind placebo-controlled study. Acta Psychiatr Scand 94(3): 175–180, 1996.

Schelosky L et al.: Kava and dopamine antagonism. J Neurol Neurosurg Psychiatry 58(5): 639–640, 1995.

Schotte A et al.: Risperidone compared with new and reference antipsychotic drugs: in vitro and in vivo receptor binding. Psychopharmacology (Berl) 124(1–2): 57–73, 1996.

Schou M: Long-lasting neurological sequelae after lithium intoxication. Acta Psychiatr Scand 70(6): 594–602, 1984.

Seeman P, Tallerico T: Rapid release of antipsychotic drugs from dopamine D2 receptors: an explanation for low receptor occupancy and early clinical relapse upon withdrawal of clozapine or quetiapine. Am J Psychiatry 156(6): 876–884, 1999.

Shale JH et al.: A review of the safety and efficacy of droperidol for the rapid sedation of severely agitated and violent patients. J Clin Psychiatry 64(5): 500–505, 2003.

Sharma ND et al.: Torsade de pointes associated with intravenous haloperidol in critically ill patients. Am J Cardiol 81(2): 238–240, 1998.

Shin JG et al.: Effect of antipsychotic drugs on human liver cytochrome P-450 (CYP) isoforms in vitro: preferential inhibition of CYP2D6. Drug Metab Dispos 27(9): 1078–1084, 1999.

Shin JG et al.: Potent inhibition of CYP2D6 by haloperidol metabolites: stereoselective inhibition by reduced haloperidol. Br J Clin Pharmacol 51(1): 45–52, 2001.

Shoaf SE, Linnoila M: Interaction of ethanol and smoking on the pharmacokinetics and pharmacodynamics of psychotropic medications. Psychopharmacol Bull 27(4): 577–594, 1991.

Silver JM et al.: Elevation of thioridazine plasma levels by propranolol. Am J Psychiatry 143(10): 1290–1292, 1986.

Silverstone PH: Prevention of clozapine-induced neutropenia by pretreatment with lithium [letter]. J Clin Psychopharmacol 18(1): 86–88, 1998.

Simpson GM et al.: Effect of antiparkinsonian medication on plasma levels of chlorpromazine. Arch Gen Psychiatry 37(2): 205–208, 1980.

Simpson GM, Lindenmayer JP: Extrapyramidal symptoms in patients treated with risperidone. J Clin Psychopharmacol 17(3): 194–201, 1997.

Singh MM, Kay SR: A comparative study of haloperidol and chlorpromazine in terms of clinical effects and therapeutic reversal with benztropine in schizophrenia. Theoretical implications for potency differences among neuroleptics. Psychopharmacologia 43(2): 103–113, 1975a.

Singh MM, Kay SR: Therapeutic reversal with benztropine in schizophrenics. Practical and theoretical significance. J Nerv Ment Dis 160(4): 258–266, 1975b.

Singh MM, Smith JM: Reversal of some therapeutic effects of an antipsychotic agent by an antiparkinsonism drug. J Nerv Ment Dis 157(1): 50–58, 1973.

Siris SG et al.: Adjunctive imipramine in the treatment of postpsychotic depression. A controlled trial. Arch Gen Psychiatry 44(6): 533–539, 1987.

Siris SG et al.: Plasma imipramine concentrations in patients receiving concomitant fluphenazine decanoate. Am J Psychiatry 139(1): 104–106, 1982a.

Siris SG et al.: Response of postpsychotic depression to adjunctive imipramine or amitriptyline. J Clin Psychiatry 43(12): 485–486, 1982b.

Siris SG et al.: The use of antidepressants for negative symptoms in a subset of schizophrenic patients. Psychopharmacol Bull 27(3): 331–335, 1991.

Sirota P et al.: An open study of buspirone augmentation of neuroleptics in patients with schizophrenia. J Clin Psychopharmacol 21(4): 454–455, 2001.

Sjoqvist F: Psychotropic drugs (2). Interaction between monoamine oxidase (MAO) inhibitors and other substances. Proc R Soc Med 58(11 Part 2): 967–978, 1965.

Skogh E et al.: Therapeutic drug monitoring data on olanzapine and its N-dimethyl metabolite in the naturalistic clinical setting. Ther Drug Monit 24(4): 518–526, 2002.

Small JG et al.: Tolerability and efficacy of clozapine combined with lithium in schizophrenia and schizoaffective disorder. J Clin Psychopharmacol 23(3): 223–228, 2003.

Sorby DL, Liu G: Effects of absorbents on drug absorption: II. effect of an antidiarrheal mixture on promazine absorption. J Pharm Sci 55: 504, 1966.

Spiker DG et al.: The pharmacological treatment of delusional depression. Am J Psychiatry 142(4): 430–436, 1985.

Spina E et al.: Inhibition of risperidone metabolism by fluoxetine in patients with schizophrenia: a clinically relevant pharmacokinetic drug interaction. J Clin Psychopharmacol 22(4): 419–423, 2002.

Spina E et al.: Plasma concentrations of risperidone and 9-hydroxyrisperidone during combined treatment with paroxetine. Ther Drug Monit 23(3): 223–227, 2001a.

Spina E et al.: Adverse drug interaction between risperidone and carbamazepine in a patient with chronic schizophrenia and deficient CYP2D6 activity [letter]. J Clin Psychopharmacol 21(1): 108–109, 2001b.

Spina E et al.: Plasma concentrations of clozapine and its major metabolites during combined treatment with paroxetine or sertraline. Pharmacopsychiatry 33(6): 213–217, 2000a.

Spina E et al.: Plasma concentrations of risperidone and 9-hydroxyrisperidone: effect of comedication with carbamazepine or valproate. Ther Drug Monit 22(4): 481–485, 2000b.

Spina E et al.: Effect of fluoxetine on the plasma concentrations of clozapine and its major metabolites in patients with schizophrenia. Int Clin Psychopharmacol 13(3): 141–145, 1998.

Spina E et al.: Adjunctive fluoxetine in the treatment of negative symptoms in chronic schizophrenic patients. Int Clin Psychopharmacol 9(4): 281–285, 1994.

Spring GK: Neurotoxicity with combined use of lithium and thioridazine. J Clin Psychiatry 40(3): 135–138, 1979.

Sproule BA et al.: Selective serotonin reuptake inhibitors and CNS drug interactions. A critical review of the evidence. Clin Pharmacokinet 33(6): 454–471, 1997.

Sternbach H: The serotonin syndrome. American Journal of Psychiatry 148(6): 705–713, 1991.

Stimmel GL, Falloon IR: Chlorpromazine plasma levels, adverse effects, and tobacco smoking: case report. J Clin Psychiatry 44(11): 420–422, 1983.

Strakowski SM et al.: The effect of multiple doses of cimetidine on the steady-state pharmacokinetics of quetiapine in men with selected psychotic disorders. J Clin Psychopharmacol 22(2): 201–205, 2002.

Strauss ME et al.: Effects of anticholinergic medication on memory in schizophrenia. Schizophr Res 3(2): 127–129, 1990.

Sullivan RJ et al.: Effects of chewing betel nut (*Areca catechu*) on the symptoms of people with schizophrenia in Palau, Micronesia. Br J Psychiatry 177(8): 174–178, 2000.

Sunderland T, Cohen BM: Blood to brain distribution of neuroleptics. Psychiatry Res 20(4): 299–305, 1987.

Susman VL, Addonizio G: Reinduction of neuroleptic malignant syndrome by lithium. J Clin Psychopharmacol 7(5): 339–341, 1987.

Swanson CL, Jr. et al.: Effects of concomitant risperidone and lithium treatment [letter]. Am J Psychiatry 152(7): 1096, 1995.

Swartz CM: Olanzapine-lithium encephalopathy [letter]. Psychosomatics 42(4): 370, 2001.

Szymanski S et al.: A case report of cimetidine-induced clozapine toxicity. J Clin Psychiatry 52(1): 21–22, 1991.

Takeda M et al.: Serum haloperidol levels of schizophrenics receiving treatment for tuberculosis. Clin Neuropharmacol 9(4): 386–397, 1986.

Tandon R et al.: Cholinergic syndrome following anticholinergic withdrawal in a schizophrenic patient abusing marijuana. Br J Psychiatry 154: 712–714, 1989.

Tandon R et al.: Effect of anticholinergic medication on positive and negative symptoms in medication-free schizophrenic patients. Psychiatry Res 31(3): 235–241, 1990.

Taylor D et al.: The effect of nefazodone on clozapine plasma concentrations. Int Clin Psychopharmacol 14(3): 185–187, 1999.

Taylor D et al.: Co-administration of citalopram and clozapine: effect on plasma clozapine levels. Int Clin Psychopharmacol 13(1): 19–21, 1998.

Taylor D: Pharmacokinetic interactions involving clozapine. Br J Psychiatry 171: 109–112, 1997.

Thornton WE: Dementia induced by methyldopa with haloperidol. N Engl J Med 294(22): 1222, 1976.

Tseng AL, Foisy MM: Significant interactions with new antiretrovirals and psychotropic drugs. Ann Pharmacother 33(4): 461–473, 1999.

Tune LE et al.: Serum levels of anticholinergic drugs and impaired recent memory in chronic schizophrenic patients. Am J Psychiatry 139(11): 1460–1462, 1982.

Tupala E et al.: Transient syncope and ECG changes associated with the concurrent administration of clozapine and diazepam [letter]. J Clin Psychiatry 60(9): 619–620, 1999.

Tyson SC et al.: Pharmacokinetic interaction between risperidone and clozapine [letter]. Am J Psychiatry 152(9): 1401–1402, 1995.

Upadhyaya MP, Chaturvedi SK: Psychosis and anti-tuberculosis therapy [letter]. Lancet 2(8665): 735–736, 1989.

Usiskin SI et al.: Retreatment with clozapine after erythromycin-induced neutropenia [letter]. Am J Psychiatry 157(6): 1021, 2000.

van Harten PN et al.: Cocaine as a risk factor for neuroleptic-induced acute dystonia. J Clin Psychiatry 59(3): 128–130, 1998.

Vandel B et al.: Interaction between amitriptyline and phenothiazine in man: effect on plasma concentration of amitriptyline and its metabolite nortriptyline and the correlation with clinical response. Psychopharmacology (Berl) 65(2): 187–190, 1979.

Verghese C et al.: Pharmacokinetics of neuroleptics. Psychopharmacol Bull 27(4): 551–563, 1991.

Vestal RE et al.: Inhibition of propranolol metabolism by chlorpromazine. Clin Pharmacol Ther 25(1): 19–24, 1979.

von Bahr C et al.: Plasma levels of thioridazine and metabolites are influenced by the debrisoquin hydroxylation phenotype. Clin Pharmacol Ther 49(3): 234–240, 1991.

von Moltke LL et al.: Protease inhibitors as inhibitors of human cytochromes P450: high risk associated with ritonavir. J Clin Pharmacol 38(2): 106–111, 1998.

Waehrens J, Gerlach J: Antidepressant drugs in anergic schizophrenia. A double-blind cross-over study with maprotiline and placebo. Acta Psychiatr Scand 61(5): 438–444, 1980.

Wallace SM et al.: Oral fluphenazine and tea and coffee drinking. Lancet 2: 691, 1981.

Wassef AA et al.: Randomized, placebo-controlled pilot study of divalproex sodium in the treatment of acute exacerbation of chronic schizophrenia. J Clin Psychopharmacol 20(3): 357–361, 2000.

White WB: Hypotension with postural syncope secondary to the combination of chlorpromazine and captopril. Arch Intern Med 146(9): 1833–1834, 1986.

Wilner KD et al.: The pharmacokinetics of ziprasidone in healthy volunteers treated with cimetidine or antacid. Br J Clin Pharmacol 49 Suppl 1: 57S–60S, 2000.

Winslow RS et al.: Prevention of acute dystonic reactions in patients beginning high-potency neuroleptics. Am J Psychiatry 143(6): 706–710, 1986.

Witchel HJ et al.: Psychotropic drugs, cardiac arrhythmia, and sudden death. J Clin Psychopharmacol 23(1): 58–77, 2003.

Wolkowitz OM et al.: Alprazolam augmentation of the antipsychotic effects of fluphenazine in schizophrenic patients. Preliminary results. Arch Gen Psychiatry 45(7): 664–671, 1988.

Wolkowitz OM, Pickar D: Benzodiazepines in the treatment of schizophrenia: a review and reappraisal. Am J Psychiatry 148(6): 714–726, 1991.

Wong AH et al.: Herbal remedies in psychiatric practice. Arch Gen Psychiatry 55(11): 1033–1044, 1998.

Wong YW et al.: The effects of concomitant phenytoin administration on the steady-state pharmacokinetics of quetiapine. J Clin Psychopharmacol 21(1): 89–93, 2001.

World Health Organization: Prophylactic use of anticholinergics in patients on long-term neuroleptic treatment. Br J Psychiatry 156: 412, 1990.

Wozniak KM et al.: Focal application of alcohols elevates extracellular dopamine in rat brain: a microdialysis study. Brain Res 540(1–2): 31–40, 1991.

Yasuda K et al.: Interaction of cytochrome P450 3A inhibitors with P-glyco-protein. J Pharmacol Exp Ther 303(1): 323–332, 2002.

Yasui N et al.: Effects of itraconazole on the steady-state plasma concentrations of haloperidol and its reduced metabolite in schizophrenic patients: in vivo evidence of the involvement of CYP3A4 for haloperidol metabolism. J Clin Psychopharmacol 19(2): 149–154, 1999a.

Yasui N et al.: Lack of significant pharmacokinetic interaction between haloperidol and grapefruit juice. Int Clin Psychopharmacol 14(2): 113–118, 1999b.

Yasui-Furukori N et al.: Effects of CYP2D6 genotypes on plasma concentrations of risperidone and enantiomers of 9-hydroxyrisperidone in Japanese patients with schizophrenia. J Clin Pharmacol 43(2): 122–127, 2003.

Yeung PK et al.: Pharmacokinetics of chlorpromazine and key metabolites. Eur J Clin Pharmacol 45(6): 563–569, 1993.

Yoon MS, Han J,: Effects of thioridazine (Mellaril) on ventricular electro-physiologic properties. Am J Cardiol 43(6): 1155–1158, 1979.

Yorkston NJ et al.: Propranolol as an adjunct to the treatment of schizophre-nia. Lancet 2(8038): 575–578, 1977.

Zaslove MO et al.: Change in behaviors of inpatients after a ban on the sale of caffeinated drinks. Hosp Community Psychiatry 42(1): 84–85, 1991.

Zelman S, Guillan R: Heat stroke in phenothiazine-treated patients: a report of three fatalities. Am J Psychiatry 126(12): 1787–1790, 1970.

Zhang W et al.: Synergistic effects of olanzapine and other antipsychotic agents in combination with fluoxetine on norepinephrine and dopamine release in rat prefrontal cortex. Neuropsychopharmacology 23(3): 250–262, 2000.

Zhao Q et al.: Pharmacokinetic and safety assessments of concurrent administration of risperidone and donepezil. J Clin Pharmacol 43(2): 180–186, 2003.

Ziemba T et al.: Do anticholinergics antagonize antipsychotic drug action? Schizophr Bull 4(1): 7–12, 1978.

Zullino DF et al.: Tobacco and cannabis smoking cessation can lead to intoxication with clozapine or olanzapine. Int Clin Psychopharmacol 17(3): 141–143, 2002.

4

Lithium

OFRA SARID-SEGAL
WAYNE L. CREELMAN
DOMENIC A. CIRAULO
RICHARD I. SHADER

Lithium is rapidly absorbed after oral administration, with peak levels occurring 2 to 4 hours after the dose, although slow release formulations also are available. Lithium elimination is primarily through renal excretion, so that drug interactions involving hepatic metabolism do not occur. Lithium does not bind to plasma proteins. Pharmacokinetic interactions therefore usually involve the altered renal clearance of lithium, with some drugs increasing clearance and lowering serum lithium (e.g., theophylline) and others drugs decreasing renal clearance and leading to toxic levels of lithium (e.g., thiazide diuretics). Lithium has a low therapeutic index, which means that only a small difference exists between therapeutic and toxic levels. Symptoms and signs associated with toxic lithium levels include nausea, vomiting, diarrhea, tremor, headache, sedation, confusion, hyperreflexia, cardiac arrhythmias, hypotension, and, in the most severe cases, coma and death. Severe lithium toxicity is usually associated with serum levels above 2.5 mEq/L; serum levels above 3.0 mEq/L require hemodialysis, and those above 3.5 mEq/L are life threatening. In elderly or medically compromised patients, much lower levels, even those typically considered therapeutic, may lead to toxicity.

Pharmacodynamic or receptor site interactions produce toxicity, with lithium levels that are often in the therapeutic range, and the clinical presentation is usually a combination of lithium toxicity with the adverse effects of the co-administered drug. The interaction of lithium with carbamazepine and some calcium channel blockers are examples of drug interactions in which neurotoxicity develops with moderate serum lithium levels.

Acetylcholinesterase Inhibitors

EVIDENCE OF INTERACTION

In 90% of laboratory animals, the combination of lithium and the acetylcholinesterase inhibitor tacrine led to seizures and brain injury. No studies or case reports were published of the treatment combination in humans (Amante et al. 2002). Similarly, physostigmine used with lithium in laboratory animals resulted in limbic seizures and brain damage (Honchar et al. 1983). A report of the use of rivastigmine in lithium-induced delirium had no adverse effect, but the patient's lithium level in this report was very low (Fischer 2001).

MECHANISM

Lithium and tacrine increase the activity of nitric oxide synthase in the hippocampus, resulting in high levels of nitric oxide in the brain.

CLINICAL IMPLICATION

The use of lithium with acetylcholinesterase inhibitors, tacrine, donepezil, rivastigmine, or galantamine should be observed carefully, despite no demonstrated evidence of the interaction in human studies.

Aminophylline/Theophylline

EVIDENCE OF INTERACTION

Aminophylline and theophylline increase lithium excretion (Thomsen et al. 1968) and have been used to treat lithium toxicity. Perry et al. (1984) studied 10 normal subjects on 12 mg/kg per day of theophylline with up to 900 mg/day of lithium. The subjects received first lithium alone, then lithium with theophylline, then lithium alone, for a total of 23 days. During the intermediate period of co-administration, lithium clearance rose from 20.1 to 26.1 mL/min, with theophylline serum levels ranging from 5.4 to 12.7 μmg/mL in a linear dose-dependent relationship with lithium clearance. Holstad et al. (1988) also reported enhanced clearance of lithium after theophylline infusion in normal volunteers. In a separate case report, increasing doses of theophylline led to clinical deterioration with decreased lithium levels (Cook et al. 1985).

MECHANISM

Aminophylline and theophylline enhance the renal excretion of lithium.

CLINICAL IMPLICATIONS

The interaction of aminophylline and theophylline with lithium may create a problem in the treatment of manic patients who require these medications for chronic obstructive pulmonary disease. A careful titration of dosages and judicious monitoring of blood levels should permit physicians to administer aminophylline or theophylline to patients taking lithium (Sierles et al. 1982). As with any interaction of this type, the closest surveillance is required for several days after starting or stopping one of the drugs.

Antiarrhythmias

EVIDENCE OF INTERACTION

Amiodarone and lithium in combination may lead to sudden hypothyroidism. Amiodarone alone has been associated with multiple side effects, including hypothyroidism and hyperthyroidism. Ahmad (1995) reported two cases in which patients developed sudden hypothyroidism 2 to 3 weeks after the initiation of a combination of lithium and amiodarone. The first case, in a man who was receiving amiodarone, started lithium treatment for acute mania. Prior to the initiation of lithium treatment, his thyrotropin (TSH) serum level was within normal range. Two weeks after beginning lithium, the patient presented with lethargy, depression, weight gain, weakness, and hoarse voice. The serum lithium level was 0.6m Eq/L, and the TSH level was 25 μU/mL, leading to the diagnosis of hypothyroidism. Amiodarone therapy was discontinued; thyroid functions normalized and a TSH level of 4 μU/mL was reported. The second patient was a 52-year-old man who had congestive cardiomyopathy and an implantable defibrillator. The patient was being treated with enalapril, lovastatin, furosemide, and amiodarone 400 mg a day, respectively. He had routine laboratory evaluations showing a normal TSH every 6 months. The patient developed an acute mania and started treatment with lithium at 75 mg due to the concern about the enalapril and furosemide drug interaction. His lithium level was 4 mEq/L, and his mania stabilized within 3 weeks. The patient then presented with depressive symptoms and severe lethargy. His TSH level was 50 μU/mL. Amiodarone was discontinued, and TSH levels dropped to 2μU/mL within 4 weeks.

MECHANISM

Amiodarone therapy leads to iodine excess, which can account for the sudden onset of hypothyroidism following the initiation of lithium treatment.

CLINICAL IMPLICATION

Close thyroid monitoring for sudden hypothyroidism is necessary when combined amiodarone and lithium treatment is used.

Antimicrobials

EVIDENCE OF INTERACTION

Antimicrobials (including oral tetracycline, parenteral spectinomycin, and metronidazole) may raise serum lithium levels and result in toxicity. These antibiotics impair renal lithium excretion (Ayd 1978, Jefferson 1987, McGennis 1978).

In an animal study, rats receiving a single dose of 10 mL/kg of lithium chloride 150 mEq combined with 33.5 mg/10 mL of tetracycline hydrochloride, 33.5 mg/10 mL ampicillin, or 15 mg/10 mL metronidazole all experienced reduced urinary lithium excretion, whereas renal lithium clearance remained unchanged. Tetracycline increased distal sodium reabsorption and reduced renal sodium clearance. Tetracycline and metronidazole both reduced serum lithium levels 6 hours following administration, but increased these levels 24 hours after administration (Lassen 1985). In another study evaluating the relationship of the interaction between lithium and tetracycline, Fankhauser et al. (1988) found a decrease in steady-state lithium levels, suggesting that some variability may exist in the response to coadministration of these drugs.

A number of case reports also document lithium–antibiotic reactions. A woman who had been taking lithium carbonate for 3 years took an initial 500 mg dose of tetracycline, followed by 250 mg 3 times a day. Serum lithium concentration rose from 0.81 mEq/L to 2.75 mEq/L over 4 days, and she suffered clinical symptoms of lithium intoxication (McGennis 1978). Another case of doxycycline-induced lithium toxicity was reported by Miller in 1997. The patient was a 68-year-old man who was started on doxycycline for the treatment of bronchitis, in addition to a stable dose of lithium. Two days after the addition of the antibiotics, he presented with signs of lithium toxicity and a lithium level of 1.8 mEq/L. He recovered after his lithium dose was decreased.

A 40-year-old woman taking lithium carbonate 1,800 mg/day, propranolol 60 mg/day, and levothyroxine 0.15 mg/day, took metronidazole 500 mg/day for 7 days. Serum lithium concentration rose from 1.3 to 1.9 mEq/L (Ayd 1982a). Two other case reports of metronidazole-induced lithium toxicity have been reported (Teicher et al. 1987). In both cases, serum creatinine rose concomitantly with serum lithium. In one case, serum creatinine increased from 1.01 to 1.6 mg/dL after 2 days of metronidazole 250 mg 3 times per day and to 1.9 mg/dL after 2 weeks. During that same period, the lithium level increased from 1.09 to 1.3 mEq/L, with symptoms of polyuria.

A man taking spectinomycin to treat gonorrhea experienced a rise in serum lithium level from 0.8 to 3.2 mEq/L (Conroy 1978). Two patients taking both lithium and sulfamethoxazole-trimethoprim experienced a 30% to 40% decrease in serum lithium level in a paradoxical reaction (Desvilles and Sevestre 1982). Twelve patients treated with ticarcillin and lithium experienced no adverse effects.

Acyclovir interaction with lithium was reported in a 42-year-old woman who was taking lithium and was admitted to the hospital for the treatment of herpes zoster. She received intravenous acyclovir at a dose of 10 mg/kg; in 6 days, her lithium level rose fourfold and she exhibited signs of lithium toxicity (Sylvester et al. 1996).

Levofloxacin is a fluoroquinolone antibiotic. A case of severe toxicity was reported in combining levofloxacin and lithium in a 56-year-old man who was treated for bipolar disorder. His lithium dose had been stable for 5 years at 1,200 mg/day. He was also treated with chlorpromazine, 50 mg/day. His lithium blood levels were approximately 0.92 mEq/L, and his creatinine level was 0.91 mg/dL. He stopped his medications and had them restarted as a result of a manic episode. For the following 5 months, his lithium level was stable. While in the hospital, he developed bronchitis and was treated with levofloxacin 300 mg/day. Two days after the start of treatment, he developed ataxia, dysarthria, tremor, confusion, emesis, and dizziness with frequent falls. His lithium blood level at that time was 2.53 mEq/L, and his plasma creatinine level increased to 1.6 mg/dL. Both drugs were discontinued, on assumption of a drug interaction. Four days after the drug discontinuation, his clinical presentation normalized; his lithium level decreased to 1.2 mEq/L, and his creatinine level returned to 1.0 mg/dL (Takahashi et al. 2000).

MECHANISM

Antimicrobial-induced renal impairment, reflected by a decrease in creatinine clearance and increase in creatinine levels, may be the mechanism responsible for increased lithium levels (Halaris 1983).

Both lithium and acyclovir are cleared by the kidneys, thus leading to the supposition that acyclovir reduces the clearance of lithium.

CLINICAL IMPLICATIONS

Because lithium intoxication has occurred while patients were receiving spectinomycin, tetracycline, metronidazole, or levofloxacin, the clinician's index of suspicion should remain high when co-prescribing lithium with these or other antimicrobials that affect renal function. Serial lithium levels may be helpful when antimicrobials with known renal effects are added to lithium.

Lithium levels and symptoms of toxicity should be monitored every 2 to 3 days after starting intravenous acyclovir.

Anticonvulsants: Carbamazepine

EVIDENCE OF INTERACTION

Carbamazepine alone and in combination with lithium may be of benefit in the treatment of mania. In one study, 3 patients with acute mania who responded poorly to either lithium or carbamazepine alone all appeared to respond very well to a combination of the medications (Lipinski et al. 1982). Some investigators have suggested that carbamazepine used in conjunction with other medications, such as neuroleptic agents or lithium, affords additional benefit beyond the use of these traditional treatments alone (Okuma et al. 1973, Ballenger et al. 1980).

On the other hand, neurotoxicity may result from the combination of lithium and carbamazepine. A case has been reported involving a possible neurotoxic interaction between carbamazepine and lithium in a 22-year-old woman hospitalized for her third manic episode in 2 years (Ayd 1982b). After an unsuccessful 4-week trial of combined lithium–neuroleptic therapy, carbamazepine at a dosage of 600 mg/day was instituted. Within 72 hours, the patient began to manifest signs of a severe neurotoxic reaction, with generalized truncal tremors, ataxia, horizontal nystagmus, marked hyperreflexia of both arms and legs, and occasional muscle fasciculation despite therapeutic blood levels of both drugs.

Asterixis has been reported as a result of the combination of carbamazepine and lithium treatment (Rittmannsberger and Leblhuber 1992, Rittmannsberger et al. 1991). Because all the patients in this series were receiving multiple medications in addition to lithium and carbamazepine, the asterixis could have been triggered by the combination of several psychotropic medications. Despite the possible induction of neutropenia by carbamazepine therapy, lithium may increase the total white blood cell (WBC) count and neutrophil count during co-treatment with carbamazepine (Mastrosimone et al. 1979, Joffe 1988, Brewerton 1986). In a placebo-controlled study of the addition of lithium carbonate to carbamazepine (Kramlinger et al. 1990) lithium reversed the leukopenia induced by carbamazepine.

The thyroid effects of both medications were observed to be additive, resulting in an increase in TSH and a decrease in peripheral thyroid hormones. The increase in TSH during combination treatment of carbamazepine and lithium is less robust than with treatment with either medication alone.

Vieweg et al. (1987) reported that lithium and carbamazepine had opposing effects in the regulation of water and electrolytes: Carbamazepine can prevent the hyponatremia that occurs with abrupt discontinuation of lithium.

Lithium and carbamazepine can induce sinus node dysfunction. In five patients who had lithium-associated sinus node dysfunction, four were treated with carbamazepine as well, but all had elevated or toxic lithium levels, thus complicating interpretation of the finding (Steckler 1994).

Tardive dyskinesia–like syndrome was reported by Lazarus (1994) in a patient who was treated with carbamazepine for a seizure disorder. Lithium was added for the treatment of bipolar disorder. She developed a movement disorder 5 years after beginning the combined treatment. The abnormal involuntary movement was increased when she was anxious and disappeared when she was asleep, and it worsened with an addition of lithium. Both medications were discontinued after the onset of the severe movement disorder. The patient was treated for three weeks using haloperidol several years earlier.

A case of acute renal failure induced by carbamazepine leading to lithium toxicity was reported by Mayan et al. (2001).

MECHANISM

The mechanism of potentiated therapeutic effect or additive neurotoxicity with carbamazepine is not known. Predisposing factors to neurotoxicity may be medical or neurologic disease, or a prior history of lithium toxicity.

With respect to myelopoiesis, carbamazepine inhibits granulocyte-macrophage stem cells (Gallicchio and Hulette 1989). Lithium increases the production of granulocytes by stimulating the stem cells (Rossof et al. 1978, Rossof et al. 1979, Stein et al. 1979, Stein et al. 1978) or by inducing the production of colony stimulating factors (Richman et al. 1981, Kramlinger et al. 1990, Harker et al. 1977).

Lithium affects thyroid function by inhibiting the release of thyroxine and liothyronine and inhibiting iodine uptake into the gland (Sedvall et al. 1968, Bakker 1977, Berens et al. 1970). Carbamazepine may increase the metabolism of thyroid hormones by the induction of liver enzymes (Aanderud et al. 1981, De Luca et al. 1986, Visser et al. 1976).

The occurrence of sinus node dysfunction with combined treatment is not surprising, because it is a well-recognized adverse effect of lithium (Brady et al. 1988). Sinus node dysfunction usually is reversible, although the dysrhythmia may be evidence of preexisting sinus node disease (Rodney et al. 1983). Carbamazepine can prolong cardiac conduction and decrease automaticity (Kasarskis et al. 1992, Steiner et al. 1970).

The mechanism of action that causes abnormal movement is unclear. The authors of the case report speculated that the movement disorder was related to an impairment of striatal dopaminergic transmission that co-occurs with lithium and carbamazepine treatment (Lazarus 1994).

CLINICAL IMPLICATIONS

Combined lithium–carbamazepine treatment may enhance the clinical response in acute mania. In some cases, however, their concurrent use may lead to neurotoxicity. The use of combined treatment may be considered in individuals with acute manic symptoms that remain unresponsive to either drug alone, although clinicians should remain alert for signs of neurotoxicity, including ataxia, tremors, muscle fasciculations, hyperreflexia, and nystagmus (Okuma et al. 1973, Chaudry et al. 1983).

It is not known how frequently neurotoxicity occurs with the combination. In one series, 5 of 10 unipolar and bipolar patients on carbamazepine and lithium suffered central nervous system (CNS) side effects (Ghose 1978). In another study, five bipolar patients on carbamazepine and lithium who suffered neurotoxicity had a history of underlying asymptomatic CNS or systemic disease. Three had previously been neurotoxic to lithium alone, and two were previously neurotoxic to lithium with neuroleptics. The researchers concluded that those with underlying CNS or metabolic disorders may be predisposed to neurotoxicity, and that carbamazepine could enhance this tendency (Shukla et al. 1984). Haloperidol also may interact with lithium and carbamazepine, even when doses are within the normal therapeutic range, producing confusion, disorientation, visual hallucinations, other perceptual disturbances, and diplopia (Andrus 1984).

In patients with a carbamazepine-induced decrease in white blood count (WBC), the addition of lithium may be of benefit (Kramlinger et al. 1990).

The periodic monitoring of the electrocardiogram (ECG) is required when using these medications alone or in combination to treat patients at risk for conduction abnormalities.

Evidence is mounting that the combination of lithium and carbamazepine is effective in both acute mania and prophylaxis (Peselow et al. 1994). The major risk of the drug combination is neurotoxicity, although cardiac effects also should be monitored.

Lithium blood levels and kidney function tests should be monitored more closely when lithium treatment is combined with carbamazepine.

Anticonvulsants: Phenytoin

EVIDENCE OF INTERACTION

Several cases of phenytoin-induced lithium toxicity have been published in the psychiatric literature. In these cases, patients had coarse tremor, drowsiness, gastrointestinal symptoms, and coma, which in some cases persisted after lithium had been discontinued (Speirs et al. 1978). Preexisting organic brain damage may increase the susceptibility to intoxication at typically nontoxic plasma concentrations. In one case report, lithium toxicity developed during combined lithium and phenytoin treatment despite therapeutic serum concentrations of both drugs; toxic symptoms (polydipsia, polyuria, and tremor) abated when carbamazepine was substituted for phenytoin (MacCallum 1980). In another case report, in a 49-year-old man treated with phenytoin 500 mg/day for bipolar disorder, a bilateral coarse tremor of the extremities and subjective anxiety developed within 3 days of starting the medications, despite therapeutic lithium and phenytoin levels. Forty-eight hours after the patient's lithium was discontinued, the symptoms disappeared (Raskin 1984).

MECHANISM
The mechanism is unknown.

CLINICAL IMPLICATIONS
Only a few reported cases document adverse interactions between lithium and phenytoin. The clinician should be aware that toxicity may occur with the combination, despite therapeutic lithium and phenytoin levels. In many, if not most cases, the drugs can be safely co-administered under careful supervision.

Anticonvulsants: Valproic Acid
EVIDENCE OF INTERACTION
The combination of lithium and valproic acid may be useful in treatment-resistant bipolar patients, and this combination appears to be well tolerated (Schaff et al. 1993).

MECHANISM
The mechanism is unknown.

CLINICAL IMPLICATION
In treatment-resistant bipolar disorder, a combined regimen using valproic acid and lithium may be appropriate, although data are limited.

Anticonvulsants: Topiramate
EVIDENCE OF INTERACTION
A case was reported of a 26-year-old woman with bipolar disorder who had topiramate added to her medication regiment of lithium,

valproic acid, and clonazepam. After a week of treatment, her lithium level increased initially to 1.24 mEq/L and continued to rise to 1.97 mEq/L, with signs of toxicity. The lithium was discontinued; the patient normalized and was later given a lower dose of lithium with therapeutic levels. This report (Abraham et al. 2004) contrasts with previous reports of no interaction between topiramate and lithium. Other reports have ruled out an interaction between lithium and topiramate. (Bialer et al. 2002)

MECHANISM
Unknown

CLINICAL IMPLICATION
Lithium levels should be carefully monitored following the beginning of treatment with topiramate.

Antidepressants: Monoamine Oxidase Inhibitors

EVIDENCE OF INTERACTIONS
Several cases of individuals with depression refractory to traditional treatment regimens have responded to the combination of lithium and tranylcypromine or phenelzine (Himmelhoch et al. 1972, Jefferson et al. 1983, Louie et al. 1984, Nelson et al. 1982, Price et al. 1985, Zall 1971). Himmelhoch et al. (1972) reported that the addition of lithium to tranylcypromine led to "modest but definite improvement" in treatment-resistant depression. They also noted that Zall (1971) had made similar observations in three patients taking isocarboxazid and lithium. Price et al. (1985) studied 12 inpatients with major depression who were refractory to at least two controlled antidepressant trials. Depending on the criteria used, between 8 and 11 of the 12 patients improved on a lithium–tranylcypromine combination. Louie et al. (1984), studying the addition of lithium to a number of antidepressants, reported much less predictable results, including a manic episode in a 36-year-old man taking phenelzine 60 mg daily.

MECHANISM
The mechanism of enhanced antidepressant response is unknown, although some attribute it to the fact that antidepressants normalize presynaptic serotonergic activity, whereas lithium acts via pre- and/or postsynaptic mechanisms. Phenelzine does not alter lithium influx into red blood cells or the lithium red blood cell-to-plasma ratio (Pandey et al. 1979).

CLINICAL IMPLICATIONS

The combination of lithium and monoamine oxidase inhibitors (MAOIs) is one of several therapeutic regimens for depression refractory to conventional antidepressant treatment. Adverse consequences from the combination are rare, although clinicians should be aware of a report of two patients taking lithium and tranylcypromine in whom tardive dyskinesia developed (Stancer 1979), and another report of an elderly man with dementia suffering significant ataxia and urinary retention while on combined therapy (Cowdry et al. 1983). Although mania has been reported using the combination, and paranoid symptoms may appear in patients with a schizoaffective disorder, these all may occur with the use of a MAOI alone and are quite unlikely to be attributable to a drug interaction.

Antidepressants: Cyclics and Related Antidepressants

EVIDENCE OF INTERACTION

A number of reports suggest that the addition of lithium to cyclic antidepressants in patients with treatment-resistant depression leads to improvement within several days. De Montigny et al. (1981) added lithium to tricyclic antidepressants in eight patients with nonresponsive depression (nonpsychotic, unipolar). Substantial decreases were seen in depression rating scale scores within 2 days, and improvement continued whether or not lithium was continued. A study comparing lithium and triiodothyronine in the augmentation of tricyclic antidepressant in a placebo-controlled design found them both to be equally effective and more effective than placebo (Joffe et al. 1993). In a review of controlled trials, Austin et al. (1990) found a highly statistically significant effect for lithium augmentation.

Other reports describe the antidepressant effect of lithium when added to a neuroleptic–desipramine combination in the treatment of refractory psychotically depressed patients (Louie et al. 1984, Price et al. 1985). Louie et al. (1984) described highly variable results when adding lithium to an antidepressant in nine patients. Two showed sustained improvement, two showed transient improvement and then relapse, two with bipolar illness became manic, and three did not improve.

De Montigny et al. (1983) reported that in 30 of 42 instances involving 39 unipolar depressed patients unresponsive to a 3-week trial of tricyclic antidepressants, the addition of lithium brought about a greater than 50% reduction in depression scores within 48 hours. Heninger et al. (1983) studied the addition of lithium to a tricyclic antidepressant (desipramine or amitriptyline) or mianserin in patients ($N = 15$) with major depression who had been unresponsive to a 3-week drug trial. A greater improvement in depression was observed in the lithium group than in the placebo group. Furthermore, the subsequent substitution of lithium for placebo in the control group resulted in improvement. Rapid improvement (within 24 to 48 hours) was noted in five patients, whereas the remaining patients did not show a clear improvement until approximately 5 to 8 days later. In patients whose depression was treatment resistant and who failed a prospective treatment trial of nortriptyline, lithium augmentation of nortriptyline was not significantly better than placebo (Nierenberg et al. 2003). Although one case report suggested that the combination of lithium, maprotiline 50 mg twice a day, and L-iodothyronine 25 μmg was effective in a depressed 73-year-old woman (Weaver 1983), others report toxicity characterized by myoclonic jerks and tremor (Kettl et al. 1983) when using the combination. Joyce et al. (1983) gave mianserin plus lithium to a 64-year-old man with a recurrent major depression that had been unresponsive to maprotiline, chlorpromazine, and electroconvulsive therapy. Within 2 days of adding lithium to mianserin, the patient improved. On the other hand, other authors have reported therapeutic failures with the combination (Gray, 1983 Graham 1984).

One case report describes the effectiveness of a trazodone–lithium combination in a 45-year-old man with depression (Birkhimer et al. 1983), and another report documents the unsuccessful treatment of a bulimic patient with the drug combination (Pope et al. 1983).

Three of six depressed patients who failed to respond to bupropion alone improved when lithium was added (Price et al. 1985). Bupropion was observed to promote weight loss even in the presence of lithium, which when given alone leads to weight gain (Gardner 1983).

Increased toxicity has been reported with the combination of antidepressants and lithium. Generalized tonic-clonic (grand mal) seizures occurred after the addition of 900 mg/day of lithium to amitriptyline 300 mg/day (Solomon 1979). Seizures recurred following rechallenge. The issue of cardiac toxicity has been raised by the report of an adolescent taking lithium and imipramine in whom cardiomyopathy and hypothyroidism developed after 6 months of treatment (Dietrich et al. 1993). After lithium and imipramine were discontinued, thyroid replacement therapy resulted in cardiac dysrhythmias.

Underactive thyroid function has been reported in 12 patients receiving lithium and tricyclic antidepressants, which led investigators to speculate that these two drugs have an additive antithyroid effect (Rogers et al. 1971).

A case report of two elderly patients who were treated with the combination of tricyclic antidepressant and lithium showed an increase in neurotoxicity with therapeutic doses. The symptoms experienced were tremors, severe memory difficulties, distractibility, and disorganized thinking (Austin et al. 1990).

Limited evidence suggests that the combination of lithium and tricyclic antidepressants may be of value in treating tardive dyskinesia in depressed patients, as documented in 19 patients, 58% of whom experienced either moderate or marked improvement in both dyskinesia and depression with combined tricyclic antidepressant and lithium therapy (Rosenbaum et al. 1980).

MECHANISM

The mechanism of lithium potentiation of antidepressant effects is unknown but may involve enhanced CNS serotonergic activity. In a study exploring the serotonergic function in lithium augmentation, McCance-Katz et al. (1992) measured the prolactin response to intravenous L-tryptophan in patients with refractory major depression. Lithium augmentation resulted in statistically significant greater increases in the prolactin response to tryptophan challenge. With regard to adverse effects, both lithium and antidepressants lower the seizure threshold, thus their combination may have had an additive effect in the occurrence of generalized tonic-clonic (grand mal) seizures as reported in the published cases. On the other hand, lithium is commonly prescribed with antidepressants without adverse consequences. Although the antithyroid effect of lithium is well known, the reported additive antithyroid effects of the combination are not proven.

CLINICAL IMPLICATIONS

In general, the combination of lithium and antidepressants appears to be well tolerated, and lithium is an effective addition to antidepressants in the treatment of patients with refractory depression. Apparently, it does not offer improved prophylaxis of recurrent manic episodes compared with lithium alone, and some have suggested that the frequency of cycling increases in bipolar patients on antidepressants. Neurotoxicity is possible when antidepressants and lithium are prescribed concurrently, and seizures have been reported. Special caution should be used in the elderly due to the increased risk of neurotoxicity, and in children and adolescents who may be more susceptible to the cardiac conduction effects of both medications. Frequent monitoring of signs of neurotoxicity such as tremors, disorientation, headaches, or confusion is necessary. Baseline and periodic EKGs are also necessary.

Antidepressants: Selective Serotonin Reuptake Inhibitors

EVIDENCE OF INTERACTION

Case reports of severe lithium toxicity resulting from the combination of lithium and fluoxetine have been published. A 44-year-old woman who had been taking lithium for 20 years without problems was given fluoxetine to treat an episode of depression (Salama et al. 1989). A few days following the initiation of treatment, dizziness, unsteadiness, and stiffness of arms and legs developed. Her gait became ataxic and her speech dysarthric, with a corresponding increase in her lithium level to 1.70 mEq/L. The patient's lithium dose was decreased, and the fluoxetine was discontinued with resolution of the neurologic symptoms. In another case report, a 53-year-old woman with a major depressive episode treated with fluoxetine and lorazepam was placed on lithium augmentation and, within 48 hours, she exhibited confusion, ataxia, and inability to follow commands (Noveske et al. 1989). She demonstrated a coarse tremor, poor coordination, and held her legs in a flexed position, extending them randomly. She could not sit, walk, or stand without help. In addition to these toxic symptoms, she had a leukocyte count of 17,300/mm^3. Her symptoms improved over several days after both medications were discontinued. In another case, the serum lithium level increased to 1.38m Eq/L in a 38-year-old woman after the addition of fluoxetine (Hadley et al. 1989). A month after her lithium dose was decreased, her serum lithium level was 0.8 mEq/L, but she became acutely manic. In another report, a 36-year-old woman taking fluoxetine 40 mg/day had an exacerbation of depression when lithium was added to her treatment (Muly et al. 1993). She was given lithium 300 mg twice daily for 5 days (serum level 0.65 mEq/L prior to increasing the lithium dose to 300 mg three times daily). Two days later, signs and symptoms consistent with a serotonin syndrome developed (e.g., akathisia, myoclonus, hyperreflexia, shivering, tremor, diarrhea, and incoordination) with a serum lithium level of 0.88 mEq/L. Lithium was discontinued, and cyproheptadine 12 mg was administered. Subsequently, the patient was able to tolerate fluoxetine alone (40 mg daily) with no adverse effects.

A case has been reported of absence seizures resulting from the combination of lithium and fluoxetine (Sacristan et al. 1991). A 44-year-old man was treated with lithium for depression. Forty-two days after the addition of fluoxetine, he had discrete episodes of immobility and staring into space, which lasted a few seconds prior to resuming his previous activity. He had no recollection of these events. When his lithium dose was reduced, no further episodes occurred. Unfortunately, no EEG recording was done during these episodes, but a recording made later showed no seizure activity.

In another report, somnolence was observed after the addition of lithium to fluvoxamine, without any other neurologic symptoms and normal laboratory results (Evans et al. 1990a). The British Committee on the Safety of Medicines has reported neurotoxicity, characterized by tremors and seizure, with the combination of fluvoxamine and lithium.

In an open, parallel randomized study, 16 volunteers received lithium 600 mg twice daily for 9 days. Ten and 20 days prior to the last lithium dose, sertraline 100 mg or placebo was administered. Sertraline did not affect the renal clearance or the serum level of lithium. The subjects who received sertraline were more likely to experience adverse events, primarily tremor (Warrington 1991). In another study of the effect of sertraline on the renal clearance of lithium, an open-label, placebo-controlled study of 20 healthy subjects did not find any statistically significant changes in the clearance or serum levels of lithium. Compared with control subjects receiving placebo, subjects taking the combination experienced more adverse effects, primarily tremors (Apseloff et al. 1992). In a study in which lithium was co-administered with fluoxetine in 10 young healthy volunteers, an initial pharmacokinetic interaction was noted in lower C_{max} and lower lithium concentrations. No clinically significant differences were observed in the serum concentrations, half life of either medication, and renal clearance of the drugs. There were also no homodynamic differences or in EKG (Breuel et al. 1995).

Dinan (1993) used lithium augmentation with sertraline in 11 patients with treatment-resistant depression. Seven of the patients responded within a week without significant side effects. No correlation of response occurred with lithium levels. Lithium augmentation was observed in a study of 12 depressed patients who were treated with fluvoxamine alone or in combination with lithium. The six patients who were treated with the combination of lithium and fluvoxamine showed a greater improvement. No pharmacokinetic differences were observed between the groups, and there were no differences in fluvoxamine blood levels (Miljkovic et al. 1997). Similar results were demonstrated by Bauer et al. (1999). In this study, the co-administration of lithium and paroxetine or amitriptyline in breakthrough depression yielded better results in the paroxetine group.

Serotonin syndrome was reported after lithium was added to paroxetine (Sobanski et al. 1997), fluvoxamine (Ohman et al. 1993), and venlafaxine (Mekler et al. 1997). In all these cases, no evidence suggested a pharmacokinetic interaction, and medications levels were within acceptable range.

MECHANISM

The mechanism of the interaction leading to seizures has not been established. Some have suggested that toxicity is a consequence of altered distribution of lithium in the brain tissue as reflected by an increased ratio of erythrocyte to plasma levels or altered receptor sensitivity (Elizur et al. 1972, Francis et al. 1970, Salama et al. 1989, Sacristan et al. 1991). Concomitant use of these medications also has an additive or synergistic effect on serotonin activity, which may be responsible for both increased efficacy and neurotoxicity (Evans et al. 1990a).

Because lithium and the different selective serotonin reuptake inhibitors (SSRIs) individually enhance the serotonin system, the combined treatment may lead to serotonin syndrome and to the increased efficacy of the drug combination.

CLINICAL IMPLICATIONS

Lithium is frequently given to patients taking SSRIs to improve antidepressant response (Fava et al. 1994). The most common adverse effect appears to be tremor, which can progress in some cases to severe neurotoxicity with ataxia, confusion, and seizures. Serum lithium level may not be elevated in all cases of neurotoxicity.

The patient should be warned of the risk of serotonin syndrome and the increased neurotoxicity when lithium and SSRI are used in conjunction, and he should be monitored for early signs.

Antidepressants: Clomipramine

EVIDENCE OF INTERACTION

A 59-year-old man suffered from depression and lacunar infarction of the basal ganglia. He was treated with clomipramine 25 mg/day (gradually increased to 175 mg/day), levomepromazine 25 mg/day, and flunitrazepam 2 mg/day. Because of an incomplete response, lithium 600 mg/day was added. After lithium was increased to 1,000 mg/day, myoclonus, shivering, tremors, incoordination, and elated mood developed, which was consistent with serotonin syndrome, with the exception of only a mild increase in temperature to 37.2°C. The lithium was stopped, followed by a dramatic reduction of symptoms. The clomipramine dose was later reduced, causing further improvement, and all symptoms abated when it was discontinued (Kojima et al. 1993).

MECHANISM

Both lithium and clomipramine enhance serotonergic activity.

CLINICAL IMPLICATIONS

A serotonin syndrome may occur with the combination of lithium and clomipramine. This is a potentially serious interaction and, if these drugs are used together, low doses and close monitoring are advised.

Antihypertensives (*See also* Calcium Channel Blockers and Diuretics, *this chapter*)

EVIDENCE OF INTERACTION

Methyldopa

Several case reports have documented increased toxicity when lithium is given with methyldopa (O'Regan 1976, Byrd 1975). One case report involved a 45-year-old woman with a 25-year history of manic depressive illness who, when discharged from inpatient hospitalization on a regimen of 1,800 mg of lithium carbonate and 1 g of methyldopa daily (serum lithium levels ranging between 0.5 and 0.7 mEq/L), began to show signs of toxicity, including blurred vision, hand tremors, mild diarrhea, confusion, and slurring of speech. Ten days after the discontinuation of methyldopa, the patient's serum lithium level was 1.4 mEq/L. As the lithium dosage was decreased to 900 mg/day, stable serum lithium levels were achieved (1.0 mEq/L), with a reversal of toxic symptoms (Byrd 1975). A second case report involved a 72-year-old man who also exhibited toxic symptoms as a result of the co-administration of lithium and methyldopa (Osanloo et al. 1980). In a study of three subjects on lithium and methyldopa, lithium levels did not change; however, confusion, sedation, and dysphoria increased (Walker et al. 1980).

Prazosin

Two patients with the diagnosis of schizophrenia who were taking neuroleptics, lithium, and prazosin did not suffer significant adverse effects (Hommer et al. 1984). This combination may be useful when thiazides and β-blockers are not effective (Schwarcz 1982).

Propranolol

Propranolol may have antimanic properties in doses considerably larger than those used in treating hypertension (Schwarcz 1982, Jefferson et al. 1981). All β-adrenergic blockers are effective in treating lithium-induced tremors. When administered with lithium, propranolol may increase lithium levels (Schou et al. 1987), although data are limited. The addition of β-blocking agents to lithium may induce bradycardia (Becker 1989).

Clonidine

Bipolar patients had smaller decreases in blood pressure in response to clonidine when taking chronic doses of lithium compared with blood pressure when lithium was withdrawn (Goodnick et al. 1984). Acute doses of lithium potentiate clonidine-induced aggressive behavior in mice (Ozawa et al. 1975).

Angiotensin-Converting Enzyme Inhibitors and Angiotensin-2 Receptor Antagonist

Several reports document patients on enalapril (Vasotec) in whom lithium intoxication developed (3.3 mEq/L), with mild impairment of kidney function, which returned to normal after discontinuation of the medications (Douste-Blazy et al. 1986). Navis et al. (1989) reported a 65-year-old woman who was admitted after 6 months of lithium and enalapril treatment with frequent monitoring of blood levels. At the time of admission, she was dehydrated, hypotensive, and oliguric, with a serum lithium level of 2.35 mEq/L. Volume restoration resulted in eventual normalization of blood pressure and laboratory values. The authors explain the change in lithium level as resulting from volume depletion due to any cause such as gastrointestinal (GI) loss and the drug combination. Other case reports (Drouet and Bouvet 1990, Correa et al. 1992) described toxic lithium levels that occurred when renal function was decreased. DasGupta et al. (1992) studied the drug interaction in a crossover study of nine healthy volunteers who took lithium alone, lithium and enalapril, and lithium alone again. No significant differences were observed between lithium serum levels when lithium was administered alone compared with administration with enalapril. Lisinopril (Prinivil) 20 mg/day led to lithium toxicity in a 49-year-old woman taking lithium 1,500 mg/day (Baldwin et al. 1990). In a retrospective longitudinal case control study, 20 hypertensive patients who were treated with lithium and maintained at stable levels had an angiotensin-converting enzyme (ACE) inhibitor treatment initiated. Lithium steady-state concentration was increased by 36.1%, and lithium clearance was reduced by 25.5%. Four patients experienced lithium toxicity. The changes in lithium clearance were correlated with serum creatinine levels. These changes were more likely to happen in the geriatric population (Finley et al. 1996). In multiple anecdotal observations of the co-administration of lithium and ACE inhibitors, lithium interaction with these drugs appears to have led to renal dysfunction. Lithium can lead to volume depletion secondary to the polyuria, and the laboratory findings of patients receiving lithium treatment may be consistent with dehydration. In the combined use of ACE inhibitors and lithium, the deterioration of the kidney function developed gradually and was fully reversible upon discontinuation of treatment (Lehmann et al. 1995).

In a case reported by Blanche et al. (1997), an angiotensin-2 receptor (AT_2 receptor) antagonist, losartan (Cozaar) co-administered with lithium led to lithium toxicity. The case reported a 77-year-old woman, who had been treated with a stable dose of lithium for bipolar disorder at 625 mg daily with a plasma level of 0.63 mEq/L and serum creatinine level of 0.9 mg/dL. She was treated with nifedipine with unsatisfactory results; losartan was added at 50 mg daily. Five weeks later, she was hospitalized with signs of lithium toxicity and lithium blood level of 2 mEq/L and serum creatinine levels of 1.08 mg/dL. No other cause for lithium intoxication was observed. Both medications were discontinued initially, with lithium restarted and nicardipine 100 mg replacing the losartan. Kidney function tests remained unchanged, but the lithium level stabilized. In another case of an AT_2 receptor antagonist, valsartan (Diovan) was concomitantly used with lithium, leading to lithium toxicity (Leung et al. 2000). Lithium levels stabilized when valsartan was replaced by diltiazem.

In a population-based nested case control study in Ontario, Canada, residents age 66 and above who were treated with lithium were assessed for the risk of hospital admissions for lithium toxicity. Loop diuretics and ACE inhibitors were the medications associated with increased risk for lithium toxicity when co-administered with lithium. For both medications, the admission to the hospital for lithium toxicity occurred within a month of initiation of treatment (Juurlink et al. 2004). In this study, neither thiazide diuretics nor nonsteroidal antiinflammatory drug (NSAID) concomitant treatment led to an admission for lithium intoxication.

MECHANISM

The mechanism of the methyldopa–lithium interaction is not clear. Methyldopa may increase serum lithium levels and thus induce toxicity; however, toxicity has been reported with normal serum lithium levels. Methyldopa may exaggerate the CNS response to lithium or increase the cellular uptake of lithium. Propranolol may reduce renal clearance of lithium.

Chronic lithium treatment may decrease α_2-adrenergic receptor sensitivity, decreasing the antihypertensive response to clonidine.

Lithium toxicity in the presence of enalapril, lisinopril, or other ACE inhibitors may be due to altered renal function secondary to the

ACE inhibition and/or the natriuretic effect of the drug. In DasGupta's study, the enalapril dose was lower than those used in the clinical cases reported. Abnormalities in hydration, renal function, and cardiovascular status all may predispose to lithium toxicity when ACE inhibitors are used concomitantly. AT_2-receptor antagonists inhibit aldosterone secretion, leading to natriuresis, which may increase renal lithium reabsorption. This effect could cause lithium toxicity when losartan treatment is combined with lithium administration.

CLINICAL IMPLICATIONS

The signs of lithium intoxication may occur during methyldopa treatment even though lithium levels are within therapeutic range. Serum lithium levels alone, therefore, cannot be used to predict or diagnose this drug interaction. Patients taking both methyldopa and lithium should be carefully monitored upon the initiation or discontinuation of methyldopa. Electroencephalograms may reflect toxicity in the presence of levels that are usually considered therapeutic.

The effectiveness of clonidine may be reduced in the presence of lithium.

Enalapril (Vasotec) may increase serum lithium levels and lead to toxicity. Other ACE inhibitors such as ramipril (Altace), captopril (Capoten), lisinopril (Prinivil, Zestril), fosinopril (Monopril), and benazepril (Lotensin) have similar risk. Although some authorities have recommended against the concurrent use of lithium and enalapril (Baldwin et al. 1990), most evidence at this time does not support complete avoidance of lithium and ACE inhibitors. Caution should be used when treating patients with these drugs by initiating treatment using small doses of lithium (e.g., we have seen patients taking ACE inhibitors reach prophylactic lithium levels at doses as low as 300 mg/day). Lithium levels and serum creatinine should be monitored frequently. The use of an AT_2-receptor antagonist together with lithium should lead to lithium dose reduction or careful monitoring of lithium levels.

Some authorities recommend that β-blockers are the preferred antihypertensive agents for patients taking lithium, although interactions are possible with this combination as well, with isolated reports of increased lithium levels and bradycardia.

Antiinflammatory Drugs

EVIDENCE OF INTERACTION

Several case reports have documented reduced renal lithium clearance, leading to 30% to 60% increases in plasma lithium levels as a result of the co-prescription of antiinflammatory medications that inhibit prostaglandin synthesis (Singer et al. 1978, Ragheb 1990). In one case report, the effects of indomethacin on renal lithium excretion and plasma lithium levels were studied in four volunteers with normal renal function. A decrease in renal lithium excretion and an increase in plasma lithium levels were found in all subjects. Increases in plasma lithium levels averaged 48% above baseline, with a range of 25% to 63% (Frolich et al. 1979). In another investigation, the influence of the nonsteroidal antiinflammatory drug diclofenac (Voltaren) on lithium kinetics was studied in five normal women. Diclofenac decreased lithium renal clearance by 23% and increased lithium plasma levels by 26% (Reimann et al. 1981). An interaction was also found in three manic patients who were given indomethacin 150 mg/day for 6 days (Ragheb et al. 1980), as were volunteers given diclofenac 150 mg/day for 8 days. In the latter study, urinary clearance decreased and plasma lithium levels rose 25% (Reimann et al. 1981). Similar results have been seen with mefenamic acid (Ponstel), clomethacin, and niflumic acid (MacDonald et al. 1988, Gay et al. 1985, Colonna 1979, Shelley 1987). Another case report found that ibuprofen (Advil, Motrin) had inconsistent effects on plasma lithium levels and lithium clearance (Ragheb et al. 1980, Ragheb 1987b). Studies on rats have documented an interaction between phenylbutazone and indomethacin and lithium urinary elimination (Imbs et al. 1980, Singer et al. 1978). Sulindac (Clinoril) increased lithium clearance but did not affect lithium levels (Furnell et al. 1985); nor have others found any changes in lithium level when sulindac was added to treatment (Ragheb et al. 1986b, Ragheb et al. 1986a). Jones et al. (2000) reported two cases of increased lithium levels following treatment with sulindac. The first is of a 23-year-old man who was treated with sulindac for shoulder pain while admitted to a state psychiatric facility. The sulindac was added to lithium 1,500 mg/day, divalproex sodium 3,500 mg/day, olanzapine 25 mg/day, and tetracycline 250 mg/day. All medications were unchanged for a period of 4 months, and serum lithium concentration was recorded as 1.0 mEq/L. Lithium concentration increased to 1.3 mEq/L 3 days after the initiation of sulindac, and to 2.0 mEq/L 19 days following the initiation of treatment. Lithium concentration decreased to 0.8 mEq/L 5 days after discontinuation of sulindac. The patient exhibited lithium toxicity signs while his levels were elevated. The second case, in a 27-year-old woman, sulindac was added to her treatment of lithium 1,800 mg/day, nefazodone 500 mg/day, fluphenazine decanoate 37.5 mg every two weeks, and lorazepam 0.5 mg 3 times a day. The treatment continued for 5 months before the initiation of sulindac. Lithium concentration prior to starting sulindac was 0.9 mEq/L and increased to 1.7 mEq/L 5 days after sulindac was added. The lithium dose was gradually decreased to 1.0 mEq/L.

Ketorolac (Toradol), a NSAID that is available in both oral and parenteral form and in wide clinical use for the treatment of acute and chronic pain may also increase serum lithium levels. When ketorolac in oral doses of 30 mg/day was given to an 80-year-old man who had been stabilized on lithium with serum levels of 0.5 to 0.7 mEq/L, his level rose to 1.1 mEq/L in 6 days (Langlois et al. 1994). Lithium serum and red blood cell (RBC) levels were monitored in five healthy volunteers taking 1,200 mg of lithium daily for 13 days. Ketorolac was added to their medication treatment at 40 mg daily on days 8 through 12. Blood samples were obtained to evaluate serum and RBC lithium levels. The lithium area under the concentration-time curve (AUC) was increased by 24%, and RBC lithium concentration was increased by 27% with the co-administration of the medications. The increase in levels also was associated with an increase in adverse events (Cold et al. 1998). Piroxicam (Feldene) also may be associated with lithium toxicity during combined therapy (Harrison et al. 1986, Kerry et al. 1983, Nadarajah et al. 1985, Walbridge et al. 1985).

Allen et al. (1989) reported successful treatment of a case of lithium-induced diabetes insipidus with indomethacin, although this is not a generally accepted treatment for the condition.

In an open controlled study exploring the effect of meloxicam on lithium pharmacokinetics, 16 healthy volunteers received lithium in combination with meloxicam to achieve a level of 0.3 to 0.7 mEq/L. At day 14, meloxicam was withdrawn, and lithium remained unchanged until day 22. Meloxicam increased lithium C_{max} values by 16%, and the total plasma clearance of lithium was reduced by meloxicam to 82.5% of lithium alone (Türck et al. 2000).

The interaction between lithium and cyclooxygenase-2 (COX-2) selective inhibitors has been reported repeatedly. Lundmark et al. (2002) described a case of a 73-year-old man who was on ongoing lithium treatment since 1969, having a lithium concentration ranging between 0.6 to 0.9 mEq/L and a creatinine level of 1.0 and 1.2 mg/dL. Other medications were lofepramine, warfarin, furosemide, and captopril, all used for two years. Nine days after rofecoxib 12.5 mg daily was initiated, the patient reported somnolence, mild confusion, irritability, tremor, and gait disturbances. The lithium serum level was 1.5 mEq/L and the creatinine level was 1.43 mg/dL. Lithium and rofecoxib were withdrawn, with resolution of the symptoms in a week and a return of lithium level to the previously recorded levels. The lithium dose was decreased following this episode. A case of life-threatening lithium toxicity was reported by Slørdal et al. (2003) in a 58-year-old woman who was treated with lithium 210 mg daily and maintained blood levels of 0.5 to 0.9m Eq/L, sertraline 100 mg, levomepromazine 25 mg/day, esomeprazole 20 mg/day, tibolone 2.5 mg/day, and ibuprofen 400 mg as needed. Five days before her admission, she started treatment with celecoxib 400 mg twice daily. Following the initiation of treatment, she developed malaise, nausea, abdominal pain, and drowsiness. On admission, she had bradycardia of 20 beats/min and hypotension. Her lithium level was 4.0 mEq/L, and her creatinine level was 2.18 mg/dL. She was treated with hemodialysis, which normalized her lithium and creatinine levels. She was found to have a preexisting condition of sinoatrial conduction block and was not restarted on the medication combination. A third case reported a 68-year-old woman treated with ongoing lithium, carbamazepine, pipamperone, and mirtazapine who started rofecoxib 25 mg twice daily for leg pain. A week following the addition of rofecoxib, she developed tremor and hypokinesia that was treated with propranolol. She developed bradycardia and was treated with isoproterenol. The patient's lithium blood concentration doubled from prior to the rofecoxib treatment, and her kidney function worsened. All findings and laboratory values tests improved after the medication combination was discontinued (Rätz Bravo et al. 2004).

MECHANISM

NSAIDs, which inhibit prostaglandin synthesis, also reduce the renal clearance of lithium by affecting a prostaglandin-dependent mechanism located in the renal tubule. Another possible mechanism is that NSAIDs compete with lithium for the transport mechanism at the proximal tubule (Brater 1986, Brater 1988, Gobe et al. 1983, Johnson et al. 1993, Tonkin et al. 1988).

In cases documenting an interaction between COX-2 inhibitors and lithium, all patients were elderly and treated with multiple medication. COX-2 inhibitors may affect kidney function as well as prostaglandins (primarily prostaglandin E_2), leading to vasodilation. These functions may play a role in the kidney's blood flow. In elderly patients, who may already be sodium and volume depleted, the use of a COX-2 inhibitor may lead to a decline in kidney function due to a decrease in blood flow and an accumulation of lithium (Rätz Bravo et al. 2004).

CLINICAL IMPLICATIONS

Many published reports document an interaction between lithium and NSAIDs, suggesting that the simultaneous administration of these drugs is potentially hazardous. Lithium levels should be monitored frequently when patients are taking this drug combination. Preliminary evidence suggests that aspirin may be less likely to interact with lithium, but data are limited (Ragheb 1987b).

The use of COX-2 inhibitors in patients treated with lithium should be avoided, especially in the elderly, who may be on multiple other medications. If lithium treatment cannot be avoided, the medication dose should be reduced and blood levels should be monitored frequently.

Antipsychotic Agents (*See* Chapter 3)

Antithyroid Drugs

EVIDENCE OF INTERACTION

Hypothyroidism, and less commonly hyperthyroidism and thyrotoxicosis, have been documented in patients taking prophylactic lithium therapy for manic depressive illness (Barclay et al. 1994, Chow et al. 1993, Jefferson and Sen 1994, Persad et al. 1993). An interaction between ambient iodine and lithium has been suggested as influencing lithium-induced hypothyroidism. Lithium-induced hypothyroidism appears more prevalent in countries in which dietary iodine is highly available (Canada), as compared to countries in which dietary iodine is relatively deficient (Italy, Germany, Spain). This appears to indicate that iodine deficiency may have a thyroid protective role in lithium treated patients (Leutgeb 2000).

Some evidence supports the efficacy of lithium in thyrotoxicosis. Serum thyroid hormone levels are consistently decreased in thyrotoxic patients receiving lithium. In one study, decreases ranging from 30% to 85% of the rate of iodine and hormonal iodine secretion occurred within 12 hours of patients' reaching lithium serum levels as low as 0.5 mEq/L. The addition of methimazole resulted in greater drops in thyroid hormone levels (Temple et al. 1972). In another study, thyrotoxic patients were treated with (a) carbimazole and lithium, (b) carbimazole and iodine, or (c) carbimazole alone. Serum thyroxine level fell almost 50% in the first two groups, compared with 18% in the third group. Mean serum level was 0.63 mEq/L (Turner 1975, Turner et al. 1976). A fall of approximately 30% in serum thyroxine level in 20 thyrotoxic patients taking lithium was reported by Gerdes et al. (1973). In a comparison of lithium and methimazole, investigators found no significant difference in the reduction of serum thyroxine iodine or free thyroxine index at 3 and 10 days (Kristensen et al. 1976).

Lithium has been used preoperatively to prevent thyroid storms in the surgical treatment of Graves disease when conventional antithyroid drugs such as methimazole, propylthiouracil, or thionamide were not well tolerated (Mochinaga et al. 1994, Takami 1994).

Carbimazole treatment was effective in treating hyperthyroidism in a 68-year-old man with bipolar disorder who had been taking lithium 1,000 mg/day for 5 years (Sadoul et al. 1994). The patient developed transient hypothyroidism followed by signs and symptoms of hyperthyroidism several months later (e.g., tremor, exophthalmus, ocular muscle enlargement, increased free thyroxine, and triiodothyronine) that responded to carbimazole therapy.

Lithium has also been used as an adjunct to radioactive iodine (^{131}I) in the treatment of thyrotoxicosis (Turner et al. 1976). Patients who had been receiving lithium carbonate 400 mg for 5 days were given the standard therapeutic dose of ^{131}I and continued on lithium for another 5 days. The lithium-treated patients had increased retention of thyroidal ^{131}I compared with control subjects. The investigators suggested that this therapeutic regimen concentrates radioactive iodine in the gland and allows for a lower total body exposure to radioactivity.

MECHANISM

Lithium rapidly blocks the release of thyroxine and triiodothyronine from the thyroid gland, resulting in a decrease in circulating hormone.

CLINICAL IMPLICATIONS

Lithium enhances the action of thyroid suppressing drugs, and combination treatment may have some clinical value in the therapy of thyrotoxicosis, especially in individuals in whom standard therapy is contraindicated.

Benzodiazepines

EVIDENCE OF INTERACTION

A few anecdotal case reports describe patients who had difficulty with the combined use of lithium and a benzodiazepine. Diazepam and oxazepam in particular were reported to produce an increase in depression that was not apparent in patients receiving lithium alone. This is most probably the effect of diazepam and oxazepam alone in patients who were particularly sensitive to benzodiazepines, and no definite drug interaction has been established (Rosenbaum et al. 1979).

A single case report of profound hypothermia resulting from the combined use of lithium and diazepam clearly implicates lithium as the causative agent. Lithium resulted in hypothermia, a comatose state with reduced reflexes, dilated pupils, a systolic blood pressure between 40 and 60 mm Hg, pulse rate of 40 beats/min, and absence of piloerection response (Naylor et al. 1977). On the removal of lithium, the patient's temperature rose progressively to normal range and, on rechallenge with lithium, again fell to similar hypothermic levels with the above-noted symptoms.

Koczerginski et al. (1989) reported five cases in which the combination of lithium and clonazepam resulted in neurotoxicity, with symptoms of ataxia and dysarthria. In all of these cases, the lithium level was increased and the symptoms were completely reversed when lithium was stopped. All of these patients were also taking neuroleptic medications at the same time, which probably contributed to the development of the neurotoxicity (see Chapter 3) (West et al. 1979). In a study of 104 outpatients taking lithium in combination with other psychoactive medications, an association was found between the use of combination treatment with lithium and benzodiazepines and sexual dysfunction (Ghadirian et al. 1992). The incidence of dysfunction was significantly higher than with any other combination or with lithium alone.

The pharmacokinetic interaction of alprazolam and lithium was studied by Evans et al. (1990b). Ten healthy volunteers were given lithium in doses of 900 to 1,500 mg/day. Although alprazolam administration (1 mg twice daily) decreased lithium clearance, steady-state lithium concentrations were increased only slightly, and the change was not of clinical significance.

In one isolated case, addition of 18 mg/day of bromazepam to a stable lithium regimen caused lithium plasma concentration to rise from 1.12 to 1.40 mEq/L with pretoxic symptoms (Raudino 1981). In another case, an unspecified benzodiazepine and lithium allegedly caused neuroleptic malignant syndrome (NMS) (Levenson 1985).

Flumazenil, a benzodiazepine antagonist, can lead to seizures when administered to patients with a seizure disorder or on medications, such as lithium, that lower the seizure threshold (Spivey 1992).

Animal studies have also examined the interaction of benzodiazepines and lithium. Rats receiving lithium for 4 weeks had a 10% to 20% decrease in benzodiazepine receptor number in the frontal cortex (Hetmar et al. 1983). Another study found an 11% decrease in rat receptor binding (Kafka et al. 1982). The effect of benzodiazepine on the midbrain and cerebellum of the rat is unchanged by chronic lithium doses (Reilly et al. 1983). A combination of lithium and phenazepam caused a statistically significant increase in lithium in the liver and mesencephalon of mice, and rapid increases in lithium in the cerebral cortex, cerebellum, mesencephalon, and liver (Samoilov et al. 1980). The sedative effects of diazepam in mice were potentiated by lithium (Mannisto et al. 1976).

MECHANISM

Hypothermia associated with combined lithium and diazepam treatment is most probably an idiosyncratic reaction.

It is possible that the increase in lithium level in the presence of clonazepam is a pharmacokinetic interaction involving renal excretion (Freinhar et al. 1985, Koczerginski et al. 1989), although neurotoxicity in the reported cases probably involved the concurrent use of neuroleptics.

CLINICAL IMPLICATIONS

Considering the wide use of benzodiazepines to sedate acutely manic patients taking lithium, and the infrequent reports of adverse consequences, the likelihood that this is a common drug interaction is remote. The possibility does exist that in some patients lithium levels may be altered slightly. The clinician should be aware that more frequent serum lithium monitoring may be advisable in some cases.

Caffeine

EVIDENCE OF INTERACTION

A caffeine-free diet study documented 11 patients who were in complete remission, were maintained on 600 to 1,200 mg of lithium, and were heavy caffeine users. Lithium blood levels increased in 8 out of the 11 patients during the caffeine-free phase of the diet. The lithium levels decreased back to pre-study levels upon resumption of regular caffeine use (Mester et al. 1995).

MECHANISM

Caffeine is a methylxanthine that increases urine production and may lead to the renal clearance of lithium.

CLINICAL IMPLICATIONS

When lithium-maintained patients attempt to reduce their caffeine intake, they should be warned of the risk of increased lithium levels.

Calcitonin

EVIDENCE OF INTERACTION

Women treated for osteoporosis with calcitonin showed a significant reduction in lithium levels (Passiu et al. 1998).

MECHANISM

Calcitonin may increase the renal clearance of lithium.

CLINICAL IMPLICATION

When starting calcitonin treatment in patients who are treated with lithium, lithium doses should be adjusted up and monitored.

Calcium Channel Blockers

EVIDENCE OF INTERACTION

A number of case reports have documented interactions between verapamil (Calan) and diltiazem (Cardizem) with lithium (Dubovsky et al. 1987, Price et al. 1986, Price et al. 1987, Wright et al. 1991, Valdiserri 1985). The primary symptoms of toxicity were ataxia, dysarthria, tremor, and nausea. In one case, rechallenge with verapamil after symptoms abated led to recurrence (Wright et al. 1991). Treatment with nifedipine, however, did not produce neurotoxicity. Neurotoxicity with psychotic symptoms were reported in a 66-year-old woman with a long-standing history of bipolar disorder who was treated with diltiazem for hypertension (Binder et al. 1991).

Another case report described a reversible choreoathetosis of the neck, trunk, and all four extremities during treatment with verapamil and lithium (Helmuth 1989). In another patient, stiffness and rigidity were reported during combined therapy with lithium and diltiazem (Valdiserri 1985).

MECHANISM

The mechanism of the interaction in not known; however, several possibilities have been proposed. Verapamil crosses the blood–brain barrier, and a risk for neurotoxicity exists, with delirium noted as related to its use alone (Jacobsen et al. 1987, Wright et al. 1991). Lithium alone can lead to neurotoxicity, and the combination of lithium and calcium channel blockers may be additive or synergistic.

In rats, verapamil increased 5HT2 receptors in the frontal cortex, whereas lithium did not (Baba et al. 1991). This animal model also suggested that lithium levels were elevated using the drug combination. Lithium increases dopamine in the striatum, where regulation of dopamine release is controlled by inhibitory D2-autoreceptors that are calcium dependent. The blockade of these receptors by verapamil can lead to increased dopamine release and result in choreoathetosis (Gudelsky et al. 1988, Helmuth et al. 1989).

CLINICAL IMPLICATIONS

The risk of neurotoxicity is increased with the concurrent use of lithium with verapamil, diltiazem, and possibly other calcium channel blockers. Nifedipine did not interact in one case. Clinicians may expect to encounter this drug combination not only in lithium-treated patients with cardiovascular disease, but also in patients for whom verapamil has been prescribed as a primary or adjunctive treatment for bipolar disorder.

Cisplatin Chemotherapy

EVIDENCE OF INTERACTION

A 33-year-old patient, who was treated with lithium at a dose of 1,000 mg/day for bipolar disorder, with blood levels well controlled for several years and monitored monthly, developed metastatic testicular cancer. He received a combination chemotherapy of bleomycin, etoposide, and cisplatin. He was hydrated and supplemented with magnesium, potassium, and calcium as well as ondansetron for emesis. Lithium levels were monitored daily. Lithium levels dropped during the first course of treatment. The drop in levels was less dramatic with further treatment cycles.

MECHANISM

Because cisplatin treatment is nephrotoxic, it requires hydration for kidney protection and the supplementation of sodium and other electrolytes. The combined effects of treatment and hydration can lead to changes in lithium clearance (Beijnen et al. 1994, Vincent et al. 1995).

CLINICAL IMPLICATIONS

To prevent toxicity, prophylactic pretreatment with diuretics should be avoided in patients who are treated with lithium. Lithium concentration must be monitored carefully.

Digoxin

EVIDENCE OF INTERACTION

A single case report described a patient in whom tremulousness, confusion, and nodal bradycardia developed, alternating with slow atrial fibrillation when the digoxin level was in the lower range of therapeutic effect (0.7 ng/mL) (Winters et al. 1977). Upon admission, the patient had a junctional bradycardia with a rate of 52 beats/min that fell to 30 beats/min the following day, despite discontinuation of both medications. A temporary pacemaker was required for 6 days, after which the patient reverted to normal sinus rhythm.

MECHANISM

The authors of the case report suggested that the combination of lithium and digoxin lowered intracellular potassium, predisposing the patient to cardiac arrhythmias.

CLINICAL IMPLICATIONS

We are aware of only one report citing toxicity using the combination of lithium and digoxin. In that case, lithium alone at a level of 2.0 mEq/L could have resulted in toxicity. Nonetheless, this is a potentially serious interaction, and close EKG monitoring may be necessary. Although one report suggested that the therapeutic response to lithium was impaired during digoxin therapy (Chambers et al. 1982), confirmatory evidence is lacking. Furthermore, a study in six healthy volunteers found no significant pharmacokinetic interaction between lithium and digoxin and no alterations in sodium pump activity or electrolyte concentrations (Cooper et al. 1984).

Disulfiram

EVIDENCE OF INTERACTION

Alcoholism is not uncommon in bipolar illness. Case reports, as well as unpublished observations, indicate that no clinically significant adverse interaction occurs between lithium and disulfiram (Ziegler-Driscoll 1977, Rothstein et al. 1971). In one case report, disulfiram appeared to precipitate hyperactive behavior that was treated very effectively with lithium at the usual therapeutic level. Although rats given lithium and disulfiram had increased mortality compared with either drug given alone, the clinical implications of this finding are not known (Millard et al. 1969).

CLINICAL IMPLICATIONS

Lithium and disulfiram appear to be compatible medications, and no theoretical or clinical reason supports withholding disulfiram administration in combination with lithium therapy.

Diuretics

Diuretics are generally divided into seven classes (Ciraulo et al. 1994): (a) osmotic diuretics, such as urea; (b) carbonic anhydrase inhibitors, such as acetazolamide (Diamox); (c) thiazide diuretics and drugs that are chemically distinct but work via similar mechanisms (e.g., the sulfonamide derivatives chlorthalidone, quinethazone [Hydromox], metolazone [Mykrox], and indapamide [Lozol]); (d) loop diuretics, such as furosemide (Lasix) and bumetanide (Bumex); (e) aldosterone antagonists, such as ethacrynic acid (Edecrin) and spironolactone (Aldactone); (f) potassium-sparing diuretics, such as triamterene (Dyrenium, or with hydrochlorothiazide, Dyazide); and (g) methylxanthines (also see the section on Aminophylline/Theophylline).

Diuretics: Acetazolamide (Diamox)

EVIDENCE OF INTERACTION

Renal lithium excretion was assessed in six healthy human subjects to determine the best methods for the treatment of lithium poisoning (Thomsen et al. 1968). Lithium excretion was not significantly affected by water diuresis or the administration of furosemide, ethacrynic acid, spironolactone, or potassium chloride. With administration of sodium bicarbonate and acetazolamide, urinary pH values rose into the 7.0 to 8.0 range, and urine flow, sodium, and potassium output were also increased, resulting in a 27% to 31% rise in lithium excretion.

MECHANISM

Osmotic diuresis and the administration of sodium bicarbonate or acetazolamide will produce a significant increase in lithium excretion. The increase following sodium bicarbonate and acetazolamide may be the result of increased urinary pH levels, but this is unlikely. It is probable that the increased lithium excretion is due to an obligatory excretion of cation with bicarbonate anion, and impairment of lithium resorption in the proximal tubule.

CLINICAL IMPLICATIONS

The clinical importance of this interaction is uncertain, although close monitoring of lithium level is advisable when adding or discontinuing acetazolamide in patients taking lithium.

Diuretics: Aldosterone Antagonists

Ethacrynic acid and spironolactone do not usually affect serum lithium concentrations. Large doses that may cause rapid volume depletion are sometimes associated with toxic serum lithium levels.

Diuretics: Loop Diuretics

EVIDENCE OF INTERACTION

A 65-year-old woman who had been stable on lithium with levels of 0.7 to 0.9 mEq/L was treated with bumetanide 0.5 mg/day for ankle edema. A month after the treatment was started, increasing tremulousness, ataxia, and confusion developed in the patient, with a lithium level of 2.3 mEq/L (Huang 1990). Another case of an increase in lithium serum level following the addition of bumetanide was reported by Kerry et al. (1980). Previous reports exist as to the potential increase in lithium level as a result of treatment with furosemide (Hurtig et al. 1974, Thornton et al. 1975).

Other investigators, in single-dose studies, have not found that loop diuretics increase serum lithium levels (Steele et al. 1975, Thomsen et al. 1968). Studies looking at the changes in lithium level as a result of an interaction with furosemide did not find significant elevation of lithium level (Saffer et al. 1983, Jefferson et al. 1979). In another study comparing the effect of furosemide, hydrochlorothiazide, and placebo on lithium blood levels in 13 healthy volunteers, furosemide had no effect on serum lithium levels, whereas hydrochlorothiazide produced a small but significant elevation of the serum lithium level (Crabtree et al. 1991).

MECHANISM

Loop diuretics act rapidly by inhibiting sodium reabsorption in the loop of Henle. As a consequence, the compensatory reabsorption of lithium may occur. It is possible that the site of action of furosemide at the ascending limb affects both lithium and sodium transport, causing loss of lithium as well (Crabtree et al. 1991). It is possible that when used in higher doses furosemide will cause lithium retention, but the effects seem highly variable.

CLINICAL IMPLICATIONS

Although the use of loop diuretics can be safe with lithium, it is important to monitor lithium levels.

Diuretics: Potassium-Sparing Diuretics

EVIDENCE OF INTERACTION

The interaction of lithium with potassium-sparing diuretics has not been studied extensively. A case report documents a modest elevation of lithium levels after triamterene was added (lithium levels rose from 0.65 to 0.95 mEq/L). In a study of amiloride treatment of lithium-induced polyuria, one patient had an increase in lithium level from 0.8 to 2.0 mEq/L.

MECHANISM

Large-volume contractions and reduced glomerular filtration may result in impaired lithium clearance.

CLINICAL IMPLICATIONS

When potassium-sparing diuretics are used in high doses or produce large-volume contractions, close monitoring of serum lithium levels is necessary.

Diuretics: Thiazide Diuretics

EVIDENCE OF INTERACTION

Some authorities believe that the lithium–thiazide combination usually leads to toxicity, despite careful supervision (Coppen 1982). Others suggest that with appropriate reductions in lithium doses thiazide diuretics may be used safely in the treatment of lithium-induced nephrogenic diabetes insipidus (Himmelhoch et al. 1977a, Levy et al. 1973). Several authors have documented that lithium and thiazide diuretics interact adversely, usually leading to diuretic-induced lithium retention and an increase in lithium serum levels (Macfie 1980, Himmelhoch et al. 1977b, Hurtig et al. 1974, Jefferson et al. 1979, Macfie 1975, Solomon 1980).

One case report also documents lithium toxicity in a 64-year-old man when indapamide was added to his regular medications for the treatment of pedal edema. A week after beginning treatment, the patient presented to the emergency room with lethargy, staggering gait, and confusion. His serum lithium level was 3.93 mEq/L (Hanna et al. 1990).

MECHANISM

Lithium is excreted by the kidneys, and a significant reabsorption of lithium occurs both in the proximal tubules and probably in the loop of Henle but not at more distal areas. Thiazide diuretics block sodium reabsorption at the distal tubules, which results in sodium depletion; this in turn stimulates proximal tubular reabsorption of both sodium and lithium. As a result, renal lithium clearance decreases and lithium plasma levels increase. Treatment with thiazide diuretics results in a compensatory increase in sodium reabsorption in the proximal renal tubule. Because lithium is reabsorbed with sodium in the proximal tubule, toxicity may result. Boer et al. (1989) demonstrated that the effect of acute administration of thiazide diuretics on lithium clearance differed depending on their level of carbonic anhydrase-inhibiting activity, with the higher activity drugs increasing lithium clearance in humans.

CLINICAL IMPLICATIONS

The frequent appearance of reversible lithium toxicity emphasizes that very close monitoring must be exercised when using a thiazide–lithium combination. However, minor toxicity is clearly not a contraindication to the use of thiazides with lithium. In two particular circumstances, the concomitant use of lithium and thiazide diuretics· may actually be beneficial. The first is when moderate to large doses of lithium have induced nephrogenic diabetes insipidus, an illness in which thiazide diuretics reduce polyuria and polydipsia, thereby allowing continuation of lithium (Himmelhoch et al. 1977a, Jakobsson et al. 1994). The second circumstance involves patients in whom large doses of lithium do not produce therapeutic plasma levels, and mood stabilization is not achieved. Some authorities recommend the addition of a thiazide diuretic in these patients to achieve clinically effective lithium concentrations at much lower lithium doses. A 50% reduction in lithium dosage is typical when hydrochlorothiazide 50 mg is used with lithium. Individuals vary, however, and this recommendation should serve only as a guideline. In some cases it is preferable to use furosemide instead of thiazide diuretics.

Ethanol

EVIDENCE OF INTERACTION

Several studies have been conducted regarding the co-administration of lithium and ethanol. One study evaluated the responses of 23 normal male subjects after pretreating these individuals with lithium prior to ethanol ingestion. Results indicated that pretreatment with lithium neither blocked nor dampened the alcohol-induced subjective "high" (Judd et al. 1977). The study did suggest that lithium may attenuate alcohol-induced cognitive inefficiency and, possibly, that alcohol may reverse some aspects of lithium-induced dysphoria. In a follow-up study (Judd et al. 1984) 35 male alcoholics who had been drug and alcohol free for a minimum of 21 days were studied in a repeated-measures, split-half crossover design. They were given lithium carbonate (mean 0.89 mEq/L) or placebo for 14 days in a double-blind randomized fashion. Ethanol was administered in a dose of 1.32 mL/kg of 95% ethanol in 4 divided doses over 60 minutes (a mean blood alcohol concentration of 104 mg/100 mL). Lithium subjects reported less intoxication, a decreased desire to continue drinking, and less cognitive dysfunction after ethanol than placebo subjects. Other studies have evaluated lithium in the treatment of alcoholic withdrawal. In one study involving 18 hospitalized chronic alcoholics, lithium decreased the amplitude of tremor during alcohol withdrawal but did not control the tremor or the subjective symptoms of alcohol withdrawal to a significant degree (Sellers 1974). In another study, lithium treatment diminished the subjective symptoms of withdrawal and normalized performance on a motor-tracking task. It was also determined that lithium did not in any significant way alter patterns of catecholamine excretion, blood pressure, heart rate, serum cyclic adenosine monophosphate, serum dopamine-β-hydroxylase, sleep patterns, or tremor amplitude during withdrawal (Sellers et al. 1976).

Still other studies have investigated the efficacy of lithium in producing abstinence in alcoholics. The first study comparing lithium to placebo in alcoholics was that of Kline et al. (1974). Seventy-three male veterans with high scores on the Zung Self-Rating Scale for Depression entered the study, but at the conclusion of the 48-week double-blind period only 30 subjects remained. Lithium patients experienced significantly fewer days of pathologic drinking and hospitalization for alcoholism.

Another study of 60 male and 11 female alcoholics, 48% of whom had Beck Depression Inventory scores greater than 15, compared lithium treatment to placebo (Merry et al. 1976). At the end of 41 weeks of treatment, both groups had improved Beck scores, with the lithium group doing slightly better. Among those classified as depressed at the start of the study, those taking lithium had significantly fewer days drinking and fewer days of incapacitating drinking than placebo patients. The conclusions are based on a very small sample size: nine depressed lithium patients and seven depressed placebo patients.

A study by Pond et al. (1981) using a 3-month crossover design of lithium and placebo studied 47 alcoholic patients. Nineteen subjects completed the study. No significant differences in Minnesota Multiphasic Personality Inventory scores or drinking patterns were found.

In a double-blind placebo-controlled study, 104 men and women with alcoholism were treated with lithium or placebo and observed for 12 months (Fawcett et al. 1987). Compliance (defined as at least 15 days of compliance to the prescribed regimen for 4 months of the first 6-month follow-up) was assessed by patient self-report and interviews of significant others, when possible. The lithium group was divided into high-blood level ($\geq$0.4 mEq/L), low-blood level (<0.4 mEq/L), and lithium noncompliant. The placebo group was classified either as compliant or noncompliant. The high-blood level group had the highest abstinence rates: 79% at 6 months and 63% at 12 months when all dropouts were considered to have relapsed, or 79% at 6 months and 67% at 12 months by survival analysis. These findings suggest that a therapeutic lithium level is an important factor in the positive outcome, which, contrary to earlier studies, did not appear to be related to lithium's effects on affective symptoms.

MECHANISM

Lithium may reduce sympathetic activity during alcoholic withdrawal. It decreases the pressor effect of infused norepinephrine and might therefore decrease catechol-mediated increases in blood pressure, thus alleviating the symptoms and clinical signs associated with alcoholic withdrawal (Sellers et al. 1976). The mechanism by which lithium may reduce ethanol consumption is unknown, although the serotonergic system has been implicated.

CLINICAL IMPLICATIONS

The implication of lithium use in alcohol withdrawal is of theoretical rather than clinical importance. Lithium–alcohol adverse interactions having clinical significance are not documented. Although some alcoholics appear to benefit from lithium treatment, this has not been a consistent or robust finding. Even if some subgroups of alcoholics do benefit from lithium treatment, the clinical characteristics of responders (other than in bipolar patients) have not as yet been identified. Depressive symptoms, in most studies, do not predict response.

Herbal Diuretics

EVIDENCE OF INTERACTION

A 26-year-old woman on a treatment regimen that included lithium 1,800 mg/day, risperidone 4mg/day, propranolol 40mg/day, lorazepam 1mg/day, sertraline 100mg/day, and hydroxyzine 50 mg/day presented with emergent symptoms of dizziness, "grogginess," and loose bowel movements after taking sinus medication, which she had discontinued 2 days earlier. She presented for treatment two more times. At the final visit, she had diarrhea, nausea, unsteady gait, tremor, and drowsiness; she reported taking for 2 to 3 weeks an over-the-counter preparation of herbal diuretics to lose weight. Lithium blood concentration on her third visit was 4.5 mEq/L. The patient was admitted to the coronary care unit. The herbal preparation the patient used contained multiple ingredients, making the identification of the cause of the lithium toxicity impossible (Pyevich et al. 2001).

MECHANISM

Unknown.

CLINICAL IMPLICATION

It is important to ask all patients receiving treatment with lithium about any use of herbal preparation, especially a diuretic. It is also important to warn them of the risk of the use.

Levodopa

EVIDENCE OF INTERACTION

Lithium has been used to treat the psychiatric and dyskinetic side effects induced by levodopa. It is widely recognized that psychoses have been induced by levodopa therapy in the treatment of Parkinson disease. One case report describes a 64-year-old man in whom a levodopa-induced psychosis developed and who responded well to treatment with lithium (Braden 1977). Another case report of a 69-year-old man suggests that lithium may be useful not only in the treatment of manic behavior but also in depressive reactions occurring as a consequence of levodopa therapy (Ryback et al. 1971). Dalen et al. (1973) successfully treated levodopa-induced dyskinesias with lithium in two patients with Parkinson disease. Another study of 21 patients with Parkinson disease and levodopa-induced dyskinesias, however, found lithium ineffective in all patients (McCaul et al. 1974). Five patients had adverse reactions to lithium. Poor therapeutic responses in other studies of lithium's effect on both the mental and motor side effects of levodopa have led clinicians to urge caution with respect to the use of lithium in patients with Parkinson disease (Van Woert et al. 1973).

MECHANISM

Lithium and levodopa may interact by affecting the noradrenergic, dopaminergic, and/or functionally related areas of the brain (Braden 1977).

CLINICAL IMPLICATIONS

Although a few case reports have found lithium to be of no value, other reports suggest that lithium may be useful in the treatment of psychiatric and motor side effects resulting from levodopa therapy.

Marijuana

EVIDENCE OF INTERACTION

One case report suggests a possible interaction between marijuana and lithium that may result in elevated serum lithium levels. The patient's serum lithium level was stable for at least 1 month during an inpatient hospitalization in which a dose of lithium 2,100 mg/day was given. When the patient began to surreptitiously use marijuana, his serum lithium level rose to toxic range (Ratey et al. 1981).

MECHANISM

The anticholinergic properties of marijuana may result in a decrease in gut motility, thus enhancing lithium absorption.

CLINICAL IMPLICATIONS

Although no additional interactions have been reported, clinicians should consider the possibility of concurrent marijuana use in patients with a history of marijuana use who have been taking regular doses of lithium but have been unable to achieve stable serum lithium levels.

Neuromuscular Blocking Agents

EVIDENCE OF INTERACTION

Several case reports have documented that lithium significantly prolongs both succinylcholine and pancuronium bromide neuromuscular blockade. These agents are used extensively in surgery and electroconvulsive treatment (Reimherr et al. 1977, Rubin et al. 1982). Neuromuscular blocking agents can be classified into two categories: the depolarizing group, including succinylcholine, and the nondepolarizing group, including pancuronium. Investigators have reported the potentiation of succinylcholine by lithium carbonate (Hill et al. 1976) as well as pancuronium (Reimherr et al. 1977), resulting in prolonged recovery from anesthesia (hours). One animal study did not confirm the interaction (Waud et al. 1982).

MECHANISM

It has been postulated that lithium may inhibit acetylcholine synthesis as well as the release of acetylcholine from nerve terminals, thus potentiating the neuromuscular blocking action.

CLINICAL IMPLICATIONS

Several reports have documented the fact that lithium potentiates the action of muscle relaxants; however, other studies have not found an adverse interaction. Until the matter is clarified, doses of lithium should be withheld prior to the use of these agents, or alternative relaxing agents should be used. Close monitoring of patients and appropriate ventilatory assistance should be available (Havdala et al. 1979). For therapeutic guidelines relative to electroconvulsive therapy, the reader is referred to Chapter 9.

Psyllium (Metamucil)

EVIDENCE OF INTERACTION

In a study of six normal volunteers who received lithium alone and lithium with psyllium, urine elimination of lithium was decreased with the use of psyllium, suggesting decreased absorption of lithium in the gut (Toutoungi et al. 1990).

MECHANISM

Psyllium causes retention of water and electrolytes in the colon.

CLINICAL IMPLICATIONS

In patients taking lithium and psyllium in combination, lithium requirements may be elevated. When psyllium treatment is initiated or discontinued, it is important to monitor lithium levels.

Zidovudine (AZT)

EVIDENCE OF INTERACTION

Lithium was used in five patients to reverse zidovudine-induced neutropenia (Roberts et al. 1988). Lithium levels were maintained between 0.6 and 1.2 mEq/L. Neutrophil counts fell when lithium was discontinued in two patients, and in another patient, tolerance to the effect of lithium developed after 10 weeks.

MECHANISM

Lithium has a myelostimulatory effect.

CLINICAL IMPLICATIONS

It is possible that lithium use will permit continued treatment with zidovudine even when neutropenia is present; however, insufficient studies exist to endorse this approach.

REFERENCES

Aanderud S et al.: The influence of carbamazepine on thyroid hormones and thyroxine binding globulin in hypothyroid patients substituted with thyroxine. Clin Endocrinol 15: 247, 1981.

Abraham G et al.: Topiramate can cause lithium toxicity. J Clin Psychopharmacol 24: 565, 2004.

Ahmad S: Sudden hypothyroidism and amiodarone-lithium combination: an interaction. Cardiovasc Drugs Ther 9: 827–828, 1995.

Allen HM et al.: Indomethacin in the treatment of lithium-induced nephrogenic diabetes insipidus. Arch Intern Med 149: 1123, 1989.

Amante AA et al.: Risk from lithium with acetylcholinesterase inhibitor. Ann Clin Psychiatry 14: 253, 2002.

Andrus PF: Lithium and carbamazepine. J Clin Psychiatry 45: 525, 1984.

Apseloff G et al.: Sertraline does not alter steady-state concentrations or renal clearance of lithium in healthy volunteers. J Clin Pharmacol 32: 643, 1992.

Austin LS et al.: Toxicity resulting from lithium augmentation of antidepressant treatment in elderly patients. J Clin Psychiatry 51: 344, 1990.

Ayd FJ: Possible adverse drug–drug interaction report: lithium intoxication in a spectinomycin-treated patient. Int Drug Ther Newslett 13: 15, 1978.

Ayd FJ: Metronidazole-induced lithium intoxication. Int Drug Ther Newslett 17: 15, 1982a.

Ayd FJ: Lithium-mefenamic acid interaction. Int Drug Ther Newslett 17: 16, 1982b.

Baba S et al.: Changes in dopamine2 and serotonin2 receptors in rat brain after long-term verapamil treatment: comparison of verapamil and lithium. Jpn J Psychiatry Neurol 45: 95, 1991.

Bakker K: The influence of lithium carbonate on the thalamo-pituitary axis: studies in patients with affective disorders, thyrotoxicosis, and hypothyroidism (MD thesis), 1977.

Baldwin CM et al.: A case of lisinopril-induced lithium toxicity. Dicp 24: 946, 1990.

Ballenger JC et al.: Carbamazepine in manic-depressive illness: a new treatment. Am J Psychiatry 137: 782, 1980.

Barclay ML et al.: Lithium associated thyrotoxicosis: a report of 14 cases, with statistical analysis of incidence. Clin Endocrinol 40: 759, 1994.

Bauer M et al.: Paroxetine and amitriptyline augmentation of lithium in the treatment of major depression: a double-blind study. J Clin Psychopharmacol 19: 164, 1999.

Becker D: Lithium and propranolol: possible synergism? J Clin Psychiatry 50: 473, 1989.

Beijnen JH et al.: Lithium pharmacokinetics during cisplatin-based chemotherapy: a case report. Cancer Chemother Pharmacol 33: 523, 1994.

Berens SC et al.: Antithyroid effects of lithium. J Clin Invest 49: 1357–1367, 1970.

Bialer M et al.: Progress report on new antiepileptic drugs: a summary of the Sixth Eilat Conference (EILAT VI). Epilepsy Res 51: 31, 2002.

Binder EF et al.: Diltiazem-induced psychosis and a possible diltiazem-lithium interaction. Arch Intern Med 151: 373, 1991.

Birkhimer LJ et al.: Combined trazodone-lithium therapy for refractory depression. Am J Psychiatry 140: 1382, 1983.

Blanche P: Lithium intoxication in an elderly patient after combined treatment with losartan. Eur J Clin Pharmacol 52: 501, 1997.

Boer WH et al.: Acute effects of thiazides, with and without carbonic anhydrase inhibiting activity, on lithium and free water clearance in man. Clin Sci (Lond) 76: 539, 1989.

Braden W: Response to lithium in a case of L-dopa-induced psychosis. Am J Psychiatry 134: 808, 1977.

Brady HR et al.: Lithium and the heart. Unanswered questions. Chest 93: 166, 1988.

Brater DC: Drug–drug and drug–disease interactions with nonsteroidal antiinflammatory drugs. Am J Med 80: 62, 1986.

Brater DC: Clinical pharmacology of NSAIDs. J Clin Pharmacol 28: 518, 1988.

Breuel HP et al.: Pharmacokinetic interactions between lithium and fluoxetine after single and repeated fluoxetine administration in young healthy volunteers. Int J Clin Pharmacol Ther 33: 415, 1995.

Brewerton TD: Lithium counteracts carbamazepine-induced leukopenia while increasing its therapeutic effect. Biol Psychiatry 21: 677, 1986.

Byrd GJ: Methyldopa and lithium carbonate: suspected interaction (Letter). JAMA 233: 320, 1975.

Chambers CA et al.: The effect of digoxin on the response to lithium therapy in mania. Psychol Med 12: 57, 1982.

Chaudry RP et al.: Lithium and carbamazepine interaction: possible neurotoxicity. J Clin Psychiatry 44: 30, 1983.

Chow CC et al.: Lithium-associated transient thyrotoxicosis in 4 Chinese women with autoimmune thyroiditis. Aust N Z J Psychiatry 27: 246, 1993.

Ciraulo DA et al.: Drug interactions in psychopharmacology. 1994.

Cold JA et al.: Increased lithium serum and red blood cell concentrations during ketorolac co-administration. J Clin Psychopharmacol 18: 33, 1998.

Colonna L et al.: Association carbonate de lithium-clometacine et lithiemie. Gaz Med France 86: 4095, 1979.

Conroy RW: Possible adverse drug-drug interaction report: lithium intoxication in a spectinomycin-treated patient. Int Drug Ther Newslett 13:15, 1978.

Cook BL et al.: Theophylline-lithium interaction. J Clin Psychiatry 46: 278, 1985.

Cooper SJ et al.: Pharmacodynamics and pharmacokinetics of digoxin in the presence of lithium. Br J Clin Pharmacol 18: 21, 1984.

Coppen A et al.: Lithium. In Paykel ES (ed): Handbook of Affective Disorders. New York, Guilford, p. 276, 1982.

Correa FJ et al.: Angiotensin-converting enzyme inhibitors and lithium toxicity. Am J Med 93: 108, 1992.

Cowdry RW et al.: Thyroid abnormalities associated with rapid-cycling bipolar illness. Arch Gen Psychiatry 40: 414, 1983.

Crabtree BL et al.: Comparison of the effects of hydrochlorothiazide and furosemide on lithium disposition. Am J Psychiatry 148: 1060, 1991.

Dalen P et al.: Lithium and levodopa in parkinsonism. Lancet 1: 936, 1973.

DasGupta K et al.: The effect of enalapril on serum lithium levels in healthy men. J Clin Psychiatry 53: 398, 1992.

De Luca F et al.: Changes in thyroid function tests induced by 2 month carbamazepine treatment in L-thyroxine-substituted hypothyroid children. Eur J Pediatr 145: 77, 1986.

De Montigny C et al.: Lithium carbonate addition in tricyclic antidepressant-resistant unipolar depression. Correlations with the neurobiologic actions of tricyclic antidepressant drugs and lithium ion on the serotonin system. Arch Gen Psychiatry 40: 1327, 1983.

De Montigny C: Lithium induces rapid relief of depression in tricyclic antidepressant drug non-responders. Br J Psychiatry 138: 252, 1981.

Desvilles M: [Paradoxical effect of the combination of lithium and sulfamethoxazole-trimethoprim]. Nouv Presse Med 11: 3267, 1982.

Dietrich A et al.: Cardiac toxicity in an adolescent following chronic lithium and imipramine therapy. J Adolesc Health 14: 394, 1993.

Dinan TG: Lithium augmentation in sertraline-resistant depression: a preliminary dose-response study. Acta Psychiatr Scand 88: 300, 1993.

Douste-Blazy P et al.: Angiotensin converting enzyme inhibitors and lithium treatment. Lancet 1: 1448, 1986.

Drouet A, Bouvet O: [Lithium and converting enzyme inhibitors]. Encephale 16: 51–52, 1990.

Dubovsky SL et al.: A new antimanic drug with potential interactions with lithium. J Clin Psychiatry 48: 371, 1987.

Elizur A et al.: Intra: extracellular lithium ratios and clinical course in affective states. Clin Pharmacol Ther 13: 947, 1972.

Evans M et al.: Fluvoxamine and lithium: an unusual interaction. Br J Psychiatry 156: 286, 1990a.

Evans RL et al.: Evaluation of the interaction of lithium and alprazolam. J Clin Psychopharmacol 10: 355, 1990b.

Fankhauser MP et al.: Evaluation of lithium-tetracycline interaction. Clin Pharm 7: 314, 1988.

Fava M et al.: Lithium and tricyclic augmentation of fluoxetine treatment for resistant major depression: a double-blind, controlled study. Am J Psychiatry 151: 1372, 1994.

Fawcett J et al.: A double-blind, placebo-controlled trial of lithium carbonate therapy for alcoholism. Arch Gen Psychiatry 44: 248, 1987.

Finley PR et al.: Lithium and angiotensin-converting enzyme inhibitors: evaluation of a potential interaction. J Clin Psychopharmacol 16: 68, 1996.

Fischer P: Successful treatment of nonanticholinergic delirium with a cholinesterase inhibitor. J Clin Psychopharmacol 21: 118, 2001.

Francis RI et al.: Lithium distribution in the brains of two manic patients. Lancet 2: 523, 1970.

Freinhar JP et al.: Use of clonazepam in two cases of acute mania. J Clin Psychiatry 46: 29, 1985.

Frolich JC et al.: Indomethacin increases plasma lithium. Br Med J 1: 1979.

Furnell MM et al.: The effect of sulindac on lithium therapy. Drug Intell Clin Pharm 19: 374, 1985.

Gallicchio VS: In vitro effect of lithium on carbamazepine-induced inhibition of murine and human bone marrow-derived granulocyte-macrophage, erythroid, and megakaryocyte progenitor stem cells. Proc Soc Exp Biol Med 190: 109, 1989.

Gardner EA: Long-term preventive care in depression: the use of bupropion in patients intolerant of other antidepressants. J Clin Psychiatry 44: 157, 1983.

Gay C et al.: [Lithium poisoning. 2 unpublished interactions: acetazolamide and niflumic acid]. Encephale 11: 261, 1985.

Gerdes H et al.: Successful treatment of thyrotoxicosis by lithium. Acta Endocrinol Suppl (Copenh) 173: 23, 1973.

Ghadirian AM et al.: Lithium, benzodiazepines, and sexual function in bipolar patients. Am J Psychiatry 149: 801, 1992.

Ghose K: Effect of carbamazepine in polyuria associated with lithium therapy. Pharmakopsychiatr Neuropsychopharmakol 11: 241, 1978.

Gobe GC et al.: Effects of indomethacin on renal concentrating capacity in lithium-treated rats. Res Commun Chem Pathol Pharmacol 39: 11, 1983.

Goodnick PJ et al.: Neurochemical changes during discontinuation of lithium prophylaxis. I. Increases in clonidine-induced hypotension. Biol Psychiatry 19: 883, 1984.

Graham PM: Drug combinations for chronic depression. Br J Psychiatry 145: 214, 1984.

Gray EG: Severe depression: a patient's thoughts. Br J Psychiatry 143: 319, 1983.

Gudelsky GA et al.: Activity of tuberoinfundibular dopaminergic neurons and concentrations of serum prolactin in the rat following lithium administration. Psychopharmacology (Berl) 94: 92, 1988.

Hadley A et al.: Mania resulting from lithium-fluoxetine combination. Am J Psychiatry 146: 1637, 1989.

Halaris AE: The use of lithium in psychiatric practice. Psychiatr Ann 13: 53, 1983.

Hanna ME et al.: Severe lithium toxicity associated with indapamide therapy. J Clin Psychopharmacol 10: 379, 1990.

Harker WG et al.: Enhancement of colony-stimulating activity production by lithium. Blood 49: 263, 1977.

Harrison TM: Lithium carbonate and piroxicam. Br J Psychiatry 149: 124, 1986.

Havdala HS et al.: Potential hazards and applications of lithium in anesthesiology. Anesthesiology 50: 534, 1979.

Helmuth D: Choreoathetosis induced by verapamil and lithium treatment. J Clin Psychopharmacol 9: 454, 1989.

Heninger GR et al.: Lithium carbonate augmentation of antidepressant treatment. An effective prescription for treatment-refractory depression. Arch Gen Psychiatry 40: 1335, 1983.

Hetmar O et al.: Decreased number of benzodiazepine receptors in frontal cortex of rat brain following long-term lithium treatment. J Neurochem 41: 217, 1983.

Hill GE et al.: Potentiation of succinylcholine neuromuscular blockade by lithium carbonate. Anesthesiology 44: 439, 1976.

Himmelhoch JM et al.: Treatment of previously intractable depressions with tranylcypromine and lithium. J Nerv Ment Dis 155: 216, 1972.

Himmelhoch JM et al.: Thiazide-lithium synergy in refractory mood swings. Am J Psychiatry 134: 149, 1977a.

Himmelhoch JM et al.: Adjustment of lithium dose during lithium-chlorothiazide therapy. Clin Pharmacol Ther 22: 225, 1977b.

Holstad SG et al.: The effects of intravenous theophylline infusion versus intravenous sodium bicarbonate infusion on lithium clearance in normal subjects. Psychiatry Res 25: 203, 1988.

Hommer DW et al.: Prazosin, a specific alpha 1-noradrenergic receptor antagonist, has no effect on symptoms but increases autonomic arousal in schizophrenic patients. Psychiatry Res 11: 193, 1984.

Honchar MP et al.: Systemic cholinergic agents induce seizures and brain damage in lithium-treated rats. Science 220: 323, 1983.

Huang LG: Lithium intoxication with co-administration of a loop-diuretic. J Clin Psychopharmacol 10: 228, 1990.

Hurtig HI et al.: Letter: Lithium toxicity enhanced by diuresis. N Engl J Med 290: 748, 1974.

Imbs JL et al.: Effects of indomethacin and methylprednisolone on renal elimination of lithium in the rat. Int Pharmacopsychiatry 15: 143, 1980.

Jacobsen FM et al.: Delirium induced by verapamil. Am J Psychiatry 144: 248, 1987.

Jakobsson B et al.: Effect of hydrochlorothiazide and indomethacin treatment on renal function in nephrogenic diabetes insipidus. Acta Paediatr 83: 522, 1994.

Jefferson JW et al.: Combining lithium and antidepressants. J Clin Psychopharmacol 3: 303, 1983.

Jefferson JW et al.: Antibiotics: In Jefferson JW et al. (eds): Lithium Encyclopedia for Clinical Practice, 2nd ed. Washington, DC, American Psychiatric Press, p. 69, 1987.

Jefferson JW et al.: Lithium: interactions with other drugs. J Clin Psychopharmacol 1: 124, 1981.

Jefferson JW et al.: Serum lithium levels and long-term diuretic use. JAMA 241: 1134, 1979.

Jefferson JW: Manic depressive disorder and lithium over the decades: the very educational case of Mrs. L. J Clin Psychiatry 55: 340, 1994.

Jefferson JW et al.: Antibiotics. 69, 1987.

Joffe RT: Hematological effects of lithium potentiation of carbamazepine in patients with affective illness. Int Clin Psychopharmacol 3: 53, 1988.

Joffe RT et al.: A placebo-controlled comparison of lithium and triiodothyronine augmentation of tricyclic antidepressants in unipolar refractory depression. Arch Gen Psychiatry 50: 387, 1993.

Johnson AG et al.: Adverse drug interactions with nonsteroidal antiinflammatory drugs (NSAIDs). Recognition, management and avoidance. Drug Saf 8: 99, 1993.

Jones MT et al.: Increased lithium concentrations reported in patients treated with sulindac. J Clin Psychiatry 61: 527, 2000.

Joyce PR et al.: Rapid response to lithium in treatment-resistant depression. Br J Psychiatry 142: 204, 1983.

Judd LL et al.: Lithium carbonate and ethanol induced "highs" in normal subjects. Arch Gen Psychiatry 34: 463, 1977.

Judd LL et al.: Lithium antagonizes ethanol intoxication in alcoholics. Am J Psychiatry 141: 1517, 1984.

Juurlink DN et al.: Drug-induced lithium toxicity in the elderly: a population-based study. J Am Geriatr Soc 52: 794, 2004.

Kafka MS et al.: Effect of lithium on circadian neurotransmitter receptor rhythms. Neuropsychobiology 8: 41, 1982.

Kasarskis EJ et al.: Carbamazepine-induced cardiac dysfunction. Characterization of two distinct clinical syndromes. Arch Intern Med 152: 186, 1992.

Kerry RJ et al.: Diuretics are dangerous with lithium. Br Med J 281: 371, 1980.

Kerry RJ et al.: Possible toxic interaction between lithium and piroxicam. Lancet 1: 418, 1983.

Kettl P et al.: Maprotiline-induced myoclonus. J Clin Psychopharmacol 3: 264–265, 1983.

Kline NS et al.: Evaluation of lithium therapy in chronic and periodic alcoholism. Am J Med Sci 268: 15, 1974.

Koczerginski D et al.: Clonazepam and lithium—a toxic combination in the treatment of mania? Int Clin Psychopharmacol 4: 195, 1989.

Kojima H et al.: Serotonin syndrome during clomipramine and lithium treatment. Am J Psychiatry 150: 1897, 1993.

Kramlinger KG et al.: Addition of lithium carbonate to carbamazepine: hematological and thyroid effects. Am J Psychiatry 147: 615, 1990.

Kristensen O et al.: Lithium carbonate in the treatment of thyrotoxicosis. A controlled trial. Lancet 1: 603, 1976.

Langlois R et al.: Increased serum lithium levels due to ketorolac therapy. Cmaj 150: 1455, 1994.

Lassen E: Effects of acute and short-time antibiotic treatment on renal lithium elimination and serum lithium levels in the rat. Acta Pharmacol Toxicol (Copenh) 56: 273, 1985.

Lazarus A: Tardive dyskinesia-like syndrome associated with lithium and carbamazepine. J Clin Psychopharmacol 14: 146, 1994.

Lehmann K et al.: Angiotensin-converting enzyme inhibitors may cause renal dysfunction in patients on long-term lithium treatment. Am J Kidney Dis 25: 82, 1995.

Leung M et al.: Potential drug interaction between lithium and valsartan. J Clin Psychopharmacol 20: 392, 2000.

Leutgeb U: Ambient iodine and lithium-associated with clinical hypothyroidism. Br J Psychiatry 176: 495, 2000.

Levenson JL: Neuroleptic malignant syndrome. Am J Psychiatry 142: 1137, 1985.

Levy ST et al.: Lithium-induced diabetes insipidus: manic symptoms, brain and electrolyte correlates, and chlorothiazide treatment. Am J Psychiatry 130: 1014, 1973.

Lipinski JF et al.: Possible synergistic action between carbamazepine and lithium carbonate in the treatment of three acutely manic patients. Am J Psychiatry 139: 948, 1982.

Louie AK et al.: Lithium potentiation of antidepressant treatment. J Clin Psychopharmacol 4: 316, 1984.

Lundmark J et al.: A possible interaction between lithium and rofecoxib. Br J Clin Pharmacol 53: 403, 2002.

MacCallum WA: Interaction of lithium and phenytoin. Br Med J 280: 610, 1980.

MacDonald J et al.: Toxic interaction of lithium carbonate and mefenamic acid. Br Med J 297: 1339, 1988.

Macfie AC: Lithium poisoning precipitated by diuretics. (Letter) Br Med J 1: 516, 1975.

Macfie AC: Lithium toxicity precipitated by diuretics. Psychosomatics 21: 425, 1980.

Mannisto PT et al.: Effect of lithium and rubidium on the sleeping time caused by various intravenous anaesthetics in the mouse. Br J Anaesth 48: 185, 1976.

Mastrosimone F et al.: [The use of lithium salts in trigeminal neuralgia in prevention of neutropenia due to carbamazepine. Preliminary considerations]. Acta Neurol [Quad] (Napoli) 39: 149, 1979.

Mayan H et al.: Lithium intoxication due to carbamazepine-induced renal failure. Ann Pharmacother 35: 560, 2001.

McCance-Katz E et al.: Serotonergic function during lithium augmentation of refractory depression. Psychopharmacology (Berl) 108: 93, 1992.

McCaul JA et al.: Lithium in Parkinson's disease. (Letter) Lancet 1: 1117, 1974.

McGennis AJ: Lithium carbonate and tetracycline interaction. Br Med J 1: 1183, 1978.

Mekler G et al.: A case of serotonin syndrome caused by venlafaxine and lithium. Pharmacopsychiatry 30: 272, 1997.

Merry J et al.: Prophylactic treatment of alcoholism by lithium carbonate. A controlled study. Lancet 1: 481, 1976.

Mester R et al.: Caffeine withdrawal increases lithium blood levels. Biol Psychiatry 37: 348, 1995.

Miljkovic BR et al.: The influence of lithium on fluvoxamine therapeutic efficacy and pharmacokinetics in depressed patients on combined fluvoxamine-lithium therapy. Int Clin Psychopharmacol 12: 207, 1997.

Millard SA et al.: Biochemical effects due to interaction of lithium ions and disulfiram in rats. Proc Soc Exp Biol Med 131: 1210, 1969.

Miller SC: Doxycycline-induced lithium toxicity. J Clin Psychopharmacol 17: 54, 1997.

Mochinaga N et al.: Successful preoperative preparation for thyroidectomy in Graves' disease using lithium alone: report of two cases. Surg Today 24: 464, 1994.

Muly EC et al.: Serotonin syndrome produced by a combination of fluoxetine and lithium. Am J Psychiatry 150: 1565, 1993.

Nadarajah J et al.: Piroxicam induced lithium toxicity. Ann Rheum Dis 44: 502, 1985.

Navis GJ et al.: Volume homeostasis, angiotensin converting enzyme inhibition, and lithium therapy. Am J Med 86: 621, 1989.

Naylor GJ et al.: Profound hypothermia on combined lithium carbonate and diazepam treatment. Br Med J 2: 22, 1977.

Nelson JC et al.: Rapid response to lithium in phenelzine non-responders. Br J Psychiatry 141: 85, 1982.

Nierenberg AA et al.: Lithium augmentation of nortriptyline for subjects resistant to multiple antidepressants. J Clin Psychopharmacol 23: 92, 2003.

Noveske FG et al.: Possible toxicity of combined fluoxetine and lithium. Am J Psychiatry 146: 1515, 1989.

Ohman R et al.: Serotonin syndrome induced by fluvoxamine-lithium interaction. Pharmacopsychiatry 26: 263, 1993.

Okuma T et al.: Anti-manic and prophylactic effects of carbamazepine (Tegretol) on manic depressive psychosis. A preliminary report. Folia Psychiatr Neurol Jpn 27: 283, 1973.

O'Regan JB: Adverse interaction of lithium carbonate and methyldopa. (Letter) Can Med Assoc J 115: 385–386, 1976.

Osanloo E et al.: Interaction of lithium and methyldopa. Ann Intern Med 92: 433, 1980.

Ozawa H et al.: Potentiating effect of lithium chloride on aggressive behavior induced in mice by nialamide plus L-DOPA and by clonidine. Eur J Pharmacol 34: 169, 1975.

Pandey GN et al.: Effect of neuroleptic drugs on lithium uptake by the human erythrocyte. Clin Pharmacol Ther 26: 96, 1979.

Passiu G et al.: Calcitonin decreases lithium plasma levels in man. Preliminary report. Int J Clin Pharmacol Res 18: 179, 1998.

Perry PJ: Theophylline precipitated alterations of lithium clearance. Acta Psychiatr Scand 69: 528, 1984.

Persad E et al.: Hyperthyroidism after treatment with lithium. Can J Psychiatry 38: 599, 1993.

Peselow ED et al.: Lithium prophylaxis of bipolar illness. The value of combination treatment. Br J Psychiatry 164: 208, 1994.

Pond SM et al.: An evaluation of the effects of lithium in the treatment of chronic alcoholism. I. Clinical results. Alcohol Clin Exp Res 5: 247, 1981.

Pope HG, Jr. et al.: Antidepressant treatment of bulimia: preliminary experience and practical recommendations. J Clin Psychopharmacol 3: 274, 1983.

Price LH et al.: Efficacy of lithium-tranylcypromine treatment in refractory depression. Am J Psychiatry 142: 619, 1985.

Price WA et al.: Neurotoxicity caused by lithium-verapamil synergism. J Clin Pharmacol 26: 717, 1986.

Price WA et al.: Lithium-verapamil toxicity in the elderly. J Am Geriatr Soc 35: 177, 1987.

Pyevich D et al.: Herbal diuretics and lithium toxicity. Am J Psychiatry 158: 1329, 2001.

Ragheb M: Ibuprofen can increase serum lithium level in lithium-treated patients. J Clin Psychiatry 48: 161, 1987a.

Ragheb M: The clinical significance of lithium-nonsteroidal antiinflammatory drug interactions. J Clin Psychopharmacol 10: 350, 1990.

Ragheb M et al.: Interaction of indomethacin and ibuprofen with lithium in manic patients under a steady-state lithium level. J Clin Psychiatry 41: 397, 1980.

Ragheb M et al.: Lithium interaction with sulindac and naproxen. J Clin Psychopharmacol 6: 150, 1986b.

Ragheb MA: Aspirin does not significantly affect patients' serum lithium levels. J Clin Psychiatry 48: 425, 1987b.

Ragheb MA et al.: Failure of sulindac to increase serum lithium levels. J Clin Psychiatry 47: 33, 1986a.

Raskin DE: Lithium and phenytoin interaction. J Clin Psychopharmacol 4: 120, 1984.

Ratey JJ et al.: Lithium and marijuana. J Clin Psychopharmacol 1: 32, 1981.

Rätz Bravo AE et al.: Lithium intoxication as a result of an interaction with rofecoxib. Ann Pharmacother 38: 1189, 2004.

Raudino F: [Interaction between benzodiazepines and blood levels of lithium salts]. Clin Ter 98: 683, 1981.

Reilly MA et al.: Influence of chronic lithium administration on binding to benzodiazepine- and histamine H1-receptors in rat brain. J Recept Res 3: 703, 1983.

Reimann IW et al.: Effects of diclofenac on lithium kinetics. Clin Pharmacol Ther 30: 348, 1981.

Reimherr FW et al.: Prolongation of muscle relaxant effects by lithium carbonate. Am J Psychiatry 134: 205, 1977.

Richman CM et al.: Granulopoietic effects of lithium on human bone marrow in vitro. Exp Hematol 9: 449, 1981.

Rittmannsberger H, Leblhuber F: Asterixis induced by carbamazepine therapy. Biol Psychiatry 32: 364–368, 1992.

Rittmannsberger H et al.: Asterixis as a side effect of carbamazepine therapy. Klin Wochenschr 69: 279, 1991.

Roberts DE et al.: Effect of lithium carbonate on zidovudine-associated neutropenia in the acquired immunodeficiency syndrome. Am J Med 85: 428, 1988.

Rodney WM et al.: Lithium-induced dysrhythmias as a marker for sick sinus syndrome. J Fam Pract 16: 797, 1983.

Rogers MP et al.: Clinical hypothyroidism occurring during lithium treatment: two case histories and a review of thyroid function in 19 patients. Am J Psychiatry 128: 158, 1971.

Rosenbaum AH et al.: Tardive dyskinesia in depressed patients: successful therapy with antidepressants and lithium. Psychosomatics 21: 715, 1980.

Rosenbaum AH et al.: Series on pharmacology in practice. 1. Drugs that alter mood. II. Lithium. Mayo Clin Proc 54: 401, 1979.

Rossof AH et al.: Lithium stimulation of granulopoiesis. N Engl J Med 298: 280, 1978.

Rossof AH et al.: Lithium carbonate increases marrow granulocyte-committed colony-forming units and peripheral blood granulocytes in a canine model. Exp Hematol 7: 255, 1979.

Rothstein E et al.: Combined use of lithium and disulfiram. N Engl J Med 285: 238, 1971.

Rubin EH et al.: Lithium-ketamine interaction: an animal study of potential clinical and theoretical interest. J Clin Psychopharmacol 2: 211, 1982.

Ryback RS et al.: Manic response to levodopa therapy. Report of a case. N Engl J Med 285: 788, 1971.

Sacristan JA et al.: Absence seizures induced by lithium: possible interaction with fluoxetine. Am J Psychiatry 148: 146, 1991.

Sadoul JL et al.: [Lithium therapy and hyperthyroidism: disease caused or facilitated by lithium? Review of the literature apropos of a case of hyperthyroidism preceded by transient hypothyroidism]. Ann Endocrinol (Paris) 54: 353, 1994.

Saffer D et al.: Frusemide: a safe diuretic during lithium therapy? J Affect Disord 5: 289, 1983.

Salama AA et al.: A case of severe lithium toxicity induced by combined fluoxetine and lithium carbonate. Am J Psychiatry 146: 278, 1989.

Samoilov NN et al.: [Effect of psychotropic drugs on the pharmacokinetics of lithium]. Biull Eksp Biol Med 89: 696, 1980.

Schaff MR et al.: Divalproex sodium in the treatment of refractory affective disorders. J Clin Psychiatry 54: 380, 1993.

Schou M et al.: Use of propranolol during lithium treatment: an enquiry and a suggestion. Pharmacopsychiatry 20: 131, 1987.

Schwarcz G: The problem of antihypertensive treatment in lithium patients. Compr Psychiatry 23: 50, 1982.

Sedvall G et al.: Effects of lithium salts on plasma protein bound iodine and uptake of I131 in thyroid gland of man and rat. Life Sciences 7: 1257, 1968.

Sellers EM et al.: Lithium treatment during alcoholic withdrawal. Clin Pharmacol Ther 20: 199, 1976.

Sellers EM et al.: Lithium treatment of alcoholic withdrawal. Clin Pharmacol Ther 15: 218, 1974.

Shelley RK: Lithium toxicity and mefenamic acid. A possible interaction and the role of prostaglandin inhibition. Br J Psychiatry 151: 847, 1987.

Shukla S et al.: Lithium-carbamazepine neurotoxicity and risk factors. Am J Psychiatry 141: 1604, 1984.

Sierles FS et al.: Concurrent use of theophylline and lithium in a patient with chronic obstructive lung disease and bipolar disorder. Am J Psychiatry 139: 117, 1982.

Singer L et al.: [The effects of phenylbutazone on the decrease of lithium clearance]. Encephale 4: 33, 1978.

Slordal L et al.: A life-threatening interaction between lithium and celecoxib. Br J Clin Pharmacol 55: 413, 2003.

Sobanski T et al.: Serotonin syndrome after lithium add-on medication to paroxetine. Pharmacopsychiatry 30: 106, 1997.

Solomon JG: Seizures during lithium-amitriptyline therapy. Postgrad Med 66: 145, 1979.

Solomon JG: Lithium toxicity precipitated by a diuretic. Psychosomatics 21: 425, 1980.

Speirs J et al.: Severe lithium toxicity with "normal" serum concentrations. Br Med J 1: 815, 1978.

Spivey WH: Flumazenil and seizures: analysis of 43 cases. Clin Ther 14: 292, 1992.

Stancer HC: Tardive dyskinesia not associated with neuroleptics. Am J Psychiatry 136: 727, 1979.

Steckler TL: Lithium- and carbamazepine-associated sinus node dysfunction: nine-year experience in a psychiatric hospital. J Clin Psychopharmacol 14: 336, 1994.

Steele TH et al.: Renal lithium reabsorption in man: physiologic and pharmacologic determinants. Am J Med Sci 269: 349, 1975.

Stein RS et al.: Lithium and granulocytopenia during induction therapy of acute myelogenous leukemia. Blood 54: 636, 1979.

Stein RS et al.: Lithium-induced granulocytosis. Ann Intern Med 88: 809, 1978.

Steiner C et al.: The antiarrhythmic actions of carbamazepine (Tegretol). J Pharmacol Exp Ther 173: 323, 1970.

Sylvester RK et al.: Does acyclovir increase serum lithium levels? Pharmacotherapy 16: 466, 1996.

Takahashi H et al.: Severe lithium toxicity induced by combined levofloxacin administration. J Clin Psychiatry 61: 949, 2000.

Takami H: Lithium in the preoperative preparation of Graves' disease. Int Surg 79: 89–90, 1994.

Teicher MH et al.: Possible nephrotoxic interaction of lithium and metronidazole. JAMA 257: 3365–3366, 1987.

Temple R et al.: The use of lithium in the treatment of thyrotoxicosis. J Clin Invest 51: 2746, 1972.

Thomsen K et al.: Renal lithium excretion in man. Am J Physiol 215: 823, 1968.

Thornton WE et al.: Lithium intoxication: a report of two cases. Can Psychiatr Assoc J 20: 281, 1975.

Tonkin AL et al.: Interactions of non-steroidal antiinflammatory drugs. Baillieres Clin Rheumatol 2: 455, 1988.

Toutoungi M et al.: [Probable interaction of psyllium and lithium]. Therapie 45: 358, 1990.

Türck D et al.: Steady-state pharmacokinetics of lithium in healthy volunteers receiving concomitant meloxicam. Br J Clin Pharmacol 50: 197, 2000.

Turner JG et al.: Lithium and thyrotoxicosis. Lancet 2: 904, 1976.

Turner JG et al.: Use of lithium in the treatment of thyrotoxicosis. NZ Med J 82: 57, 1975.

Valdiserri EV: A possible interaction between lithium and diltiazem: case report. J Clin Psychiatry 46: 540, 1985.

Van Woert MH et al.: Lithium and levodopa in parkinsonism. Lancet 1: 1390, 1973.

Vieweg V et al.: Absence of carbamazepine-induced hyponatremia among patients also given lithium. Am J Psychiatry 144: 943, 1987.

Vincent F et al.: Lithium concentrations during cisplatin-based chemotherapy: evidence for renal interaction. Cancer Chemother Pharmacol 35: 533, 1995.

Visser TJ et al.: Subcellular localization of a rat liver enzyme converting thyroxine into tri-iodothyronine and possible involvement of essential thiol groups. Biochem J 157: 479, 1976.

Walbridge DG et al.: An interaction between lithium carbonate and piroxicam presenting as lithium toxicity. Br J Psychiatry 147: 206, 1985.

Walker N et al.: Lithium-methyldopa interactions in normal subjects. Drug Intell Clin Pharm 14: 638, 1980.

Warrington SJ: Clinical implications of the pharmacology of sertraline. Int Clin Psychopharmacol 6 Suppl 2: 11, 1991.

Waud BE et al.: Lithium and neuromuscular transmission. Anesth Analg 61: 399, 1982.

Weaver KE: Lithium for delusional depression. Am J Psychiatry 140: 962, 1983.

West AP et al.: Paradoxical lithium neurotoxicity: a report of five cases and a hypothesis about risk for neurotoxicity. Am J Psychiatry 136: 963, 1979.

Winters WD et al.: Digoxin-lithium drug interaction. Clin Toxicol 10: 487, 1977.

Wright BA et al.: Lithium and calcium channel blockers: possible neurotoxicity. Biol Psychiatry 30: 635, 1991.

Zall H: Lithium carbonate and isocarboxazid—an effective drug approach in severe depressions. Am J Psychiatry 127: 1400, 1971.

Ziegler-Driscoll G et al.: Lithium use in the treatment of affective disorders in an abstinent therapeutic community. In Seixas J (ed), Currents in Alcoholism. New York, Grune and Stratton, 2: 19–34, 1977.

5

Anticonvulsants

DOMENIC A. CIRAULO
MANUEL N. PACHECO
MICHAEL SLATTERY

The use of anticonvulsants in psychiatry has grown rapidly over the past decade. The general psychiatrist has become as familiar with prescribing mood-stabilizing anticonvulsants as with prescribing antipsychotics. In this chapter, we review in detail the drug interactions of carbamazepine (Tegretol), valproate (Depakene, Depakote), phenytoin (Dilantin), gabapentin (Neurontin), lamotrigine (Lamictal), oxcarbazepine (Trileptal), and topiramate (Topamax). In our practice, these anticonvulsants are prescribed most commonly. Somewhat less detail is presented regarding the interactions of barbiturates (Table 5.1) and primidone. For a detailed discussion of anticonvulsant interactions with antidepressants or antipsychotics refer to Chapters 2 and 3.

Carbamazepine (CBZ) is an iminostilbene derivative anticonvulsant that is used in a variety of seizures, impulse-control disorders, sedative-hypnotic withdrawal, and bipolar disorder. It has several characteristics that make it subject to drug interactions (Ketter et al 1991a,b). It is a potent inducer of the cytochrome P450 3A4 enzyme and, as a consequence, is subject to autoinduction. It is a less potent inducer of both 1A2 and 2C19. It is not known to be an inhibitor of any cytochrome P450 enzymes. Because its metabolism is exclusively hepatic, it may be affected by other drugs that induce or impair hepatic metabolism. Carbamazepine-(10-11)-epoxide (CBZ-E) is an active metabolite, and an assessment of the clinical impact of drug interactions must consider the effects of both the parent compound and its metabolite. Signs and symptoms of toxicity with elevated levels of carbamazepine include sedation, nausea, vomiting, vertigo, ataxia, blurred vision, and diplopia.

Valproic acid is a branched-chain fatty acid with antiepileptic activity against a variety of seizures and efficacy in bipolar disorder. Most

(text continues on page 299)

TABLE 5.1. BARBITURATE DRUG INTERACTIONS

Drug	Clinical Effect
Acetaminophen	Barbiturates reduce acetaminophen bioavailability and half-life. With acetaminophen overdoses, chronic phenobarbital treatment increases hepatotoxicity.
Anticoagulants	Barbiturates enhance the metabolism of coumarin anticoagulants. Gastrointestinal absorption of dicumarol, but not wararin, is decreased. Caution is required when a barbiturate is added or discontinued in patients receiving coumarin anticoagulants.
Antidepressants	Barbiturates induce metabolism of antidepressants resulting in decreased serum levels. In tricyclic overdoses, respiratory depression may occur. (*See* Chapter 2)
Antipyrine	Metabolism of antipyrine is enhanced by barbiturates.
β-Adrenergic blockers	Those β-blockers that are metabolized by the liver (propranolol, metoprolol, alprenolol) will have enhanced elimination during chronic barbiturate therapy. Those β-blockers that are primarily excreted unchanged by the kidneys (atenolol, sotalol, nadolol) will not be affected.
Carbamazepine	Barbiturates stimulate carbamazepine metabolism.
Chloramphenicol	Barbiturates stimulate chloramphenicol metabolism, Chloramphenicol inhibits barbiturate metabolism.
Cimetidine	Chronic phenobarbital treatment induces cimetidine metabolism.
Contraceptives	Barbiturates enhance the metabolism of estrogens, and low dose oral contraceptive agents may be rendered less effective.
Corticosteroids	Barbiturates enhance the metabolism of corticosteroids. Concurrent barbiturate therapy worsens the clinical condition of steroid-dependent asthmatics and decreases renal allograft survival.
Cyclophosphamide	Barbiturates enhance the metabolism of cyclophosphamide to active alkylating metabolites, but also promote elimination of these active agents. Clinical significance not known.
Digitalis glycosides	Barbiturates may lower plasma digitoxin levels and shorten its half-life. Some studies have found no interaction.
Estrogens	Barbiturates induce metabolism of estrogens.
Griseofulvin	Barbiturates impair absorption of griseofulvin.
Lidocaine	Barbiturates reduce oral bioavailability of lidocaine, although this is an uncommon clinical route of administration. They also induce hepatic metabolism of

(continued)

TABLE 5.1. BARBITURATE DRUG INTERACTIONS (CONTINUED)

Drug	Clinical Effect
	lidocaine. The two drugs given together may cause respiratory depression.
Methoxyflurane	Barbiturates induce metabolism of methoxyflurane to nephrotoxic metabolites, which may also induce renal insufficiency.
Methyldopa	Findings are contradictory, but barbiturates may reduce methyldopa plasma levels.
Metronidazole	Barbiturates induce metabolism of metronidazole and higher doses may be required.
Monoamine oxidase inhibitors	Trenylcypromine prolongs barbiturate hypnosis in animals. Sedative effects may also be potentiated in humans.
Narcotic analgesics	Barbiturates promote metabolism of meperidine to normeperidine. CNS depression is potentiated.
Phenmetrazine	Concurrent barbiturate therapy reduces weight lose associated with phenmetrazine treatment.
Phenothiazines	Barbiturates induce metabolism (See Chapter 3)
Phenylbutazone	Metabolism induced by barbiturates.
Phenytoin	Therapeutic doses of phenobarbital induce phenytoin metabolism, although large doses may actually inhibit metabolism. Phenytoin may increase plasma levels of phenobarbital. Osteomalacia may be promoted by the combination. (See Phenytoin section)
Primidone	Because primidone is converted to phenobarbital, excessive levels of the latter drug may occur if they are coadministered.
Probenecid	Probenecid may prolong thiopental anesthesia.
Propoxyphene	The addition of propoxyphene to phenobarbital may raise plasma levels of the latter drug.
Pyridoxine	May lower phenobarbital levels.
Quinidine	Barbiturates induce metabolism of quinidine.
Rifampin	Rifampin induces metabolism of hexobarbital.
Sulfonamides	Intravenous sulfisoxazole reduces minimum effective doses of thiopental and shortens wakening time, perhaps via displacement from protein binding sites. Phenobarbital may increase billary excretion and decrease urinary excretion of sulfasalazine. Acetylation of sulfapyridine is decreased while hydroxylation is

(continued)

TABLE 5.1. BARBITURATE DRUG INTERACTIONS (CONTINUED)

Drug	Clinical Effect
	increased. Phenobarbital does not affect sulfisoxazole or sulfisomidine.
Tetracycline	Metabolism of doxycycline is induced by barbiturates.
Theophylline	Metabolism is induced by barbiturates.
Valproate	Valproate inhibits phenobarbital metabolism.

interactions with valproate involve impaired metabolism, although a protein-binding interaction occurs with aspirin. Acute toxicity from elevated valproate serum levels is characterized by anorexia, nausea, vomiting, sedation, ataxia, and tremor.

Phenytoin is a hydantoin anticonvulsant that is less widely used as a primary treatment for psychiatric disorders than in years past, although it is still used in some treatment-resistant obsessive compulsive disorders (OCDs) and impulse-control disorders.

Gabapentin is approved for the adjunctive treatment of complex partial seizures with or without generalization. Off-label uses include migraine prophylaxis and neuropathic pain. Symptoms of anxiety disorders, such as social phobia, have been found to improve with gabapentin monotherapy. However, no controlled double-blind data corroborate the large open-label uncontrolled data for gabapentin as adjunctive therapy in the management of bipolar disorder. It has no active metabolites and is exclusively renally excreted. Plasma protein binding is absent, and it lacks hepatic metabolism or enzyme induction or inhibition.

Lamotrigine (LTG), a phenyltriazine, is a structurally unique compound compared to other antiepileptic drugs (AEDs). It is useful as a mood stabilizer when administered either in combination treatment or as monotherapy in bipolar disorder, especially bipolar depression. Its Food and Drug Administration (FDA) indications include the adjunctive treatment of partial seizures and generalized seizures secondary to Lennox-Gastault syndrome. It is rapidly absorbed, reaching peak plasma concentrations in 2 to 3 hours with a half-life of approximately 27 hours. LTG protein binding is approximately 50%. Hepatic UDP glucuronidation is its primary metabolic pathway, and this pathway is vulnerable to induction and inhibition. Elimination is primarily renal. Adverse effects observed with LTG administration include headache, nausea, emesis, diplopia, dizziness, and ataxia. However, the complication of greatest concern is rash, including Stevens-Johnson syndrome. Rash is much less likely to appear at or below LTG's maximum recommended daily dosage. "Start low and go slow" is good advice when beginning LTG treatment.

Oxcarbazepine (OXC), like CBZ, has efficacy in treating absence and partial seizures with or without generalization. It is also an off-label second-line treatment for bipolar disorder. OXC differs from CBZ in that it possesses a ketone group at the 10-11 position. OXC's main active metabolite, a monohydroxy derivative (MHD), is not as susceptible to hepatic enzyme induction or inhibition compared to carbamazepine-10-11-epoxide (CBZ-E). OXC is not subject to autoinduction as CBZ. OXC, compared to CBZ, is only a moderate inducer of cytochrome P450 3A4. Hyponatremia, LFT elevation, rash, gastrointestinal complaints, sedation, dizziness, and fatigue can be seen with OXC monotherapy. The majority of patients who experience rash while being administered CBZ do not exhibit the same symptoms when receiving OXC. Blood dyscrasias are less frequent in OXC than CBZ (OXC lacks the black box warning for agranulocytosis), and hematologic monitoring is not required as frequently.

Topiramate is a sulfamate-substituted monosaccharide and is roughly 70% excreted unchanged in the urine. It inhibits cytochrome P450 2C19. Topiramate's FDA-approved indications include partial and generalized tonic-clonic seizures. It is useful in off-label acute and maintenance management of treatment resistant bipolar disorder as well as alcoholism. Common side effects include cognitive dulling, dose related weight loss, dizziness, headache, somnolence, psychomotor slowing, nausea, and diplopia. Other adverse effects include nephrolithiasis and secondary angle closure glaucoma that both resolve with topiramate discontinuation.

Section 5.1   Carbamazepine

Azole Antifungal Agents

EVIDENCE OF INTERACTION

The manufacturer's product information cautions that voriconazole co-administration with CBZ is contraindicated and likely to decrease voriconazole plasma concentrations, resulting in a decrease in efficacy (Pfizer Labs 2002).

Spina et al. (1997) studied the effect of ketoconazole on plasma levels of carbamazepine and its active metabolite, carbamazepine-10,11-epoxide. All patients were stabilized on CBZ 400 to 800 mg/day and received 6 days of ketoconazole 200 mg/day. On combined therapy, serum CBZ concentrations increased from 5.6 mg/mL to 7 mg/mL. Upon discontinuation of ketoconazole, the mean CBZ level returned to baseline 5.9 mg/mL. During combined therapy, seizure frequency did not change, and no patient exhibited signs or symptoms of CBZ toxicity.

Nair (1999) found that 3 days after initiating fluconazole therapy, the CBZ plasma level increased from 11.1 to 24.5 mg/mL in a 33-year-old man on 1,200 mg/day of CBZ. The patient also exhibited stupor and required the discontinuation of fluconazole. CBZ was held for 24 hours, leading to a resolution of symptoms. Carbamazepine was restarted without incident.

MECHANISM
The inhibition of cytochrome P450 3A4 by azole antifungals.

CLINICAL IMPLICATIONS
Monitor for signs of CBZ toxicity and obtain more frequent CBZ serum levels when initiating, discontinuing, or modifying the dose of azole antifungals in patients already receiving CBZ. The CBZ dose should be adjusted as necessary.

Barbiturates

The possible interactions of barbiturates and CBZ are summarized in Table 5.1.

Benzodiazepines (BZD)

EVIDENCE OF INTERACTION
One case report noted a more than 50% reduction in plasma alprazolam concentrations and the reappearance of disabling panic attacks in a patient who was on alprazolam 7.5 mg/day and had CBZ 300 mg/day added to his medication regimen (Arana 1988).

A similar result was noted in a small study (Backman 1996) of patients receiving CBZ or phenytoin and oral midazolam. The half-life, area-under-plasma-curve (AUC) time curve and peak concentration of midazolam were decreased by 94%, 92%, and 42%, respectively, compared with control subjects. Midazolam's sedative effects were greatly reduced in the epileptic patients receiving either carbamazepine or phenytoin.

MECHANISM

The induction of cytochrome 3A4 by CBZ.

CLINICAL IMPLICATIONS

BZD dose adjustment may be necessary when initiating, discontinuing, or modifying CBZ dose.

Calcium Channel Blockers

EVIDENCE OF INTERACTION

Eimer et al. (1987) reported a case of carbamazepine (CBZ) neurotoxicity following the addition of diltiazem 30 mg every 6 hours to a patient's medication regimen. Other medications in the regimen included digoxin 0.25 mg/day orally, levothyroxine 0.15 mg daily, nitroglycerin ointment (1/2 inch every 6 hours), Coumadin 5 mg alternating with 7.5 mg daily, and KCl elixir. One month after the initiation of diltiazem therapy, the patient presented with mental slowing and increased difficulty speaking. The CBZ level was 15.5 µg/L. Diltiazem was discontinued, and a CBZ level on the 4th day of hospitalization was 7.7 µg/mL.

Another case was reported in which three calcium channel blockers—verapamil, diltiazem, and nifedipine—were co-administered at separate times to a 34-year-old man with refractory epilepsy also taking CBZ and having serum levels of 12 to 13 µg/mL (Brodie and MacPhee 1986). Verapamil 120 mg orally 3 times a day produced signs of neurotoxicity during co-administration with CBZ. After 48 hours of co-administration with CBZ, diltiazem 60 mg 3 times a day produced signs of neurotoxicity (dizziness, nausea, ataxia, and diplopia) with a coincident CBZ level of 21 µg/mL. These neurotoxic signs resolved after stopping diltiazem, with a corresponding decrease in CBZ levels. Of interest is that, 3 months later, nifedipine was given as adjunctive anticonvulsive treatment, and a substantial improvement in the control of seizures was noted without signs of neurotoxicity or change in circulating CBZ levels.

In a separate case reported by MacPhee et al. (1986), verapamil co-administered with CBZ to refractory epileptics resulted in a 94% rise in CBZ levels and coincident neurotoxic signs, which abated with verapamil withdrawal. They also noted a 36% reduction in the CBZ-E-to-CBZ ratio during the co-administration of these two medications.

Other reports confirm the potential neurotoxicity of the combination of CBZ with diltiazem or verapamil (Ahmad 1990, Bahis et al. 1991, Beattie et al. 1988, Gadde 1990, Maoz et al. 1992, Price 1988). Felodipine plasma levels were lower in patients taking a variety of anticonvulsants, including CBZ (Capewell et al. 1987).

MECHANISM

The inhibition of CBZ metabolism via 3A4 (its main metabolic pathway) by diltiazem and verapamil is the likely mechanism. Both these medications have been shown to inhibit hepatic cytochrome P450 monooxygenase activity in mice in vivo and in vitro (Renton 1985). Brodie and MacPhee (1986) make the point that, although nifedipine does undergo hepatic metabolism, it belongs to a subgroup of calcium channel blockers that are structurally and functionally dissimilar to diltiazem.

CLINICAL IMPLICATIONS

The combination of CBZ and calcium channel blockers may be used in the treatment of medical conditions, refractory epilepsy, or treatment-resistant psychotic disorders. It appears that a substantial risk of CBZ neurotoxicity is present with the use of either verapamil or diltiazem but not nifedipine. When possible, nifedipine, in contrast to diltiazem or verapamil, should be the drug of choice when considering the co-administration of CBZ with calcium channel blockers.

Cimetidine and H$_2$-Antagonists

EVIDENCE OF INTERACTION

The co-administration of a 1,200-mg daily dose of cimetidine with a single dose of CBZ resulted in a 26% increase in the AUC time-curve and 18% increase in the elimination half-life of CBZ (Dalton et al. 1985). In a subsequent study by the same authors, CBZ (300 mg orally twice a day) was administered to eight healthy volunteers for 42 days (days 1–42) and cimetidine was added to the regimen on days 29 to 35. In this study, CBZ levels increased by 17% after 2 days of cimetidine treatment but returned to premedication levels by the 7th day of co-administration, indicating a time-dependent interaction (Dalton et al. 1986). Others found no effect of cimetidine 1,200 mg/day on CBZ levels after 7 days of co-administration (Levine et al. 1985). Similarly, Sonne et al. (1983) found no effect of cimetidine 1 g daily for 7 days on CBZ or CBZ-10,11-epoxide levels in seven epileptic patients.

In another study, cimetidine 400 mg twice a day or placebo was administered to healthy males for 25 days (Macphee et al. 1984). Co-administration with CBZ 200 mg/day for 15 days resulted in a 25% and 33% rise in CBZ concentration during the 1st and 2nd weeks of CBZ administration, respectively.

Webster et al. (1984) studied the pharmacokinetics of a single dose of CBZ 400 mg or valproic acid (VPA) 400 mg after 4 weeks of a therapeutic course of either cimetidine (1 g/day, $N = 6$) or ranitidine (300 mg/day, $N = 6$). The authors found a decrease in the oral clearance of CBZ of up to 20% after cimetidine treatment (from 20.3 ± 2.2 to 18.0 ± 1.4 mL/hr per kg), with a corresponding prolongation in the elimination half-life from 35.3 (± 3.7) to 38.6 (± 1.8) hours. VPA clearance also decreased (10.9 ± 0.8 to 10.0 ± 0.4 mL/hr per kg), with a corresponding prolongation in the elimination half-life. Ranitidine-treated patients failed to show any of the above trends.

MECHANISM

Cimetidine inhibits the hepatic cytochrome P450 3A family, as well as other cytochrome P450 enzymes (2D6, 1A2).

CLINICAL IMPLICATIONS

When these medications are co-administered, transient increases in CBZ levels may result, and clinicians should monitor for CBZ toxicity. Although dosage adjustments are rarely necessary, patients should be advised of the possibility that CBZ side effects may be exacerbated 3 to 5 days after the initiation of cimetidine co-administration.

Clozapine

The possible interactions of cloapzine and CBZ are summarized in Table 5.2.

EVIDENCE OF INTERACTION

Raitasuo et al. (1993) described two patients in whom an interaction of clozapine and CBZ was suspected. The first patient was a 25-year-old schizophrenic man who had been taking a regimen of clozapine 800 mg/day and CBZ 600 mg/day for several months. After CBZ was discontinued, this patient's clozapine level rose from 1.4 to 2.4 μmol/L. The second patient was a 36-year-old schizophrenic man with epilepsy taking clozapine 600 mg/day and CBZ 800 mg/day. After CBZ was

TABLE 5.2 ANTICONVULSANT ANTIPSYCHOTIC INTERACTIONS

CARBAMAZEPINE

Haloperidol	Decreased levels of haloperidol with exacerbation of psychosis
	CBZ levels may also be decreased
	Delirium reported in two cases of rapid cycling bipolar on combination
Clozapine	Case reports of doubling of clozapine levels with combination
Aripiprazole	70% reduction in Cmax and AUC of parent and metabolite with CBZ
Ziprasidone	36% reduction in AUC with CBZ, 27% reduction in C_{max}
Olanzapine	25% reduction in C_{max}, 34% in AUC, 20% in $t_{1/2}$
Quetiapine	Elevated CBZ metabolite, CBZ-epoxide
Risperidone	Decreased levels of risperidone and 9-OH risperidone, clinical deterioration reported

VALPROIC ACID

Risperidone	Elevated VPA levels
Clozapine	Slight elevation of clozapine possible, but not established
Chlorpromazine	Slight elevation of VPA possible, but of uncertain clinical significance

LAMOTRIGINE

Clozapine	LTG may increase clozapine levels (case report)

HYDANTOIN

Quetiapine	80% decrease in steady state AUC of quetiapine
Clozapine	Decreased clozapine levels (case reports)
Phenothiazines	Phenytoin levels may be lower with concomitant use of phenothiazine antipsychotics such as thioridazine, chlorpromazine, and mesoridazine
Haloperidol	Possibility of lowered haloperidol levels, but not adequately studied

discontinued in this patient, clozapine levels rose from 1.5 to 3.0 μmol/L. In another case, a 76-year-old man with a history of bromperidol-induced neuroleptic malignant syndrome (NMS) developed NMS 3 days after the addition of clozapine to a stable carbamazepine dose (Müller et al. 1988).

MECHANISM

CBZ induces the metabolism of clozapine via induction of cytochrome P450 1A2 and 3A4.

CLINICAL IMPLICATIONS

CBZ and clozapine are sometimes co-administered in patients with seizures and/or complex psychotic disorders. If CBZ is added to clozapine, antipsychotic efficacy may be reduced. When CBZ is stopped, clozapine dosage reduction will be necessary to avoid toxicity. The combined effects of the two drugs on myelopoiesis are unknown

Corticosteroids

EVIDENCE OF INTERACTION

CBZ lowers the plasma levels of dexamethasone and invalidates the dexamethasone suppression test (Privatera et al. 1982). Prednisolone and other corticosteroids are probably similarly affected (Olivesi 1986).

MECHANISM

CBZ enhances the metabolism of corticosteroids via induction of cytochrome P450 3A4.

CLINICAL IMPLICATIONS

Patients taking CBZ should not receive a dexamethasone suppression test until CBZ has been discontinued for several weeks. Patients on corticosteroid therapy may require dosage adjustments when CBZ is started or discontinued.

Cyclosporine (Sandimmune)

EVIDENCE OF INTERACTION

CBZ decreases cyclosporine (an immunosuppressive agent) plasma levels (Soto Alvarez 1991, Hillebrand et al. 1987, Lele et al. 1985, Schofield et al. 1990, Yee et al. 1990). The onset of effect is a few days after the addition of CBZ, and persists for about 2 to 3 weeks.

In a case control study involving pediatric renal transplant patients, mean average steady-state blood concentrations of cyclosporine (CsA) per mg of CsA administered were less than 50% in those subjects co-administered CBZ compared with the control group (Cooney et al. 1995).

MECHANISMS

CBZ enhances the metabolism of cyclosporine via the induction of cytochrome P450 3A4.

CLINICAL IMPLICATIONS

Some authorities recommend the use of valproate in place of CBZ if possible. If CBZ is used, special attention must be directed to cyclosporine levels after the initiation and termination of CBZ therapy, and appropriate dosage adjustments made.

Danazol (Danocrine)

EVIDENCE OF INTERACTION

Danazol, a synthetic androgen used in the treatment of endometriosis, fibrocystic breast disease, and hereditary angioedema may cause increases in CBZ levels (Hayden et al. 1991). Six epileptic patients with fibrocystic breast disease receiving both CBZ and danazol had CBZ levels increased by almost twofold in the presence of danazol (Zielenski et al. 1987).

In a case study measuring radio-labeled CBZ levels, the steady-state plasma concentrations of CBZ increased between 50% and 100% during the co-administration of danazol and CBZ (Kramer et al. 1986).

MECHANISM

Using a stable radioactive nitrogen (^{15}N) CBZ isotope technique, danazol co-administration increased CBZ elimination half-life (11 to 24.3 hour). CBZ plasma clearance decreased from 57.7 to 23.2 mL/hour per kg. Danazol inhibits the epoxide transdiol pathway of CBZ metabolism (Kramer et al. 1986).

CLINICAL IMPLICATIONS

Danazol co-administration with CBZ appears to significantly inhibit CBZ metabolism and raise CBZ serum levels. Physicians should monitor patients for the emergence of CBZ side effects or toxicity when these drugs are administered concurrently. CBZ dosage reduction may be necessary.

Erythromycin, Troleandomycin, Other Macrolide and Ketolide Antibiotics

EVIDENCE OF INTERACTION

Numerous reports have been published of CBZ toxicity precipitated by co-administration with erythromycin (Stafstrom et al. 1995) and other macrolides such as clarithromycin (Biaxin) (Metz et al. 1995). Hedrick et al. (1983) reported four cases of epileptic children in which the addition of erythromycin to the medication regimen resulted in an increase in CBZ levels to the toxic range (16 to 19 μg/mL) and clinical signs of neurotoxicity. Signs of neurotoxicity remitted as CBZ levels decreased after erythromycin was discontinued.

Another case described a 41-year-old woman with epilepsy receiving CBZ 400 mg 3 times daily (level 9.3 to 13 μg/mL) and phenobarbital (Pb) 100 mg 4 times daily, in whom dizziness, nausea, vomiting, ataxia, and blurred vision developed 3 days after erythromycin stearate was added to her regimen for an infected forehead laceration (Carranco et al. 1985). The CBZ level was 28.2 μg/mL, and the Pb level was 17.2 μg/mL. These symptoms did not reappear when CBZ and phenobarbital were reinstituted without erythromycin.

Another case of erythromycin-induced CBZ toxicity was reported in a 6-year-old epileptic child (Zitelli et al. 1987). Within 5 days of the addition of erythromycin, vomiting, weakness, lethargy, ataxia, nystagmus, and cogwheeling movements developed with a CBZ level of 25.8 μg/mL (CBZ level was 11.9 pre-erythromycin therapy).

Wong et al. (1983) performed a controlled two-way crossover study in eight volunteers with CBZ 400 mg/day alone or with erythromycin 250 mg every 6 hours for 5 days prior to, and 3 days after, concurrent CBZ treatment. They found that the clearance of CBZ was lowered in the presence of erythromycin from 15.0 (±3.0) to 12.1 (±3.1) mL/kg per hour. The mean volume of distribution, elimination rate constant, and absorption rate constant of CBZ were not altered by erythromycin.

Azithromycin (Zithromax) is only a weak inhibitor of cytochrome P450 3A4, so its impact in CBZ levels is minimal to nonexistent.

Dirithromycin (Dynabac) does not have any known cytochrome P450 interactions and thus does not affect CBZ levels (Watkins et al. 1997).

Troleandomycin (TAO), like erythromycin, is a macrolide antibiotic that may elevate CBZ serum levels during co-administration. The addition of TAO to the medication regimen of 17 patients with epilepsy led to the development of nausea, vomiting, dizziness, and in six patients, a two- to fourfold increase in plasma CBZ was also noted, which returned to normal after TAO was withdrawn (Mesdjian et al. 1980). Sixteen of 17 patients were on combination anticonvulsant therapy. The levels of other anticonvulsants were not affected by TAO administration. Another series described symptoms of CBZ toxicity in eight epileptic patients 24 hours after receiving TAO (Dravet et al. 1977). Of eight patients, two had elevated plasma CBZ levels after TAO was added; these levels decreased after TAO was discontinued.

In the other six patients, symptoms of toxicity were reported, but CBZ plasma levels were not obtained.

Telithromycin (Ketek) is a ketolide, a new subclass of antibiotics, similar to macrolides, recently developed for use in macrolide-resistant respiratory infections. Telithromycin is known to be a potent inhibitor of cytochrome P450 3A4, so all the cautions used in co-administration of CBZ and erythromycin and clarithromycin hold true with this medication (Bearden et al. 2001).

MECHANISM

CBZ is almost entirely metabolized in the hepatic microsomal system, with only approximately 2% of the dose excreted unchanged in the urine (Bowdle et al. 1979). The primary metabolic pathway is via cytochrome P450 3A4, which is also responsible for erythromycin macrolide metabolism (Danan et al. 1981, Faigle et al. 1976). Erythromycin significantly inhibits the epoxide-diol metabolic pathway by which CBZ is transformed to carbamazepine-10,11-epoxide and thus increases it serum levels (Miles et al.1989). TAO may inhibit the hepatic metabolism of CBZ, but detailed pharmacokinetic studies have not been published (Mesdjian et al. 1980).

CLINICAL IMPLICATIONS

Patients taking CBZ who are started on erythromycin antibiotic therapy should be monitored closely for signs and symptoms of CBZ toxicity. The likelihood of the interaction increases with larger doses of erythromycin (Mitsch 1989). Other macrolide antibiotics (e.g., troleandomycin and clarithromycin) also may interact similarly with CBZ.

Felbamate

EVIDENCE OF INTERACTION

The co-administration of felbamate, an anticonvulsant, with CBZ results in a decrease in CBZ levels and an increase in the CBZ metabolite CBZ-10,11-epoxide (CBZ-E). Albani et al. (1991) examined the effect of the administration of felbamate on 22 patients receiving constant CBZ monotherapy in a double-blind controlled study. The authors found that administering felbamate to patients previously receiving CBZ monotherapy resulted in a consistent reduction in the CBZ plasma levels (average of 25% reduction). This effect was evident after 1 week of treatment and reached a plateau after 2 to 4 weeks of co-administration. In addition, the authors found a corresponding increase in the CBZ-E concentration consistently following the reduction in serum CBZ concentrations. Wagner et al. (1993) evaluated the effect of felbamate on the concentrations of carbamazepine and of its metabolites carbamazepine-10,11-epoxide and carbamazepine-trans 10,11-diol (diol) in 26 patients. These authors found that the addition of felbamate increased mean epoxide concentrations from 1.8 µg/mL during placebo or baseline levels to 2.4 µg/mL during felbamate therapy. No significant change in the diol concentration was found.

MECHANISM

The likely mechanism of the interaction is an induction of CBZ metabolism via cytochrome P450 3A4 after the addition of felbamate (Glue et al. 1997).

CLINICAL IMPLICATIONS

The addition of felbamate to patients already on CBZ may result in a reduction of CBZ levels, but a corresponding increase in the serum concentration of the active CBZ-epoxide metabolite may also occur. Thus, the CBZ-epoxide concentrations as well as CBZ concentrations should be taken into account in patients on this combination before dosage changes are made. Clinical signs of CBZ toxicity may result from increased CBZ-epoxide concentrations if the CBZ dose is increased on the basis of CBZ serum levels alone.

Haloperidol

The possible interactions of haloperidol and CBZ are summarized in Table 5.3 (also see Chapter 3).

Isoniazid

EVIDENCE OF INTERACTION

The signs of CBZ toxicity occurred in 10 of 13 patients (disorientation, listlessness, aggression, lethargy, and drowsiness) after isoniazid (INH) 200 mg daily was added to CBZ. Toxic symptoms remitted when CBZ dosage was reduced (Valsalan and Cooper 1982). CBZ levels were monitored in three of these patients; CBZ levels were elevated to 26.7, 15.2, and 13.4 µg/mL after the initiation of INH therapy (200 mg every day), respectively. The symptoms of CBZ toxicity remitted with reductions in CBZ dosage reductions.

Another case described a patient who was taking phenytoin 200 mg/day and CBZ 1,000 mg/day (with therapeutic levels of both medications). When INH 300 mg/day was added to the patient's regimen, signs of neurotoxicity developed, including ataxia, headaches, vomiting, drowsiness, and confusion (CBZ level = 15 µg/mL) (Block 1982). The phenytoin level was 18 μg/mL at the same time. Her symptoms resolved after INH was discontinued, with anticonvulsant dosages unchanged. CBZ level 1 week later was 6.1 μg/mL; phenytoin was 17.8 μg/mL.

A 35-year-old epileptic man on a regimen composed of nitrazepam 10 mg 4 times a day, CBZ 400 mg 4 times a day, and valproic acid 300 mg 4 times a day became drowsy and then stuporous with CBZ levels of 18 to 22 μg/mL 2 days after INH 400 mg/day was started. Prior to INH therapy, CBZ levels were 5 to 8 μg/mL. Valproic acid levels were not altered with INH therapy. Nitrazepam levels were not measured in this study. CBZ clearance was reduced from 6.2 L/hr before INH to 3.3 L/hr 3 days after isoniazid treatment was initiated (Wright et al. 1982).

MECHANISM

INH decreases the clearance of CBZ by inhibiting hepatic microsomal metabolism (Kutt et al. 1970). This interaction possibly could be related to INH's inhibition of cytochrome P450 2C9, one of the enzymes responsible for CBZ metabolism.

CLINICAL IMPLICATIONS

CBZ metabolism is impaired when INH is co-administered, and toxicity may result. CBZ levels should be monitored, and signs of CBZ toxicity should be checked in regular clinical assessments.

Isotretinoin (Accutane)

The plasma levels of CBZ and CBZ-E are reduced when CBZ and isotretinoin are co-administered (Marsden 1988).

Lamotrigine

EVIDENCE OF INTERACTION

Warner et al. (1992) described an interaction between lamotrigine (LTG), and CBZ. These authors reported that after the introduction of LTG to nine patients already taking CBZ, the mean CBZ-E concentration increased by 45%, and the CBZ-E : CBZ ratio increased by 19%. A variable increase or decrease occurred in concomitant serum CBZ concentration. A mean rise of the CBZ concentration of 16% was noted. In four of these patients, this change was associated with symptoms of clinical toxicity.

In another study, it was found that CBZ toxicity was more likely to occur when LTG was added to CBZ and the initial CBZ level was high, typically >8 mg/L. This study found that a reduction of the CBZ dose usually reversed the toxicity. LTG dose then could be increased to maximal effect, and it was not necessary to stop either drug (Besag et al. 1998).

The manufacturer's product information states that CBZ may decrease steady-state lamotrigine serum levels 40%. Similar decreases in LTG levels may occur with other enzyme-inducing antiepileptic agents, including phenobarbital, phenytoin, and primidone (GlaxoSmithKline Lamictal package insert 1994).

One report found a dose-dependent decrease in LTG half-life of 1.7h per 100 mg of CBZ in the range of 800 to 1,600 mg/day of CBZ (Jawad 1987). This was replicated in pediatric patients receiving enzyme-inducers, including CBZ (Vauzelle-Kervroedan 1996, Eriksson 1996, GlaxoSmithKline Lamictal package insert 1994).

MECHANISM

The authors (Warner 1992) speculate that because these patients showed a marked increase in the CBZ-E concentration without a consistent reduction in CBZ levels, the likely mechanism of this interaction is an inhibition of the CBZ-E hydrolase, the enzyme that converts CBZ-E to CBZ-10,11-dihydroxide.

CLINICAL IMPLICATIONS

These studies suggest the potential for toxic symptoms to develop with the co-administration of LTG and CBZ. Toxic CBZ symptoms such as dizziness, nausea, and diplopia may occur secondary to the active CBZ-E metabolite of CBZ. CBZ-epoxide levels should be checked if toxic symptoms develop on this drug combination, and the CBZ dosage should be adjusted as necessary.

LTG may need to be increased when initiating, discontinuing, or altering the dose of CBZ in patients receiving both LTG and CBZ.

Lithium

EVIDENCE OF INTERACTION

Neurotoxicity developed in a series of five rapid-cycling manic patients when they were treated with a regimen of CBZ and lithium, despite therapeutic plasma levels of both medications (Shukla 1984). Risk factors for developing neurotoxicity from this combination may include a history of lithium neurotoxicity or the presence of concurrent medical or neurologic illness. Neurotoxic symptoms developed in a 22-year-old woman with bipolar affective disorder when she was treated with a regimen composed of lithium carbonate and CBZ, despite therapeutic drug plasma levels (Chaudhry et al. 1983).

In other reports, similar neurotoxic effects have been observed from a few days to 2 weeks after initiating combined therapy (Marcoux 1996, Shukla et al. 1984). In most cases, neurotoxicity resolved after discontinuing all medications; however, one case of irreversible tardive dyskinesia–like syndrome has been reported after 7 years of combined lithium and carbamazepine therapy (Lazarus 1994).

MECHANISM
The mechanism is unknown.

CLINICAL IMPLICATIONS
Lithium and CBZ are frequently used in the treatment of rapid-cycling bipolar disorder, and thus the potential exists for this interaction to occur in clinical practice. Patients started on this combination should be monitored carefully for signs of neurotoxicity. Patients at high risk may be those with a previous history of lithium neurotoxicity or those with medical or neurologic disorders. In most cases, however, the combination of lithium and CBZ is well tolerated.

Levetiracetam

EVIDENCE OF INTERACTION
Sisodiya reported (2002) symptoms of CBZ toxicity (ataxia and nystagmus) in four patients following the addition of as low as 500 mg twice daily levetiracetam to a treatment regimen that included CBZ. This situation resolved when the dose of CBZ was reduced or discontinued. Interestingly, neither CBZ nor CBZ-E plasma concentrations were elevated.

MECHANISM
The mechanism of interaction is not known, but a possible pharmacodynamic interaction has been postulated.

CLINICAL IMPLICATIONS
The monitoring of clinical response and careful observation of signs of CBZ toxicity should occur when levetiracetam is added or removed from a patient's treatment regimen. A decrease in CBZ dose may be required.

Mebendazole (Vermox)

EVIDENCE OF INTERACTION
Plasma levels of mebendazole, a broad spectrum anthelmintic, may be reduced in the presence of CBZ (Luder et al. 1986, Witassek et al. 1983).

MECHANISM
CBZ induces the hepatic metabolism of mebendazole.

CLINICAL IMPLICATIONS
The effect of reduced mebendazole plasma levels is probably minimal in the treatment of intestinal organisms such as hookworm or trichuriasis (whipworm). In high-dose applications, such as in the treatment of hydatid disease, the drug interaction may take on more significance. Valproate does not affect mebendazole metabolism and may provide an alternative anticonvulsant.

Methadone

EVIDENCE OF INTERACTION
CBZ may lower methadone plasma levels and lead to opiate withdrawal symptoms (Bell et al. 1988).

MECHANISM
CBZ induces methadone metabolism via cytochrome P450 3A4.

CLINICAL IMPLICATIONS
In patients taking methadone, the addition of CBZ may lower methadone plasma levels and lead to the precipitation of opiate withdrawal. Conversely, when CBZ is discontinued, methadone levels may rise. Plasma monitoring of methadone is usually readily available and should be used to guide dosage adjustments under these circumstances.

Oral Contraceptives

EVIDENCE OF INTERACTION
Several reports have documented that the effectiveness of oral contraceptives is reduced in patients using CBZ and phenytoin (Coulam et al. 1979, Janz et al. 1974, Kenyon 1972, Laengner and Detering 1974, Rapport and Calabrese 1989). In progestin formulations, low plasma norgestrel levels were noted in patients taking anticonvulsants. CBZ also alters the single-dose pharmacokinetics of ethinylestradiol and levonorgestrel (Crawford et al. 1990).

In another randomized, open-label study, female subjects received oral doses of norethindrone and ethinyl estradiol (Ortho-Novum 1/35) alone for one menstrual cycle and then the oral contraceptive (OC) concomitant with CBZ, 600 mg/day during the next cycle. The results reinforced the above observations of decreased efficacy when CBZ and OCs are co-administered. (Doose et al. 2003)

MECHANISM

CBZ (and phenytoin) induce the metabolism of contraceptive agents via induction of cytochrome P450 3A4.

CLINICAL IMPLICATIONS

CBZ and phenytoin should be avoided in patients taking contraceptives. Oral contraceptives, levonorgestrel implants (Norplant®), Norelgestromin/Ethinyl estradiol transdermal system (Ortho Evra®), and etonogestrel/ethinyl estradiol vaginal ring (Nuva Ring®) are affected. Although patients who have breakthrough bleeding are at obvious risk, pregnancy can occur even without this warning.

Phenytoin, Phenobarbital, Primidone

EVIDENCE OF INTERACTION

The plasma levels of CBZ were significantly decreased in patients receiving phenytoin, phenobarbital, or both drugs together, when compared with CBZ alone (Christiansen and Dam 1973). The average plasma CBZ concentrations in the regimens composed of CBZ alone, CBZ plus phenytoin, CBZ plus phenobarbital, and the combination of CBZ, phenobarbital, and phenytoin were 6.7, 4.4, 5.5, and 3.7 μg/mL, respectively. In a study of 142 epileptic patients, 28 received CBZ alone, while 40, 44, and 30 patients received also phenobarbital (PB), phenytoin, or both drugs, respectively (Johannessen et al. 1975). CBZ levels were significantly decreased in patients receiving co-medication regimens, compared with those receiving CBZ alone. The mean serum concentrations of CBZ alone, CBZ + phenytoin, CBZ + PB, and CBZ + PB + phenytoin were 7.2 (±2.5), 5.7 (±2.0), 4.6 (±1.8), and 3.9 (±2.0) μg/mL, respectively.

In a large series of epileptic patients taking CBZ alone or in various combinations with phenytoin, PB, or primidone, significantly lower CBZ levels occurred in all patient groups receiving the other anticonvulsants with CBZ than in the group taking CBZ alone (Schneider 1975). A double-blind study followed 41 patients given CBZ alone for 3 days and then assigned to one of the following groups: (a) CBZ 1,200 mg + phenytoin 300 mg, (b) CBZ 1,200 mg + PB 300 mg, or (c) CBZ 1,200 mg + phenytoin 300 mg + PB 300 mg. The study found that CBZ levels were significantly decreased when CBZ was administered with either phenytoin or phenobarbital or both (Cereghino et al. 1975). This effect of phenobarbital on CBZ levels was replicated in several studies (Spina et al. 1991, Ramsey et al. 1990).

MECHANISM

CBZ levels are significantly lower in patients who are also taking phenytoin, PB, and/or primidone all via induction of cytochrome P450 3A4.

CLINICAL IMPLICATIONS

Small decreases probably do not affect seizure control, but monitoring serum drug levels may be helpful.

Effect of Carbamazepine on Phenytoin

CBZ co-administration with phenytoin has been noted by various investigators to increase, decrease, or have no effect on phenytoin levels. Zielenski (1983) reported the effect of CBZ–phenytoin co-administration in 24 epileptics. In 50% of the patients, the mean steady-state plasma phenytoin concentration rose from 12.54 (± 3.93) to 22.7 (± 5.64) μg/mL when phenytoin was given with CBZ, compared with phenytoin alone.

CBZ co-administration also has been reported to decrease phenytoin levels. Hansen et al. (1971) described five patients in whom CBZ 600 mg/day was added to phenytoin. The half-life of phenytoin decreased from 10.6 to 6.7 hours with CBZ co-administration after at least 9 days of combined therapy.

Windorfer and Sauer (1977) and Windorfer et al. (1975) found significant decreases in serum phenytoin concentrations when co-administered in long-term therapy with CBZ. Others found serum phenytoin concentrations unaffected by CBZ (Cereghino 1975). The differences among various reports might be accounted for by variations in CBZ and phenytoin doses, duration of therapy, variation in the types and sizes of the study populations, or other factors. Browne et al. (1988), studying the combinations in normal volunteers, found that CBZ increased steady-state phenytoin levels by 35%.

Lai et al. (1992) performed a three-phase trial in which 11 subjects were given 600 mg phenytoin (Dilantin capsules) in each phase after an overnight fast. In the first phase, phenytoin was given alone. In the second phase, 400 mg carbamazepine (CBZ) was given at the same time as the phenytoin; and in phase three, 200 mg CBZ 3 times a day was given for 1 week prior to the phenytoin. This group found that single and multiple doses of CBZ decreased the plasma level of phenytoin.

MECHANISM

The specific mechanism by which CBZ affects phenytoin levels is unknown, although it is generally known that CBZ induces cytochrome P450 2C19, one of the metabolic pathways of phenytoin.

Effect of Phenytoin on Carbamazepine

EVIDENCE OF INTERACTION

The effect of phenytoin on CBZ levels is well established. Phenytoin reduced CBZ levels in 144 patients, while phenobarbital, methylphenobarbital, primidone, and sulthiame did not (Lander et al. 1975). For each 2 mg/kg per day of phenytoin given, the mean plasma CBZ level fell by 0.9 μg/mL. A study of 60 patients co-administered phenytoin and CBZ also found a reduction in plasma CBZ by phenytoin (Hooper 1974).

MECHANISM

Phenytoin may induce CBZ metabolism.

CLINICAL IMPLICATIONS

When both drugs are co-administered, their plasma levels may be lowered. Effects on phenytoin levels are inconsistent among studies with increases and decreases reported when CBZ is co-administered. Clinical effects on seizure control are possible but not likely. Careful monitoring of serum levels may be required.

Phenobarbital

EVIDENCE OF INTERACTION

Several studies indicate that PB lowers CBZ plasma levels (Cereghino et al. 1975, Christiansen and Dam 1973, Rane et al. 1976).

MECHANISM

PB induces hepatic metabolism of CBZ via cytochrome P450 3A4.

CLINICAL IMPLICATIONS

CBZ levels are significantly lower in patients who are also taking phenytoin, PB, and/or primidone. Small decreases probably do not affect seizure control, but monitoring serum drug levels may be helpful.

Propoxyphene

EVIDENCE OF INTERACTION

Dextropropoxyphene and CBZ are sometimes prescribed in combination for treatment of conditions such as severe herpetic neuralgia. Yu et al. (1986) have described two cases of CBZ intoxication when used in combination with dextropropoxyphene. Two patients became comatose and another patient became confused when taking this combination for painful acute herpes zoster infection. None were on excessive doses (400, 600, and 400 mg/day) of CBZ, yet all had toxic CBZ levels.

Dam et al. (1977) evaluated the effect of propoxyphene hydrochloride (65 mg 3 times a day) on seven epileptic outpatients receiving CBZ and found that combined treatment resulted in a marked increase (44% to 77%) in plasma CBZ levels and a decrease (32% to 44%) in plasma clearance in five patients. Three patients experienced signs of CBZ toxicity. No significant changes in CBZ-10,11-epoxide (CBZ-E) were noted.

Hansen et al. (1980) evaluated the effects of dextropropoxyphene 65 mg in six patients receiving CBZ 600 to 800 mg/day for longer than 6 months. They noted a mean increase of CBZ 66% in serum levels. CBZ-E levels declined, whereas CBZ protein binding was unaffected.

Oles (1989) reported eight cases of carbamazepine toxicity associated with variable increases in levels (up to sixfold) following propoxyphene administration. In another report, it was noted that geriatric patients may be more susceptible and demonstrate signs of toxicity even with therapeutic carbamazepine serum levels (Bergendal et al. 1997).

MECHANISM

Propoxyphene inhibits the hepatic metabolism of CBZ via cytochrome P450 3A4 (Spina et al. 1996).

CLINICAL IMPLICATIONS

The risk of CBZ toxicity is increased when this combination is used; consider alternate drug regimens for therapy of such conditions as postherpetic neuralgia, or, alternatively, CBZ levels should be monitored closely, and the physician should be alert for the signs and symptoms of CBZ toxicity.

Ritonavir/Protease Inhibitors

EVIDENCE OF INTERACTION

In one case report, CBZ toxicity (CBZ levels of 17.8 and 16.3 mg/mL) was seen in a 20-year-old HIV-positive man who had ritonavir added to his anticonvulsant regimen (Kato et al. 2000). Following a one-third decrease of his CBZ dose, the level was reduced to 6.2 mg/mL.

Two other HIV-positive patients who had ritonavir and other antiretrovirals added to a medication regimen that included CBZ experienced similar supratherapeutic increases of their CBZ levels and subsequent returns to normal levels when ritonavir was discontinued (Berbel Garcia et al. 2000, Mateu-de Antonio et al. 2001).

MECHANISM

Ritonavir not only induces 3A4, the major metabolic pathway of CBZ, but it also induces most of the other P450 cytochromes as well. Thus it increases the active metabolites of CBZ, potentially to toxic levels.

CLINICAL IMPLICATIONS

In clinical scenarios necessitating the addition of an antiretroviral treatment to a patient's medication regimen that includes CBZ, substitution of other protease inhibitors, such as nelfinavir, is advised, when possible. CBZ levels should be followed closely when antiretrovirals are administered to patients on anticonvulsants.

Theophylline

EVIDENCE OF INTERACTION

An 11-year-old girl with a 2-year history of asthma treated with theophylline 23 mg/kg per day and prednisone 10 mg/day had a generalized seizure. Phenobarbital was started but discontinued because of behavioral problems, and she was then started on CBZ therapy (Rosenberry et al. 1983). During co-administration with CBZ, the theophylline elimination half-life fell from 5.25 to 2.75 hours. Theophylline levels, which had been 21 to 23 μg/mL before CBZ initiation, dropped below therapeutic range, and the patient had an exacerbation of asthmatic symptoms. CBZ was discontinued and ethotoin was started. The theophylline half-life rose to 6.25 hours within 3 weeks.

MECHANISM

CBZ induces the metabolism of theophylline.

CLINICAL IMPLICATIONS

CBZ reduces theophylline half-life and serum concentrations during co-administration. If these medications are co-administered, the physician should be prepared to increase the theophylline dosage. If CBZ is stopped, theophylline doses should be decreased. Careful monitoring of theophylline levels and pulmonary status is necessary.

Thyroid Hormone

EVIDENCE OF INTERACTION

CBZ has a hypothyroid effect, as evidenced by reductions in serum concentrations of total thyroxine, free thyroxine, and triiodothyronine (Cathro et al. 1985, Connell et al. 1984, Roy-Byrne et al. 1984). Requirements for thyroxine replacements increase in hypothyroid patients (Aanderud et al. 1981).

MECHANISM

CBZ induces the metabolism of thyroxine and triiodothyronine; it also inhibits compensatory increases in thyrotropin.

CLINICAL IMPLICATIONS

Thyroid supplementation requirements are altered during CBZ therapy.

Valproate (*See* Valproic Acid section, this chapter)

Warfarin (Coumadin)

EVIDENCE OF INTERACTION

The co-administration of CBZ with warfarin decreased warfarin half-life and serum levels (Hansen et al. 1971). In a single case study, the anticoagulant effect of warfarin was neutralized when 400 mg/day of CBZ was added to the patient's regimen (Kendall and Boivin 1981). This effect was reversed after CBZ had been discontinued for 6 weeks. Reinstitution of CBZ required an 80% increase in warfarin dose to maintain a therapeutic prothrombin time. Massey (1983) found a similar effect in three other cases.

Similarly, CBZ in doses of 300 mg/day co-administered with warfarin required an increase in the daily warfarin dose from 4 to 5.5 mg/day to maintain a therapeutic prothrombin time (Ross and Beeley 1980).

MECHANISM

CBZ induces hepatic microsomal enzymes and enhances warfarin metabolism. Although warfarin is metabolized mainly by cytochrome P450 2C9, it is also metabolized via 3A4 and 2C19, all of which are induced by CBZ.

CLINICAL IMPLICATIONS

When CBZ is administered, the dose of warfarin may need to be increased to maintain a therapeutic prothrombin time. Correspondingly, the dose of warfarin may need to be decreased when CBZ is discontinued.

Section 5.2   Valproic Acid

Antacids

EVIDENCE OF INTERACTION

A small study involving seven healthy volunteers given an aluminum hydroxide-magnesium antacid and a single 500-mg dose of valproic acid (VPA) had a 12% higher AUC with the combination than with VPA alone (May et al. 1982).

MECHANISM

Unknown.

CLINICAL IMPLICATIONS

Antacids are commonly given for the gastrointestinal side effects of VPA. Although this does not appear to be a significant interaction, it can be avoided easily by separating the dose of antacid and VPA by an hour or more.

Amitriptyline

EVIDENCE OF INTERACTION

Pisani et al. (1986) evaluated six patients during the co-administration of amitriptyline (AT) and VPA. The authors found that during AT treatment, a slight but significant increase in both the apparent volume of distribution (Vd) and elimination half-life of VPA occurred.

MECHANISM

The mechanism of the interaction is unknown.

CLINICAL IMPLICATIONS

VPA and AT are sometimes used together in the treatment of postherpetic neuralgia and in the treatment of bipolar disorder. This combination also potentially could be used in the treatment of epilepsy patients with chronic pain or headaches. VPA toxicity may occur if AT is administered concurrently.

Aspirin

EVIDENCE OF INTERACTION

Orr et al. (1982) found that in five of six epileptic children who were taking 18 to 49 mg/kg per day of VPA, the steady-state free fraction of VPA rose from 12% to 43% during co-administration of antipyretic doses of aspirin. Some evidence suggests valproate toxicity may result from the combination (Goulden et al. 1987).

MECHANISM

VPA is highly protein bound at therapeutic concentrations and has a small volume of distribution (Rotne et al. 1980). In vitro, salicylate has been reported to displace VPA from its plasma protein-binding sites (Fleitman et al. 1980, Schobben et al. 1978). In addition, salicylates have been shown to inhibit β-oxidation of VPA. Abbott et al. (1986) noted that all metabolites of VPA β-oxidation (2-ene-VPA, 3-OH-VPA, and 3-keto-VPA) were significantly decreased in the urine during ASA-VPA co-administration. Significant increase also occurred in the urinary VPA glucuronide conjugates as well as the 4-ene-VPA metabolites. 4-Ene-VPA itself may be a potent inhibitor of the hepatic fatty acid β-oxidation sequence by sequestering acetylcoenzyme A.

CLINICAL IMPLICATIONS

The above evidence suggests that the potential for VPA toxicity may be increased during the co-administration of salicylates and VPA.

Benzodiazepines

EVIDENCE OF INTERACTION

Dhillon et al. (1982) found that when 10 mg of diazepam was administered intravenously to healthy young volunteers, each receiving 1,500 mg of valproate daily, the concentration of unbound diazepam in serum increased by approximately twofold compared with diazepam administered alone. The intrinsic clearance and volume of distribution of unbound diazepam were significantly reduced during co-administration. In addition, mean serum levels of the diazepam metabolite N-desmethyldiazepam were significantly lower during valproate co-administration. Absence seizures have been reported with the combination of clonazepam and valproate, but causality has not been established (Browne 1979, Watson 1979).

MECHANISM

Valproate displaces diazepam from plasma protein-binding sites and inhibits its metabolism.

Another study (Samara 1997) found a similar effect with the co-administration of lorazepam and VPA. Valproate increases plasma concentrations and reduces the clearance of lorazepam, most likely by impairing hepatic glucuronidation.

CLINICAL IMPLICATIONS

The co-administration of diazepam and valproic acid may result in increased effects of diazepam.

Cimetidine

EVIDENCE OF INTERACTION

VPA clearance was decreased and elimination half-life was increased when VPA was co-administered with cimetidine, but not ranitidine (Webster et al. 1984).

MECHANISM

Cimetidine, a potent P450 inhibitor, inhibits the metabolism of sodium valproate via the inhibition of cytochrome P450 2C9.

CLINICAL IMPLICATIONS

Dosage adjustments in sodium valproate will be necessary when the clinician is initiating or discontinuing cimetidine therapy. Alternatively, ranitidine, famotidine, or nizatidine may be used.

Carbamazepine

EVIDENCE OF INTERACTION

The combination of VPA and carbamazepine (CBZ) resulted in higher plasma levels of the CBZ active metabolite, carbamazepine-10,11-epoxide (CBZ-E), whereas CBZ levels were not significantly affected (McKauge et al. 1982). Another study found that VPA reduced the binding of CBZ to plasma protein in vitro (Mattson et al. 1982). Levy et al. (1984) administered VPA (1 g twice a day for 1 week) to seven epileptic patients receiving CBZ therapy and found that CBZ serum levels were reduced by 3% to 59% in six of seven patients and were unchanged in one patient. The plasma concentration ratio of CBZ-E : CBZ increased in all patients by 11% to 500%. In the plasma protein-binding portion of the study, the mean CBZ free fraction was increased in three subjects, decreased in one subject, and remained unchanged in two subjects with VPA-CBZ co-administration. The same authors also found that the co-administration of CBZ with 24-hour infusions of VPA at 75 and 150 mg/hour in rhesus monkeys resulted in a decrease in the mean clearance of free CBZ from 7.96 ($\pm$1.75) to 4.84 ($\pm$1.26) liter/hour per kg (p <0.01) and 4.12 ($\pm$1.75) liter/hour per kg (p <0.01), respectively.

MECHANISM OF INTERACTION

These results suggest that VPA inhibits CBZ metabolism. Pisani et al. (1986) evaluated the comparative effects of VPA and valpromide (VPM), a prodrug of VPA, on the plasma levels and protein binding of CBZ and CBZ-E in 12 epileptic patients. The authors found that CBZ levels were not affected by either treatment. In the VPA-treated group, CBZ-E levels increased by 101% (range 29% to 238%) within 1 week of combined therapy and returned to baseline after VPA was stopped. In the VPM-treated group, levels of CBZ-E increased by an average of 330%. The plasma protein binding of CBZ and CBZ-E was not significantly affected by either VPM or VPA. The authors suggest that VPA and VPM inhibit the epoxide hydroxylase enzyme in CBZ-E metabolism.

CLINICAL IMPLICATIONS

CBZ and VPA are frequently used in combination for the treatment of epilepsy. In addition, both these drugs are used for treatment-resistant schizophrenia and for bipolar patients, making the interaction of possible clinical importance for psychiatrists. Because VPA appears to increase the level of CBZ-E, an active metabolite of CBZ, and may cause protein-binding displacement of CBZ, the possibility exists that CBZ toxicity may develop when using these medications in combination. VPA levels may be decreased by the concomitant administration of CBZ.

Patients should be monitored carefully for signs of toxicity response. The serum levels of both drugs should be determined when adding or discontinuing either one.

A pharmacodynamic synergistic interaction between VPA and CBZ, in which the psychotropic efficacy of both agents is augmented, has been reported (Ketter et al. 1992). Several studies have reported that CBZ increases VPA clearance, decreases serum levels, and prolongs VPA half-life (Jann et al. 1998, Panesar 1989 et al). CBZ may promote the formation of a hepatotoxic and teratogenic VPA metabolite. It does not appear to alter protein binding.

Ethosuximide

EVIDENCE OF INTERACTION

Pisani et al. (1984) found that, when 500 mg of ethosuximide (ESM) was administered during the course of VPA therapy (800 to 1,600 mg/day titrated to therapeutic levels), a significant increase occurred in ESM serum elimination half-life (from 44 to 54 hours). Also, ESM total body clearance was significantly decreased (from 11.2 to 9.5 mL/min on average) during co-administration with VPA. The ESM renal clearance was unchanged during co-administration.

MECHANISM
The authors suggest that VPA increases ESM's half-life and decreases total body clearance of ESM via an unknown inhibition of hepatic metabolism.

ESM decreases VPA half-life and serum levels during co-administration, and VPA serum levels rebound upon cessation of ESM. In one study, the mean valproic acid serum level before taking MSM was 85.4 mg/L (14 patients), which decreased to 58.2 mg/L while taking MSM (p <0.001). In patients who stopped taking methsuximide, the mean serum level increased from 49.8 to 71.7 mg/L (p = 0.025) (Besag et al. 2001). This effect was also observed in another study (Salke-Kellermann 1997).

CLINICAL IMPLICATIONS
VPA, when co-administered with ESM, increases the risk of ESM toxicity. A different anticonvulsant combination should be chosen or ESM doses decreased to minimize the risk of toxicity. Clinicians should monitor for signs of VPA toxicity when discontinuing ESM and adjust the dosage of each drug as necessary.

Felbamate

EVIDENCE OF INTERACTION
Wagner et al. (1994), in a random crossover study, administered felbamate 600 mg and 1,200 mg twice daily to 10 patients already maintained on VPA 9.5 to 26.2 mg/kg per day. These authors found that the addition of felbamate to VPA resulted in increased serum concentrations of VPA. The co-administration of felbamate increased average VPA steady-state concentrations and decreased VPA clearance.

Eighteen subjects received VPA 400 mg/day for 21 days in a study conducted by Hooper et al. (1996). From day 8 to day 21, subjects received placebo or FBM at the following doses (mg/day): 1,200, 2,400, 3,000, or 3,600. Higher plasma VPA levels were observed when FBM was administered concurrently (55.4 to 63.8 μg/mL), which was an increase from 32 to 42 μg/mL during VPA monotherapy. The excretion of 3-oxo-VPA in urine was significantly lower on day 21 than on day 7, whereas VPA-glucuronide was significantly increased. The effects of FBM on VPA disposition were dose dependent and were maximal at approximately 2,400 mg/day. FBM caused an inhibition of the β-oxidation pathway for VPA metabolic clearance, which had been largely compensated by increased VPA glucuronidation.

MECHANISM

Felbamate may inhibit the metabolism of VPA via inhibition of VPA β-oxidation.

CLINICAL IMPLICATIONS

The co-administration of felbamate and VPA may result in increased levels of VPA and toxicity. Thus, if this combination is prescribed, VPA levels should be monitored closely and dosage reductions of VPA should be made when appropriate.

Lamotrigine

EVIDENCE OF INTERACTION

Yuen et al. (1992) examined the effect of VPA on lamotrigine (LTG) metabolism in six male subjects. Each subject received 100 mg of LTG orally on two occasions at a minimum of 14 days apart. One of these doses was given alone and the other concomitantly with VPA at a dose of 200 mg every 8 hours, the first dose of which was given 1 hour before LTG was initiated. The authors found that co-administration of LTG and VPA resulted in the slower elimination of LTG and a 21% reduction in LTG clearance, with a corresponding increase in LTG elimination half-life. Reduced elimination occurred within the first hour after administration. Reutens et al. (1993) reported that disabling tremor developed when LTG and VPA were co-administered. The first case was a patient with complex partial seizures. On a regimen of LTG 200 mg/day and VPA 2,000 mg/day, a severe tremor developed in the patient. The corresponding random serum concentration of LTG was 628 μmol/L and that of VPA was 53 μmol/L. This patient's tremor resolved after the LTG dose was reduced to 100 mg/day. The second case was a patient with multiple seizure types including myoclonus, generalized tonic-clonic seizures, and absence seizures. Titubation and a disabling postural and action tremor developed while this patient was taking a regimen of LTG 150 mg/day and VPA 2,500 mg/day. The VPA concentration was 1,030 μmol/L. This patient's tremor resolved when the VPA dose was reduced to 2,000 mg/day. A third more complicated case was also described. In a patient taking a combination of phenytoin 425 mg/day, VPA 2,500 mg/day, and LTG 200 mg/day, ataxia and upper extremity action tremor developed only after phenytoin was discontinued from the regimen. Random plasma levels of LTG and VPA were 55 and 868 μmol/L, respectively. These symptoms resolved after LTG was decreased to 100 mg/day. Thus, the authors speculated that the withdrawal of phenytoin from this regimen induced toxic symptoms, presumably by unmasking the VPA/LTG interaction, because phenytoin induces the hepatic enzymes responsible for the metabolism of LTG and VPA (Peck 1991). Finally, Pisani et al. (1993) described seven patients with refractory partial seizures whom, when taking the combination of VPA and LTG, had high concentrations of LTG that at times resulted in toxic symptoms of sedation, ataxia, and fatigue that resolved after the LTG dosage was reduced.

Less consistent findings have been reported with respect to alterations of VPA metabolism by LTG. One report found 25% reductions in VPA levels with combined LTG therapy (Andersen et al. 1996), whereas another study found no effect (Binnie et al. 1989).

MECHANISM
Yuen et al. (1992) postulate that VPA impairs the hepatic glucuronidation of LTG via competitive inhibition of enzymes.

CLINICAL IMPLICATIONS
The co-administration of VPA and LTG may result in elevated LTG levels and clinical signs of toxicity; thus, with this combination, serum levels of both drugs must be monitored carefully and dose adjustments made if necessary. Some evidence suggests that the combination improves seizure control compared to monotherapy (Morris et al. 2000).

Phenobarbital

EVIDENCE OF INTERACTION
VPA appears to impair the metabolism of phenobarbital (PB) and increase plasma PB levels (Bruni et al. 1980a, Wilder et al. 1978). Patel et al. (1980) performed a randomized crossover study of six normal subjects and found that when steady-state VPA concentrations of 20 to 30 µg/mL were achieved, mean PB elimination half-life was prolonged from 96 to 142 hours. In addition, mean PB clearance was reduced from 4.2 to 3.0 mL/hr/kg. The renal clearance of PB, urine pH levels, and PB volume of distribution did not change significantly.

MECHANISM
Metabolic studies in four patients co-administered PB and VPA found a decrease in the hepatic conversion of phenobarbital to hydroxyphenylphenobarbital and decreased the urinary hydroxyphenylphenobarbital : PB ratio (Bruni et al. 1980a). These data imply an inhibition of the hepatic microsomal enzymes, probably cytochrome P450 2C9 and 2C19. The VPA-mediated inhibition of PB hepatic metabo-

lism may be secondary to VPA's short-chain fatty acid structures; fatty acids have been shown to nonspecifically inhibit hepatic oxidative and/or conjugative metabolic processes (Lang 1976, Patel et al. 1980).

Phenytoin (See Phenytoin section in this chapter.)

Naproxen

EVIDENCE OF INTERACTION

A single study in healthy volunteers suggested that naproxen may displace valproic acid from its protein-binding sites (Grimaldi et al. 1984).

MECHANISM

Naproxen displaces valproic acid from its protein-binding sites.

CLINICAL IMPLICATIONS

This is probably not a clinically significant interaction, although if a patient had high serum levels of VPA, a temporary increase in unbound levels could lead to transient adverse effects.

Neuroleptics

The possible interactions of other neuroleptics with valproic acid are summarized in Table 5.1 (also see Chapter 3).

EVIDENCE OF INTERACTION

Ishizaka et al. (1984) administered VPA 400 mg/day to six schizophrenic patients, measured the minimum trough levels of VPA (C_{min}), and compared these values to the C_{min} of VPA after a single 400-mg dose of chlorpromazine was co-administered. The mean C_{min} of VPA, when co-administered with chlorpromazine (33.2 ± 1.7 µg/mL), was significantly greater (p <0.01) than when VPA was administered alone (27 ± 1.4 µg/mL). With discontinuation of the chlorpromazine (after a 2-week washout period), the mean VPA elimination half-life was shortened from 15.4 (± 1.4) to 13.5 (± 1.2) hours (p <0.05), with a corresponding increase in VPA clearance from 7.18 (± 0.38) to 8.32 (± 0.34) mL/hr per kg (p <0.01). Of note is that this study was nonblind and no placebo was used. The same investigators found that haloperidol (6 to 10 mg/day) had no significant effect on the C_{min}, half-life, or clearance of VPA.

MECHANISM

Chlorpromazine may competitively inhibit the metabolism of VPA. VPA and chlorpromazine share common metabolic pathways, whereas haloperidol is metabolized primarily via oxidative dealkylation.

CLINICAL IMPLICATIONS

VPA increases endogenous brain γ-aminobutyric acid (GABA) levels (Pinder et al. 1977) and may improve psychotic symptoms (Linnoila et al. 1980). Given the possible effectiveness in schizophrenia and mania, the potential exists for valproate and chlorpromazine to be used in combination. Chlorpromazine has been shown to increase the C_{min} and elimination half-life and to decrease the clearance of VPA, which may lead to VPA toxicity. Thus, the physician should monitor VPA serum concentrations closely and make VPA dosage adjustments as necessary.

Thiopental

EVIDENCE OF INTERACTION

An increase occurs in the unbound fraction of the anesthetic agent thiopental in rabbits also receiving valproate (Aguilera et al. 1986). In the absence of VPA, the unbound fraction of thiopental was 15.2% (±0.64%), but with the concentration of VPA above the therapeutic range, the unbound fraction of thiopental was increased to 22.42% (±1.65%). In addition, the recovery time from the hypnotic effects of thiopental was increased in the presence of VPA.

MECHANISM

It would appear from Aguilera's study that VPA, which is extensively protein bound, causes the protein displacement of thiopental, thus increasing the unbound fraction.

CLINICAL IMPLICATIONS

Because unbound thiopental is more accessible to the central nervous system (CNS), thus leading to prolonged hypnotic anesthetic effects, doses of thiopental in the anesthesia of epileptic or psychiatric patients taking VPA may require downward adjustments.

Topiramate (See Topiramate section in this chapter)

Zidovudine (AZT)

EVIDENCE OF INTERACTION

In vitro studies in human liver microsomes suggest that valproic acid may impair zidovudine metabolism (Rajaonarison et al. 1992). The co-administration of zidovudine and valproic acid increased plasma AUC for zidovudine by twofold (Lertora et al. 1994).

Akula et al. (1977) found that peak plasma AZT levels increased almost threefold from 11.9 ng/mL to 344 ng/mL with valproic acid (1.5 g/day). Cerebrospinal AZT levels, drawn 30 minutes after peak plasma levels, paralleled the change in peak plasma concentrations, increasing from 27 ng/mL for the control to 47 ng/mL with valproic acid.

MECHANISM

Valproic acid impairs glucuronidation of zidovudine.

CLINICAL IMPLICATIONS

It may be necessary to alter AZT dose when initiating, discontinuing, or modifying VPA dose.

Section 5.3   Phenytoin

Acetaminophen

EVIDENCE OF INTERACTION

Some evidence suggests that patients on a combination of antiepileptic agents have reduced acetaminophen bioavailability and half-life (Perucca and Richens 1971). Phenytoin was one of a number of anticonvulsants used in this study. The addition of acetaminophen in oral doses of 1.5 g/day to nine epileptic patients on phenytoin did not affect serum levels of the latter drug (Neuvonen et al. 1979, Minton et al. 1988).

MECHANISM

Phenytoin and some other anticonvulsants may increase hepatic microsomal metabolism or reduce the bioavailability of acetaminophen.

CLINICAL IMPLICATIONS

The clinical significance of this interaction is unknown. The potential exists for decreased effectiveness of acetaminophen in this population and perhaps increased toxicity from its metabolites in circumstances in which clinicians increase the dose or in overdose situations.

Acetazolamide

EVIDENCE OF INTERACTION

Case reports have suggested that acetazolamide may accelerate the osteomalacia secondary to anticonvulsants (Mallette 1975, 1977). When acetazolamide was stopped, hyperchloremic acidosis was reversed and urinary calcium excretion decreased.

MECHANISM

The mechanism is unknown. It is well recognized that anticonvulsants can induce osteomalacia. Acetazolamide may accelerate this process by increasing calcium and phosphate excretion and causing a systemic acidosis.

CLINICAL IMPLICATIONS

The evidence supporting the interaction is limited, but caution should be used when prescribing anticonvulsants with carbonic anhydrase inhibitors. Physicians should be aware that osteomalacia may be accelerated in some patients.

Allopurinol (Zyloprim)

Allopurinol may inhibit phenytoin metabolism and increase serum phenytoin levels, but data are limited (Yokochi et al. 1982).

Amiodarone

Phenytoin levels may increase with the co-administration of amiodarone, an antiarrhythmic agent (Gore et al. 1984, McGovern et al. 1984).

Antacids

EVIDENCE OF INTERACTION

One multiple-dose and three single-dose studies have examined the interaction of antacids and phenytoin, with conflicting results. Neither aluminum hydroxide 10 mL nor magnesium hydroxide 10 mL every 6 hours administered for 3 days prior to a 100-mg oral dose of phenytoin affected maximum serum concentration, time to maximum concentration, or apparent oral clearance of phenytoin in six subjects (O'Brien et al. 1978). The simultaneous administration of an oral dose of 300 mg of phenytoin and antacids (aluminum and magnesium hydroxide 30 mL, aluminum hydroxide/magnesium trisilicate 30 mL, and calcium gluconate 2 g crossover in two subjects) showed no effect of the antacids on apparent oral clearance (Chapron et al. 1979). On the other hand, when antacids were given with an oral 600-mg dose of phenytoin and for 6 additional doses following the anticonvulsant, apparent oral clearance was reduced 30.4% and 24.6% with aluminum and magnesium hydroxide 160 mEq, reduced 24.2% and 17.6% with calcium carbonate 160 mEq, but not changed with aluminum hydroxide/magnesium trisilicate, as compared with control periods (Garnett et al. 1981). In a multiple-dose study of 12 patients taking 300 to 350 mg of oral phenytoin daily, antacid was added for 7 days. The average serum phenytoin levels were reduced by approximately 12% with aluminum hydroxide/magnesium trisilicate 30 mL but unchanged with calcium carbonate 30 mL (Kulshrestha et al. 1978). Another report describes three patients taking phenytoin who had lower serum levels when phenytoin was given alone, rather than with antacids (type unreported) (Kutt 1975). When the antacid was given 2 to 3 hours after phenytoin, levels increased. Another clinical report suggests that seizure control was impaired when antacids were ingested with phenytoin (O'Brien et al. 1978).

MECHANISM

Several mechanisms have been proposed but none adequately explain the interaction. Decreased gastrointestinal pH levels, complexation by divalent cations, and antacid-induced diarrhea have been suggested by individual investigators but are not supported by the body of data.

CLINICAL IMPLICATIONS

The evidence available on the interaction is contradictory. The clinician should be aware that the commonly used antacids may decrease phenytoin bioavailability. Clinical reports suggest that the addition of an antacid to a phenytoin regimen can lower serum levels and impair seizure control. Separating administration by 3 hours, or the use of nizatidine, ranitidine, or famotidine, when appropriate, are reasonable alternatives.

Anticoagulants

EVIDENCE OF INTERACTION

In a study of six volunteers given dicumarol (dosed to give prothrombin values of 30%) after 1 week of phenytoin 300 mg/day orally, phenytoin levels increased by 126% over 7 days (Hansen et al. 1966). Radio-labeled intravenous phenytoin was given alone and again after 1 week of dicumarol therapy in two volunteers, and the elimination half-life of phenytoin was increased in both subjects (from 9 to 36 hours and 9.75 to 44 hours). Another study examined changes in dicumarol level at oral doses of 40 to 160 mg daily and the prothrombin–proconvertin percentage during concurrent phenytoin administration (300 mg/day orally for 1 week). A decreased anticoagulant effect was found, and dicumarol levels decreased from a mean 29 µg/mL after 5 days of phenytoin treatment and fell to 21 µg/mL 5 days after phenytoin had been discontinued (Hansen et al. 1971). Other studies

(Skovsted et al. 1976) and a case report (Frantzen et al. 1967) support these findings.

The half-life and steady-state serum concentrations of phenytoin do not appear to be affected by the co-administration of warfarin (Skovsted et al. 1976), although one case report describes a patient who had been maintained on oral phenytoin 300 mg daily for over a year in whom signs of phenytoin toxicity developed shortly after warfarin was started (Rothermich 1966). Another case report describes an increase in prothrombin time (from 21 to 32 seconds) when oral phenytoin 300 mg daily was added to warfarin (2.5 mg 5 days a week, 5 mg on the other 2 days) (Nappi 1979). Serum levels of phenytoin were increased by about 40%, with an increase in elimination half-life from 9.9 to 14 hours when phenprocoumon was given concurrently (Skovsted et al. 1976), but the anticoagulant does not appear to be affected by phenytoin. Phenytoin levels are unaffected by phenindione (Skovsted et al. 1976).

MECHANISM

The mechanisms are not fully understood. The hepatic metabolism of phenytoin is probably inhibited by some anticoagulants (dicumarol, phenprocoumon). Phenytoin may displace oral anticoagulants from plasma protein-binding sites, resulting in a transient increase in anticoagulant effect. Phenytoin is known to induce hepatic enzymes and may increase the clearance of dicumarol. Phenytoin itself may prolong prothrombin time (Solomon et al. 1972).

CLINICAL IMPLICATIONS

It would seem advisable to avoid the concurrent administration of dicumarol or phenprocoumon with phenytoin when possible. Warfarin may be preferable, although initial transient increases in anticoagulant effect may be observed when phenytoin is added to warfarin. Careful clinical and laboratory monitoring should permit appropriate dosage modification to adjust for the interaction.

Antihistamines

EVIDENCE OF INTERACTION

A single case report describes the development of toxic serum phenytoin levels (>60 μg/mL) when a patient was given phenytoin 300 mg/day orally and chlorpheniramine 12 mg/day orally (Pugh 1975).

MECHANISM

Unknown.

CLINICAL IMPLICATIONS

Evidence supporting the interaction is very limited. It may be useful to monitor carefully phenytoin serum levels and observe patients for toxicity when using this drug combination.

Antineoplastics

EVIDENCE OF INTERACTION

Intravenous chemotherapy with carmustine, methotrexate, and vinblastine reduced plasma phenytoin levels and increased partial seizures (Bollini et al. 1983). Similar reductions in phenytoin levels with loss of seizure control have been reported in patients receiving bleomycin and cisplatin (Fincham et al. 1979, Sylvester et al. 1984).

Case reports have been published demonstrating elevated phenytoin levels and signs and symptoms of toxicity with fluorouracil (Gilbar 2001, Rosemergy 2002).

MECHANISM

The decreased oral bioavailability of phenytoin by carmustine, methotrexate, vinblastine, bleomycin, and cisplatin is the presumed mechanism of interaction, although altered metabolism is also possible.

Fluorouracil induces cytochrome P450 2C9.

CLINICAL IMPLICATIONS

Phenytoin plasma levels should be monitored during chemotherapy.

Barbiturates

EVIDENCE OF INTERACTION

The interaction of barbiturates with phenytoin is not straightforward. In most instances, barbiturates induce the metabolism of phenytoin; however, it also has been reported that high doses of phenobarbital competitively inhibit the metabolism of phenytoin (Hansten 1974). Five children who were maintained on phenobarbital 5 mg/kg for 28 days were given a single dose of phenytoin 10 mg/kg both before starting and at the completion of drug treatment. Phenytoin levels were 50% lower after 28 days of phenobarbital (Buchanan and Allen 1971). In another study, 12 epileptic patients were given phenytoin (3.7 to 6.8 mg/kg per day) both with and without phenobarbital (1.4 mg/kg per day). During combined therapy, phenytoin levels were depressed; in some patients, serum levels dropped as much as 70%.

After discontinuation of the phenobarbital, phenytoin levels rose and, in some instances, led to toxicity (Morselli et al. 1971). Another study of 73 patients found that those receiving combined treatment had lower levels of both drugs than those patients who were taking either alone (Sotaniemi et al. 1970). In one case, phenytoin toxicity developed after phenobarbital was discontinued (Morselli et al. 1971). Although some studies have found no interaction (Booker et al. 1971, Kutt et al. 1969, Vapaatola and Lehtinen 1971), most carefully designed studies support the observation that chronic phenobarbital treatment enhances the metabolism of phenytoin, resulting in lower serum levels during combined treatment and increases in phenytoin levels when the phenobarbital is stopped.

MECHANISM

Chronic phenobarbital treatment induces the hepatic microsomal enzyme system, particularly 2C9 and 2C19, thus increasing the metabolism of phenytoin/hydantoins.

CLINICAL IMPLICATIONS

Patients receiving phenobarbital (or other barbiturates) with phenytoin should have frequent monitoring of serum levels. With prolonged treatment, the possibility exists that serum phenytoin levels will fall below the minimal therapeutic level, causing loss of seizure control. If the barbiturate is discontinued, phenytoin toxicity could result because the enzymes will no longer be induced.

Calcium Sulfate Excipient

EVIDENCE OF INTERACTION

Phenytoin intoxication occurred in 51 patients when capsules using calcium sulfate as an excipient were replaced by capsules using a lactose excipient (Tyrer et al. 1970). In three patients for whom serum levels were available before and after the change, a three- to fourfold increase occurred. In a later study, 13 patients received either phenytoin sodium capsules with lactose or calcium sulfate excipient and then crossed-over (Bochner et al. 1972). Mean serum phenytoin concentrations were 7.7 μg/mL with lactose and 1.7 μg/mL with calcium sulfate.

MECHANISM

It has been suggested that a lipid-insoluble complex of phenytoin—calcium sulfate forms that decreases bioavailability.

CLINICAL IMPLICATIONS

This interaction is primarily of historical interest in the United States, but should serve as a caution to clinicians when different brands of phenytoin are used. Excipients may influence the completeness of absorption.

Carbamazepine

EVIDENCE OF INTERACTION

When administered concurrently, carbamazepine and phenytoin may interact to produce lower steady-state plasma levels. When phenytoin was administered intravenously to five patients before and during treatment with carbamazepine 600 mg daily, the elimination half-life of the phenytoin decreased from 10.6 to 6.4 hours after at least 9 days of carbamazepine treatment (Hansen et al. 1971). In the same study, seven patients on phenytoin treatment received 600 mg of oral carbamazepine daily after steady-state phenytoin levels were achieved. In three of these patients, the phenytoin level decreased significantly following 4 to 14 days of carbamazepine, from 15 to 7, 18 to 12, and 16 to 10 µg/mL, respectively. After the carbamazepine was withdrawn, the phenytoin level returned to the original level in 10 days. In one subject, a transient rise was seen. In general, other reports support the finding that some, but not all, patients will have lower phenytoin levels on combination therapy (Cereghino et al. 1973, Hooper et al. 1974). Carbamazepine levels also have shown to be reduced by the concurrent administration of phenytoin (Cereghino et al. 1975, Christiansen et al. 1973, Rane et al. 1976).

MECHANISM

Both phenytoin and carbamazepine induce hepatic metabolism.

CLINICAL IMPLICATIONS

Although the evidence that plasma levels fall during concurrent therapy is substantial, no evidence suggests that seizure control is compromised with the lower levels. Careful clinical monitoring and the judicious use of serum drug monitoring is recommended when this drug combination is utilized.

Chloramphenicol

EVIDENCE OF INTERACTION

Chloramphenicol can increase phenytoin serum levels and lead to toxicity. Phenytoin 250 mg/day orally was administered to two patients for a 4-day period, after which chloramphenicol 2 g/day was also given (Christensen and Skovsted 1969). Both patients showed an increase in serum phenytoin levels, although the data are reported for only one of them. In that patient, serum phenytoin rose from 2 μg/mL prior to chloramphenicol to between 7 and 11 μg/mL. In three other patients, the elimination half-life of phenytoin was increased from 11.75 to 22.75, 16.25 to 38.5, and 9.75 to 25.75 hours, respectively, when given with chloramphenicol 2 g/day than when administered alone. A single intravenous dose of 3 g of chloramphenicol caused a change in the slope of the (β-phase that corresponded to a change in half-life from 10.5 to 22 hours. In another patient, a 1.5-g dose caused a change in half-life from 9 to 12.5 hours. A case report describes a patient with a third-ventricle tumor who was taking phenytoin 400 mg/day orally and was given chloramphenicol to treat meningitis (Ballek et al. 1973). Nystagmus on lateral gaze developed in the patient, and the serum phenytoin reached 24 μg/mL. When chloramphenicol was stopped, the serum phenytoin level dropped to 3 μg/mL on 300 mg daily. A patient with a cavernous hemangioma was being treated with cortisone 2 mg, thyroid extract 3 grains, and phenytoin 300 mg (Rose et al. 1977). Fever developed, and the patient was treated with chloramphenicol and other antibiotics. After the 7th day, all the antibiotics were discontinued. On the 18th day, fever returned, and chloramphenicol 1 g every 6 hours was started. The temperature returned to normal, but the patient became stuporous. The discontinuation of chloramphenicol led to improved mental status, but return of the fever. Reinstitution of the chloramphenicol once again led to the patient being unresponsive to pain, but it was discovered that the serum phenytoin level reached 54 μg/mL. In a review of the serum phenytoin levels during the hospitalization, it was observed that they increased each time chloramphenicol was added.

MECHANISM

Chloramphenicol possibly inhibits the hepatic phase II metabolism of phenytoin.

CLINICAL IMPLICATIONS

Although not a common drug combination, the interaction appears serious and well-documented. Patients who receive the drugs concurrently may be likely to have serious medical illnesses that could be difficult to differentiate from phenytoin toxicity, as was the case in the report of Rose et al. (1979). Phenytoin serum levels must be monitored if the two drugs are given concurrently.

Cimetidine

EVIDENCE OF INTERACTION
Several studies and case reports suggest that cimetidine may impair the metabolism of phenytoin, increasing serum levels of the anticonvulsant and occasionally leading to phenytoin toxicity (Bartle et al. 1983, Hetzel et al. 1981, Iteogu 1983, Neuvonen et al. 1980, Salem et al. 1983, Watts et al. 1983).

MECHANISM
Cimetidine inhibits the hepatic metabolism of phenytoin.

CLINICAL IMPLICATIONS
Cimetidine, in the usual therapeutic doses, impairs the metabolism of phenytoin and may lead to toxicity. The effect is rapid, beginning within the first 2 days after the addition of cimetidine. After the discontinuation of cimetidine, phenytoin levels will drop within 1 to 2 weeks. Because there appears to be some variability in the magnitude of the effect, frequent serum phenytoin monitoring is recommended. When possible, ranitidine, famotidine, or nizatidine should be used instead of cimetidine.

Ciprofloxacin

Many studies have shown that ciprofloxacin (and possibly quinolone antibiotics as a class) inhibits phenytoin metabolism, leading to increased serum concentrations and possible toxicity (Dillard et al. 1992, Hull 1993, Pollack 1997, Brouwers 1997, Mcleod and Trinkle 1998, Otero 1999).

The mechanism of the interaction is unknown.

Cyclosporine

Cyclosporine serum levels are reduced by concomitant phenytoin (Freeman et al. 1984). The mechanism is induction of cytochrome 3A4 by phenytoin.

Diazoxide

EVIDENCE OF INTERACTION
Low serum phenytoin levels, increased metabolite hydroxy-phenyphenylhydantoin (HPPH) formation, and reduced phenytoin half-life have been reported when diazoxide and phenytoin are administered concurrently (Petro et al. 1986, Roe et al. 1975).

MECHANISM

Diazoxide appears to induce the metabolism of phenytoin.

CLINICAL IMPLICATIONS

Serum phenytoin concentrations should be monitored frequently during concomitant therapy.

Digitalis Glycosides

EVIDENCE OF INTERACTION

Serum levels of digoxin and digitoxin are reduced in the presence of phenytoin (Solomon et al. 1971).

MECHANISM

Phenytoin is a hepatic enzyme inducer.

CLINICAL IMPLICATIONS

Serum levels of digitalis glycosides should be monitored frequently whenever phenytoin is added to digoxin or digitoxin, or when it is discontinued after combined therapy.

Disulfiram

EVIDENCE OF INTERACTION

Serum phenytoin levels increase with concurrent disulfiram administration (Kiorboe 1966, Olesen 1967). The effect is rapid, within several hours after disulfiram administration, and long lasting, up to 3 weeks following disulfiram discontinuation.

MECHANISM

Disulfiram inhibits phenytoin metabolism.

CLINICAL IMPLICATIONS

Phenytoin serum levels should be closely monitored when disulfiram is added or discontinued. Toxicity has resulted from the administration of disulfiram to patients taking phenytoin when appropriate dosage adjustments were not made.

Enteral Feeding Products

EVIDENCE OF INTERACTION

Twenty patients received a 1-mg loading dose of phenytoin followed by 7 days of 300 mg/day of phenytoin suspension either, alone or with

125 mL/hr of Isocal (Bauer 1982). After the first 7 days, patients were crossed over to the other cell. An almost fourfold increase occurred in phenytoin levels when phenytoin was given with Isocal. A case report describes a patient who was receiving phenytoin 400 mg twice daily via nasogastric tube with Osmolite, resulting in phenytoin serum levels between 2.9 and 4.5 μg/mL (Hatton 1984). Oral phenytoin was discontinued and an intravenous loading dose of 1,000 mg was given, followed by intravenous doses of 400 mg/day. Over the next month levels ranged from 10 to 20 μg/mL.

MECHANISM

The mechanism by which Isocal and Osmolite decrease phenytoin bioavailability is unknown.

CLINICAL IMPLICATIONS

During enteral feedings, phenytoin should be administered intravenously if possible. If oral doses must be used, the frequent monitoring of serum concentrations is recommended.

Ethanol

EVIDENCE OF INTERACTION

Abstinent alcoholics metabolize phenytoin more rapidly than nonalcoholics. In a study of 15 alcoholics and 76 control subjects, the mean serum phenytoin level in alcoholics 24 hours after the last dose was half that of control subjects. Mean elimination half-life was 16.3 hours in alcoholics versus 23.5 hours in controls (Kater et al. 1969). The acute ingestion of alcohol in normal volunteers did not affect phenytoin metabolism according to one report (Schmidt 1980).

MECHANISM

Chronic ethanol ingestion induces the liver microsomal enzyme system, thus increasing phenytoin clearance. Acute alcohol ingestion usually impairs this system, making it difficult to explain the negative findings of Schmidt (1980).

CLINICAL IMPLICATIONS

Phenytoin is commonly used for alcoholic patients with a preexisting seizure disorder who require ethanol detoxification. Clinicians should anticipate the need for higher doses in this population.

Fluconazole (Diflucan)/Azole Antifungals

Fluconazole inhibits phenytoin metabolism and may lead to toxicity (Blum et al. 1991, Howitt et al. 1989). The mechanism is inhibition of cytochrome 2C9 by azole antifungals.

Folic Acid

EVIDENCE OF INTERACTION

For many patients, phenytoin treatment leads to folic acid deficiency (Mattson et al. 1973, Norris and Pratt 1974, Reynolds 1973, Wells 1968). The clinical manifestations of folate deficiency include psychiatric disturbances, neuropathy, and megaloblastic anemia. Some workers have suggested that phenytoin-induced folate deficiency may lead to congenital malformations (Janz 1975, Speidel and Meadow 1974). Replacement of folate may be associated with decreased serum phenytoin, which may lead to lack of seizure control (Baylis et al. 1971, Maxwell et al. 1972, Norris and Pratt 1971, Reynolds 1967, Strauss and Bernstein 1974). Although most patients have relatively small decreases in phenytoin levels and remain in the therapeutic range (Baylis et al. 1971, Furlanat et al. 1978, Jensen et al. 1971), reductions of 15% to 25% have been reported.

MECHANISM

Folate may increase phenytoin metabolism or reduce its bioavailability. Phenytoin may reduce folate absorption or increase folate utilization as a coenzyme for drug metabolism. Some have suggested that the transport of folate from the serum to the CNS is impaired by phenytoin. Folic acid, when given alone, may induce seizures in animals (Hommes and Obbens 1972) and may directly antagonize the action of phenytoin.

CLINICAL IMPLICATIONS

Phenytoin can reduce folate levels, and the addition of folic acid therapy can reduce serum levels of the anticonvulsant. Occasionally, this reduction may lead to impaired seizure control. Serum folate and phenytoin levels should be monitored and patients observed closely for increased seizure activity.

Furosemide

EVIDENCE OF INTERACTION

Epileptic patients on a variety of anticonvulsants had a slowed onset and a decreased intensity of diuretic effect from furosemide (Ahmad

1974). A study of five healthy volunteers found that treatment with phenytoin 300 mg daily for 10 days reduced furosemide oral bioavailability by 50% (Fine et al. 1977).

MECHANISM

Phenytoin impairs the systemic bioavailability of furosemide, probably by reducing gut absorption, although the mechanism is not fully understood. The diuretic response is inhibited, even after intravenous administration, suggesting other mechanisms are also involved.

CLINICAL IMPLICATIONS

Larger doses of furosemide may be required when phenytoin is administered concurrently.

Glucagon

EVIDENCE OF INTERACTION

Patients taking phenytoin may have false-negative glucagon stimulation tests (Kumer et al. 1974). A 44-year-old epileptic man taking phenytoin had the diagnosis of an islet-cell adenoma obscured because no elevation of insulin was observed until phenytoin was discontinued. This observation suggests that phenytoin has the ability to inhibit insulin release (Knopp et al. 1972).

MECHANISM

Phenytoin blocks insulin release from the pancreas.

CLINICAL IMPLICATIONS

Patients treated with phenytoin may have false-negative glucagon stimulation tests.

Halothane and Fluroxene (Halogenated Anesthetic Agents)

EVIDENCE OF INTERACTION

Case reports suggest that phenytoin may interact with halogenated anesthetic agents to increase the hepatotoxicity of these agents; this toxicity may in turn cause increased phenytoin levels (Karlin and Kutt 1970, Reynolds et al. 1972). The first case involved a 10-year-old child who had been treated with phenytoin 10 mg/kg per day orally without adverse effects other than gingival hyperplasia and nystagmus. Following anesthesia for 90 minutes, body temperature was elevated for 3 days, as was serum glutamic oxaloacetic transaminase (120 units/mL, normal 8 to 33 units/mL). Serum glutamic pyruvic transaminase level was normal. Intramuscular phenytoin was continued after surgery, and the serum phenytoin levels increased to 41 µg/mL. Clinical signs of nystagmus and poor muscle tone and symptoms of lethargy and blurred vision were consistent with phenytoin toxicity. Histologic examination confirmed hepatic necrosis. In the second case, a woman who had been taking phenytoin and phenobarbital died from massive necrosis after fluroxene anesthesia, and the authors speculated that phenytoin led to increased hepatotoxicity.

MECHANISM

Halothane and fluroxene may cause hepatotoxicity, which may impair phenytoin metabolism. No good evidence suggests that phenytoin increases the likelihood of hepatotoxicity with halogenated anesthetic agents, although it is possible that phenytoin enhances the metabolism of the anesthetic to a hepatotoxic metabolite.

CLINICAL IMPLICATIONS

The documentation of this interaction is limited, but common sense dictates that caution should be used when halothane or any hepatotoxic drug is administered with phenytoin.

Isoniazid

EVIDENCE OF INTERACTION

The first indication that phenytoin toxicity could develop with the concurrent administration of isoniazid was when the addition of the latter drug to phenytoin and phenobarbital resulted in the onset of drowsiness, ataxia, and incoordination in about 10% of 637 epileptic patients (Murray 1962). In a later study, 6 of 32 patients who were all classified as slow metabolizers of isoniazid showed higher mean serum levels of phenytoin; the typical signs and symptoms of toxicity developed when phenytoin levels increased to above 20 µg/mL (Brennan et al. 1970). In another study, in 6 of 36 patients phenytoin toxicity developed when they received the combination (Kutt et al. 1970). The addition of aminosalicylic acid to the phenytoin–isoniazid combination may increase the risk of phenytoin toxicity (Kutt 1975).

MECHANISM

Isoniazid impairs the parahydroxylation of phenytoin via inhibition of cytochrome P450 2C9. Because this is a dose-related phenomenon, those patients who are the slowest metabolizers of isoniazid are at highest risk.

CLINICAL IMPLICATIONS

About half the population are slow metabolizers of isoniazid. Phenytoin toxicity will develop in approximately 10% to 25% of patients taking the phenytoin–isoniazid combination. Those on other antitubercular drugs as well, such as aminosalicylic acid and cycloserine, which inhibit phenytoin metabolism to a lesser degree, may have increased chances of toxicity, although this is controversial. When patients are receiving phenytoin and isoniazid concurrently, frequent serum phenytoin levels and careful observation for signs and symptoms of phenytoin intoxication are necessary. Dosage adjustments must be made when isoniazid is started or discontinued.

Levodopa

EVIDENCE OF INTERACTION

In one study, phenytoin was successful in the treatment of levodopa-induced dyskinesia but reversed the effect of levodopa on the symptoms of Parkinson disease (Mendez et al. 1975).

MECHANISM

Unknown.

CLINICAL IMPLICATIONS

Limited data are available on this interaction. It would appear wise to avoid the combination if possible, or increase the dose of levodopa when administered with phenytoin.

Lidocaine

EVIDENCE OF INTERACTION

The combination of lidocaine and phenytoin is associated with enhanced toxicity, including a case of sinoatrial arrest that was reversed by isoproterenol (Wood 1971). The incidence of less serious side effects (diplopia, nystagmus, nausea, vertigo, hearing disturbance) is also increased (Karlsson et al. 1974).

MECHANISM

Drug clearance is not altered to a significant degree during combined therapy. There would appear to be a pharmacodynamic interaction due to enhanced depressant effect on cardiac function.

CLINICAL IMPLICATIONS

When clinicians use this drug combination, they should be aware of the possibility of toxicity.

Methadone

EVIDENCE OF INTERACTION

The addition of phenytoin to methadone maintenance therapy may induce withdrawal symptoms (Finelli 1976, Tong 1981).

MECHANISM

Phenytoin induces the hepatic metabolism of methadone via cytochrome P450 3A4.

CLINICAL IMPLICATIONS

Enzyme-inducing agents should be avoided in methadone patients. Alternatively, plasma levels of methadone should be followed and appropriate dosage adjustments made.

Methylphenidate

EVIDENCE OF INTERACTION

Anecdotal reports have suggested that phenytoin toxicity may develop in children who are treated concurrently with phenytoin and methylphenidate (Garrettson et al. 1969), but clinical studies have failed to establish this interaction. A 5-year-old child receiving phenytoin 8.9 mg/kg and primidone 17.7 mg/kg had methylphenidate added to his regimen. Phenytoin levels increased from 8 to 35 μg/mL. Primidone levels increased from 4 to 21 μg/mL, and its metabolite phenobarbital increased from 23 to 39 μg/mL. Two other children in the same report did not show elevations of anticonvulsants when methylphenidate was added. One clinical report cites the experience of more than 100 patients taking the combination without adverse consequences (Oettinger 1976). Another report describes an increase in phenytoin concentration during one period of combined administration but not in another (Mirkin and Wright 1971). In two studies, interaction was noted in 14 patients (Kupferberg et al. 1972, Mirkin and Wright 1971).

MECHANISM

In vitro studies indicate that methylphenidate generally is a competitive inhibitor of the hepatic metabolism of phenytoin and other drugs (Hunninghake 1970, Perel and Black 1970). The variability of this effect is substantial.

CLINICAL IMPLICATIONS

In isolated cases, methylphenidate has been associated with phenytoin toxicity; however, clinical experience and studies suggest the combination usually does not present problems.

Phenylbutazone

Phenylbutazone and oxyphenbutazone (its major metabolite) impair phenytoin clearance and may lead to phenytoin toxicity (Andreasen et al. 1973, Lunde 1970, Neuvonen et al. 1979, Shoeman et al. 1975).

Dosage reduction of phenytoin may be required during concurrent therapy.

Pyridoxine

Large doses of pyridoxine 200 mg/day for 4 weeks may enhance phenytoin metabolism and lower serum levels (Hansson et al. 1976).

With small doses of pyridoxine, as are found in multivitamin preparations, no special precautions appear necessary. With larger doses, such as daily doses of 200 mg or greater, the monitoring of serum phenytoin levels may be necessary.

Quinidine

EVIDENCE OF INTERACTION

The metabolism of quinidine is enhanced when given with phenytoin (Data et al. 1976, Jaillon and Kates 1980, Farringer et al. 1985).

MECHANISM

The induction of cytochrome P450 3A4 by phenytoin is likely.

CLINICAL IMPLICATIONS

Quinidine levels should be monitored whenever an enzyme-inducing agent such as phenytoin is added or withdrawn from the medication regimen.

Salicylates

Salicylates displace phenytoin from plasma protein-binding sites, which could in theory lead to toxicity (Ehrnebo et al. 1977, Fraser et al. 1980, Leonard et al. 1981, Paxton 1980).

The clinical importance of this interaction is not documented. Plasma protein-binding interactions usually cause only temporary alterations in free (unbound) drug, so that although total phenytoin concentration may decrease in patients taking high doses of aspirin, the free concentration remains relatively constant. Patients at higher therapeutic levels could experience transient toxicity.

Steroids, Corticosteroids

EVIDENCE OF INTERACTION

Phenytoin has been shown to increase the clearance and reduce the elimination half-life of several corticosteroids, including hydrocortisone (Choi et al. 1971), methylprednisolone (Stjernholm and Katz 1975), prednisone (Meikle et al. 1975), prednisolone (Petereit et al. 1977, Wassmer et al. 1976, Frey et al. 1984), dexamethasone (Brooks et al. 1972, Haque et al. 1972, Chalk et al. 1984), fludrocortisone (Keilholz et al. 1986), and metyrapone (Meikle et al. 1969). Several reports in the literature document the clinical importance of the interaction. The results of the dexamethasone and metyrapone tests are difficult to interpret in the presence of phenytoin and may yield false-positive results (Jubiz et al. 1970, Meikle et al. 1969, Werk et al. 1967, 1969). Renal transplant and graft patients taking phenytoin may have a greater rejection rate, presumably due to enhanced clearance of the corticosteroids used as immunosuppressives (Wassner et al. 1976). The effectiveness of dexamethasone in the treatment of cerebral edema also may be reduced in the presence of phenytoin (McClelland and Jack 1978).

MECHANISM

Phenytoin induces the hepatic metabolism of corticosteroids via cytochrome P450 3A4 hydroxylation.

CLINICAL IMPLICATIONS

The clinical effectiveness of steroids is reduced when they are given in combination with phenytoin. In these cases, the clinician can increase the steroid dose or replace phenytoin with another anticonvulsant that does not induce hepatic metabolism. Some have also suggested that hydrocortisone is affected to a lesser extent than other steroids. This has led to the suggestion that hydrocortisone replace dexamethasone in the suppression test for those patients taking phenytoin (Meikle et al. 1969).

Sucralfate

Sucralfate may reduce phenytoin absorption (Hall et al. 1986, Smart et al. 1985).

Sulfonamides

EVIDENCE OF INTERACTION

Phenytoin elimination half-life increased from a mean 11.3 to 20.5 hours following sulfamethizole therapy (4 g/day taken orally) (Lumholtz et al. 1975, Siersbaek-Nielsen et al. 1973). Sulfaphenazole may also inhibit phenytoin metabolism, but sulfisoxazole, sulfadimethoxine, and sulfamethoxypyridazine do not.

MECHANISM

Some sulfonamides inhibit the hepatic metabolism of phenytoin via cytochrome P450 2C9.

CLINICAL IMPLICATIONS

Serum phenytoin monitoring and reduced dosage may be required in the presence of some sulfonamides (Hansen et al. 1966, 1975, 1979, Lumholtz et al. 1975, Siersbaek-Nielsen et al. 1973).

Sulthiame

EVIDENCE OF INTERACTION

Several studies have documented an increase in plasma phenytoin when sulthiame is co-administered, and toxicity may develop (Frantzen 1967, Hansen et al. 1968, Houghton 1974, Houghton and Richens 1974, 1975, Olesen et al. 1969, Richens et al. 1973).

MECHANISM

Sulthiame inhibits hepatic metabolism of phenytoin.

CLINICAL IMPLICATIONS

Clinicians should be aware that the addition of sulthiame to phenytoin can raise serum levels of the latter drug by 75%. Sulthiame is an anticonvulsant that is not marketed in the United States.

Tetracyclines

EVIDENCE OF INTERACTION

The elimination half-life of doxycycline was approximately 50% shorter in patients taking phenytoin than in control subjects (7.1 vs. 15.1 hours) (Alestig 1974, Penttila et al. 1974, Neuvonen et al. 1974, 1975, 1979). Chlortetracycline, demeclocycline, methacycline, oxytetracycline are not affected by phenytoin.

MECHANISM

Phenytoin enhances the phase II conjugation metabolism of doxycycline.

CLINICAL IMPLICATIONS

Phenytoin may lower doxycycline levels below minimum therapeutic concentrations. Alternative antibiotics or appropriate dosage adjustments should be made.

Theophylline

EVIDENCE OF INTERACTION

Theophylline clearance is higher, and elimination half-life and clinical effect are reduced, through concomitant phenytoin administration (Marquis et al. 1982, Taylor et al. 1980).

MECHANISM

Phenytoin stimulates the hepatic metabolism of theophylline via an unknown mechanism.

CLINICAL IMPLICATIONS

Theophylline dosage adjustment and plasma-level monitoring may be necessary when phenytoin is added to or withdrawn from treatment (Marquis et al. 1982, Taylor et al. 1980).

Thyroid Hormones

EVIDENCE OF INTERACTION

Phenytoin may increase the metabolism of thyroid hormone, requiring changes in the dosage of replacement therapy (Blackshear et al. 1983). One case report of a patient with hypothyroidism who was treated with replacement therapy cites the occurrence of supraventricular tachycardia when phenytoin was administered intravenously for atrial flutter (Fulop et al. 1966).

MECHANISM

Phenytoin enhances the metabolism of thyroid hormones via an unknown mechanism.

CLINICAL IMPLICATIONS

Phenytoin administration may alter required dosage of thyroid replacement hormone.

Valproate

EVIDENCE OF INTERACTION

Clinical studies suggest that phenytoin may in some, but not all cases, increase the metabolism of valproate when the two drugs are given in combination. In addition, phenytoin levels may transiently decrease when valproate is added, although the literature is contradictory. Four adult patients with intractable seizures were stabilized on phenytoin (between 4.1 and 5.5 mg/kg per day); one patient was also taking phenobarbital 90 to 120 mg/day (Bruni et al. 1980a). The patients were then given valproate, in doses determined by their clinicians (plasma concentrations ranged from 36.8 to 56.2 µg/mL, dosages not reported) and were observed for 22 to 32 weeks. Within 2 weeks of starting the valproate, the patients had total phenytoin plasma concentrations that decreased transiently and returned to baseline in three of the four patients by about 5 weeks. In all four patients, the percentage of unbound phenytoin increased 2 weeks after valproate was started. It remained elevated in three patients over a 22-week follow-up period. Urinary concentration of the metabolite of phenytoin, HPPH, increased during weeks 2 to 5, but decreased over 5 to 22 weeks. Elimination half-life was not significantly reduced during 2 to 5 weeks and significantly increased during weeks 5 to 22. This study confirmed an earlier animal study and in vitro study of human plasma, which suggested that valproate displaced phenytoin from its protein-binding sites (Patsalos et al. 1977). This is of dubious clinical importance because the excess phenytoin is metabolized (as indicated by increased HPPH). Although total plasma phenytoin may decrease, seizure control generally is not jeopardized. In another study, 23 patients with uncontrolled seizures of a generalized or partial type were given an open clinical trial of valproate in addition to phenytoin (Mattson et al. 1978). During the initiation of valproate, a decline occurred in total serum phenytoin concentration (16.5 to 10.2 µg/mL), whereas the percentage of free phenytoin increased (10.9 to 20%). In another study of the interactions of valproate and other anticonvulsant drugs, 10 of 15 patients had a decrease in phenytoin concentrations during valproate therapy (Wilder et al. 1978). Decreases ranged from slight to greater than 50% in those patients. In a 1-year follow-up of eight patients, the phenytoin levels were similar to the prevalproate levels in seven, suggesting that any effect is merely temporary (Bruni et al. 1980b). A study of five children reported that after the addition of valproate to phenytoin, an increase occurred in the serum levels of the latter drug for the first few days, followed by a return to prevalproate levels or lower (Windorfer et al.

1975). Another study found that the administration of a single 800-mg valproate dose to patients who had been taking phenytoin for 3 months resulted in both a decrease in total serum phenytoin concentration and percentage of protein found (Monks et al. 1980). Phenytoin also may induce the metabolism of valproate. In a study of seven patients taking valproate alone (mean dose 14.8 mg/kg) and 12 patients taking the combination, the serum concentration of valproate was lower in the combined group than in the former group (205 versus 333 μmol/L, Reunanen et al. 1980).

A case report also documents a 31-year-old man taking valproate in whom delirium and increased seizure frequency developed after phenytoin (1.0 g oral loading dose followed by maintenance) was added (Hansten 1982).

MECHANISM

Phenytoin enhances the metabolism of valproate via cytochrome P450 2C9 and 2C19, whereas the latter drug may displace phenytoin from its protein-binding sites.

CLINICAL IMPLICATIONS

In most cases, this is not a clinically significant interaction. Theoretically, the displacement of phenytoin from its binding sites could lead to toxicity if a patient has a particularly high level to begin with. When valproate is added to phenytoin, it is possible that a transient increase may occur in the unbound phenytoin level, with a temporary decrease in total plasma phenytoin level for a few weeks, and a return to prevalproate levels in about 5 weeks. Caution is especially required for patients with hypoalbuminemia and antiepileptic drug polypharmacy (Mamiya 2002). Reports of the interaction affecting seizure control are not common; however, the clinician should monitor such patients carefully.

Section 5.4　Gabapentin

β-Blockers

EVIDENCE OF INTERACTION

Palomeras (2000) reported that a 68-year-old man with a 10-year history of essential tremor experienced paroxysmal dystonic movements during the co-administration of gabapentin and propranolol. The administration of propranolol 120 mg/day was mildly successful in relieving the patient's essential tremor. The tremors worsened when propranolol was replaced by gabapentin 900 mg/day. Seven months later, propranolol 80 mg/day was restarted. After 48 hours of combined therapy, the patient developed paroxysmal dystonic movements in both hands and experienced several episodes of dystonia daily. Almost 3 weeks later, the propranolol dose was reduced to 40 mg/day, and the dystonia immediately subsided. The patient was successfully maintained on gabapentin 900 mg/day and propranolol 40 mg/day.

MECHANISM
Unknown.

CLINICAL IMPLICATIONS
Patients must be monitored closely for signs of gabapentin toxicity, such as movement disorders, when β-blockers are co-administered. Doses should be adjusted as necessary.

Felbamate

EVIDENCE OF INTERACTION
Hussein et al. (1996) found that, in 11 patients who were treated with both felbamate and gabapentin, a 37% reduction occurred in felbamate clearance and a 46% prolongation occurred in the half-life.

MECHANISM
Both drugs may compete for renal excretion transporters.

CLINICAL IMPLICATIONS
Consider decreasing felbamate dose and monitor for adverse effects of felbamate during concomitant administration with gabapentin.

Phenytoin and Hydantoins

EVIDENCE OF INTERACTION
Tyndel (1994) reported increased serum phenytoin concentrations in a 31-year-old man following the addition of gabapentin to his long-standing antiepileptic regimen consisting of phenytoin 300 mg/day, carbamazepine 1,400 mg/day, and clobazam (not available in the United States) 20 mg/day. Gabapentin was added at 300 mg/day, and increased to 600 mg/day after 1 week. Because the patient complained of dizziness and imbalance, gabapentin was discontinued halfway through the second week. Nevertheless, symptoms worsened to include dysarthria, horizontal jerk nystagmus, and ataxia. The serum phenytoin concentration 1.5 weeks after stopping gabapentin

was 177 mmol/L, up from 42 mmol/L (therapeutic range, 40 to 80 mmol/L = 10 to 20 mg/mL). After stopping phenytoin for 1.5 weeks, the serum concentration decreased to 68 mmol/L, but when phenytoin and gabapentin were added back to the regimen, the serum phenytoin concentration increased to 136 mmol/L after 1 week. When gabapentin was then discontinued, the phenytoin concentration fell again (Tyndel 1994).

Another group found a dose–response relationship. Gabapentin 900 mg/day resulted in a 25% increase in the serum phenytoin concentration. However, no change in serum phenytoin concentrations were found with daily doses of 300 or 600 mg (Crawford 1987).

MECHANISM
Unknown.

CLINICAL IMPLICATIONS
When phenytoin and gabapentin are co-administered, the physician must carefully monitor serum phenytoin concentrations and watch for signs of toxicity. Adjust doses accordingly.

Section 5.5   Lamotrigine

Acetaminophen

EVIDENCE OF INTERACTION
Depot et al. (1990) studied the effect of multiple oral doses of acetaminophen totaling 2,700 mg daily, on a single 150-mg oral dose of lamotrigine in healthy volunteers. Acetaminophen administration decreased the AUC time curve of lamotrigine from 229 to 191.2 mg/hr per mL and the half-life from 35.7 to 30.2 hr (p = 0.01). Also, the percentage of lamotrigine β-glucuronidase hydrolyzable conjugate recovered in the urine was significantly higher (72.5% versus 65.9%), relative to that measured in subjects receiving acetaminophen (p = 0.05).

MECHANISM
Unknown.

CLINICAL IMPLICATIONS
Physicians should closely monitor the clinical response in patients receiving lamotrigine when they are taking multiple doses of acetaminophen on a standing daily basis. Adjust lamotrigine dosage as necessary.

Carbamazepine (*See* Carbamazepine section in this chapter)

Oral Contraceptives

EVIDENCE OF INTERACTION

Sabers et al. published two Danish studies, involving almost 30 women, which demonstrated lamotrigine plasma concentrations decreased by more than 50% during co-medication with oral contraceptives consisting of ethinyl estradiol plus desogestrel, ethinyl estradiol plus norethindrone, and norethindrone alone. Most patients either experienced increased seizure frequency or recurrence of seizures after oral contraceptives (OCs) had been added, or symptoms of LTG toxicity following the withdrawal of OCs (Sabers 2001, 2003).

MECHANISM

Oral contraceptives induce phase II glucuronidation of lamotrigine, its main metabolic pathway.

CLINICAL IMPLICATIONS

Physicians should carefully monitor clinical response and obtain more frequent serum lamotrigine levels when initiating, discontinuing, or modifying the dose of OCs in patients receiving lamotrigine. Watch for signs of lamotrigine toxicity (e.g., nausea, diplopia, and dizziness), especially when discontinuing OC. Adjust lamotrigine dosage as necessary.

Oxcarbazepine

EVIDENCE OF INTERACTION

A retrospective study (May et al. 1999) investigated the effects of oxcarbazepine (OCBZ), carbamazepine (CBZ), and methsuximide (MSM) on lamotrigine (LTG) serum levels in 222 patients with or without valproic acid (VPA) co-medication (May et al. 1999). MSM reduced the plasma levels of LTG by 70%; CBZ reduced LTG levels by 54%; OCBZ reduced LTG levels by 29%. VPA alone increased LTG levels (211%), but when given in combination with other anticonvulsants, this effect was reduced. LTG increases were 8% with VPA/MSM, 21% with VPA/CBZ, and 111% with OCBZ.

MECHANISM

CBZ is a more potent enzyme inhibitor than OCBZ.

CLINICAL IMPLICATIONS

Carefully monitor clinical response when initiating, discontinuing, or modifying the dose of lamotrigine in patients receiving both carbamazepine and lamotrigine. Adjust dosages as necessary. In patients receiving lamotrigine, if oxcarbazepine is substituted for carbamazepine, lamotrigine plasma concentrations may increase.

Rifamycins (Rifabutin, Rifampicin, Rifapentine)

EVIDENCE OF INTERACTION

Ebert et al. administered a single oral dose of 25 mg lamotrigine to ten healthy male subjects after a 5-day pretreatment with (1) cimetidine 800 mg divided into two equal doses, (2) rifampicin 600 mg, or (3) placebo. Serum and urine samples were analyzed using high-performance liquid chromatography. Changes in electroencephalographic (EEG) power were determined up to 48 h after lamotrigine administration as a pharmacodynamic assessment of drug action. Rifampicin significantly increased LTG clearance over bioavailability (CL/F) and the amount of lamotrigine excreted as glucuronide, whereas both half-life and AUC were decreased (p <0.05). Cimetidine failed to affect pharmacokinetics of lamotrigine. Lamotrigine EEG power did not change. (Ebert 2000)

MECHANISM

Rifamycins induce the phase II glucuronidation of lamotrigine.

CLINICAL IMPLICATIONS

Carefully monitor clinical response when initiating, discontinuing, or modifying the dose of rifamycins in patients receiving both rifamycins and lamotrigine. Monitor serum lamotrigine levels more frequently and adjust lamotrigine dosage as necessary.

Succinimides (Ethosuximide, Methsuximide, Phensuximide)

EVIDENCE OF INTERACTION

Analyzing 376 samples from 222 patients receiving both methsuximide (MSM) and LTG, May et al. (1999) found that methsuximide decreased LTG concentrations markedly (about 70% compared to LTG monotherapy).

Besag et al. (2004) conducted a study including 16 patients receiving both MSM and LTG and found that MSM lowered the LTG serum concentration in every patient, with a mean decrease of 53%. In some patients, this led to a deterioration in seizure control when MSM was added or an improvement in seizure control after MSM was stopped.

MECHANISM
LTG metabolism is induced by succinimides.

CLINICAL IMPLICATIONS
Carefully monitor clinical response when initiating, discontinuing, or modifying the dose of succinimides in patients receiving lamotrigine. Obtain more frequent serum lamotrigine levels and adjust dosages as necessary.

Section 5.6   Oxcarbazepine *See also* Carbamazepine

Cyclosporine

EVIDENCE OF INTERACTION
The influence of oxcarbazepine on cyclosporine trough concentrations was studied in a 32-year-old male renal transplant recipient with drug-resistant epilepsy. His initial drug regimen included valproate, gabapentin, cyclosporine (270 mg/day), prednisone, doxepin, allopurinol, levothyroxine, and pravastatin. The investigators preemptively added mycophenolate mofetil to maintain immunosuppression in the event the trough concentration of cyclosporine fell precipitously. Fourteen days after starting oxcarbazepine, the patient's cyclosporine trough levels decreased to below the lower limit of the therapeutic range (100 ng/L). Cyclosporine trough concentrations remained stable following an increase of the dose of cyclosporine to 290 mg/day and an oxcarbazepine dose reduction from 750 to 600 mg/day (Rösche 2001).

MECHANISM
The induction of cytochrome P450 3A4 by oxcarbazepine.

CLINICAL IMPLICATIONS
The physician should monitor clinical response and closely follow the cyclosporine trough concentrations of patients receiving oxcarbazepine. This especially should be done during periods of increasing or discontinuing oxcarbazepine. Adjust cyclosporine dose as necessary.

Felodipine

EVIDENCE OF INTERACTION

In seven healthy male volunteers receiving the calcium channel blocker felodipine 10 mg/day, the co-administration of 600 mg oxcarbazepine did not affect the steady-state pharmacokinetics of felodipine or its pyridine metabolite. However, when subjects received oxcarbazepine 450 mg twice daily, the felodipine AUC fell 28%, and the peak concentration dropped 34% from 9.7 to 6.4 nmol/L. It should be noted that plasma felodipine concentrations consistently remained within the therapeutic range during this study (Zaccara 1993).

The reduction in felodipine AUC with simultaneous usage of carbamazepine is 94%.

MECHANISM

It is likely that enzyme inhibition results from oxcarbazepine, although the effect is less than with carbamazepine.

CLINICAL IMPLICATIONS

The physician should closely monitor the clinical response in patients receiving felodipine when increasing or discontinuing their oxcarbazepine. Vary the dose of felodipine as necessary. The effect of oxcarbazepine is less than that seen with carbamazepine. When switching between these anticonvulsant agents, appropriate dose adjustments should be made.

Lamotrigine (*See* Lamotrigine section in this chapter)

Oral Contraceptives

EVIDENCE OF INTERACTION

In a study of the effects of oxcarbazepine on the pharmacokinetics of an oral contraceptive containing ethinyl estradiol and levonorgestrel, 10 healthy women on the contraceptive for 3 months received oxcarbazepine 300 mg on day 16 of the first study cycle, 300 mg twice daily on day 17, and 300 mg 3 times daily from day 18 of the first cycle to day 18 of the next menstrual cycle. The administration of both contraceptive and oxcarbazepine decreased the AUCs of both ethinyl estradiol 48% and levonorgestrel 32%. The incidence of breakthrough bleeding was 15%, compared with an expected rate of 0.48% with the OC alone (Klosterskov Jensen et al. 1992).

These findings were replicated in a study involving 16 women over two menstrual cycles receiving both oxcarbazepine and an OC (Fattore et al. 1999).

MECHANISM

Oxcarbazepine causes the induction of cytochrome P450 3A4, a major hepatic metabolic pathway for many OCs.

CLINICAL IMPLICATIONS

The physician should advise patients receiving oxcarbazepine of the possible decreased efficacy of OCs and suggest alternative or additional methods of contraception, such as barrier and spermicidal preparations.

Section 5.7   Primidone
Acetazolamide

EVIDENCE OF INTERACTION

Syversen et al. (1976) studied the effects of acetazolamide on primidone plasma levels in three epileptic patients. They co-administered acetazolamide 250 mg 12 hours before and concurrently with the primidone dose 500 mg. Serum and urine levels of primidone were measured under both conditions. Each patient participated in two studies, with a time interval of 2 to 17 days between studies. In one patient, primidone was not detected in the plasma when given with acetazolamide. In another patient, the peak serum primidone concentration was delayed, with corresponding delays in the urinary excretion of primidone and metabolites (phenylethylmalonamide and phenobarbital). The third patient had a higher peak concentration in the primidone-alone experiment, but had no difference in the urinary excretion of drug or metabolites.

MECHANISM

The investigators suggest that acetazolamide interferes with primidone absorption.

CLINICAL IMPLICATIONS

After the addition of acetazolamide to a medication regimen containing primidone, serum primidone levels should be checked and appropriate dosage changes made.

Phenytoin

EVIDENCE OF INTERACTION

Fincham et al. (1974) studied the effect of phenytoin on the phenobarbital (a primidone metabolite) : primidone ratio in epileptic patients.

Fifteen patients taking primidone alone had a low ratio (1.05 ± 0.2). The ratio in 44 patients taking both phenytoin and primidone was notably higher (4.35 ± 0.5). Another case study supports these findings. Porro et al. (1982) reported a case in which an interaction was found between primidone and phenytoin in an epileptic patient treated with the combination for 3 months. The addition of phenytoin (level 20.7 μg/mL ± 0.5) to the medication regimen increased steady-state levels of primidone metabolites phenobarbital and phenylethylmalonamide (pema). Serum levels of primidone decreased (9.5 μg/mL (±0.08) to 7.8 μg/mL (±0.9) as did serum levels of p-hydroxyphenobarbital, a metabolite of phenobarbital. The urinary excretion of primidone and its metabolites paralleled the changes observed in their plasma levels after the addition of phenytoin. The urinary excretion of unchanged primidone significantly decreased 271 (±21.2 mg/24 hours) to 114.7 (±21.8 mg/24 hours), and the urinary output of pema and unchanged phenobarbital significantly increased. The percentage of unconjugated p-hydroxyphenobarbital in the urine remained unchanged throughout the course of study. After withdrawal of phenytoin, plasma phenobarbital and primidone levels slowly returned to previous steady-state levels.

MECHANISM

Phenytoin induces the biotransformation of primidone to pema and phenobarbital, possibly via cytochrome P450 2C9 and 2C19.

CLINICAL IMPLICATIONS

When phenytoin is co-administered with primidone, the physician should be aware of a potential interaction, which may require frequent plasma anticonvulsant monitoring.

Isoniazid

EVIDENCE OF INTERACTION

A single case report describes a 46-year-old epileptic woman with miliary tuberculosis who was treated with a combination of isoniazid (INH) 300 mg/day and primidone 250 mg every 6 hours (Sutton et al. 1975). As a result, the steady-state serum level of primidone rose from 14.7 to 26.9 μg/mL, and the serum levels of primidone metabolites, Pb and pema, fell (Pb 36.4 to 32 μg/mL, pema 12.4 to 8.8 μg/mL). The elimination half-life of primidone increased from 8.7 to 14.0 hours and the steady-state primidone levels rose by 83%. Pb and pema levels fell by 12% and 29%, respectively.

MECHANISM

INH inhibits the hepatic metabolism of primidone, possibly via cytochrome P450 2C9 and 2C19.

CLINICAL IMPLICATIONS

Primidone toxicity may occur during administration with INH. The monitoring of primidone levels and dosage adjustments may be required.

Phenobarbital

EVIDENCE OF INTERACTION

The serum levels of phenobarbital may be elevated in patients receiving primidone plus phenobarbital therapy (Griffin et al. 1976).

MECHANISM

Because a portion of primidone is converted to phenobarbital in the body, the co-administration of these medications may lead to phenobarbital toxicity via progressive accumulation.

CLINICAL IMPLICATIONS

Because primidone is metabolized to phenobarbital, the co-prescription of these agents is unwarranted.

Nicotinamide

EVIDENCE OF INTERACTION

Nicotinamide is a water-soluble vitamin used in the treatment of pellagra. It also has been used in conjunction with primidone in cases of refractory epilepsy. A significant interaction between primidone and nicotinamide was reported in mice and three epileptic patients (Bourgeois et al. 1982). In mice, 200 mg/kg of nicotinamide increased the elimination half-life of primidone by 47.6%. The conversion of primidone to its metabolites, Pb and pema, was decreased in mice by 32.4% and 14.5%, respectively. Nicotinamide also was found to decrease the conversion of primidone to phenobarbital in three epileptic patients when added to their regimen. Nicotinamide at doses of 41 to 178 mg/kg per day increased the primidone : phenobarbital ratio and decreased the primidone clearance. The dose of nicotinamide correlated directly with the primidone : phenobarbital ratio for all patients.

MECHANISM

Nicotinamide may inhibit the hepatic cytochrome P450 enzymes involved in primidone metabolism.

CLINICAL IMPLICATIONS

Nicotinamide may be used in conjunction with primidone to improve seizure control or reduce toxicity by lowering levels of phenobarbital. In addition, nicotinamide may be useful in patients with psychiatric symptoms of pellagra (acute psychosis, violence, hallucinations, and delusions of persecution). When using the combination, the physician should be aware of the potential shifts in the primidone : Pb ratio. One group suggests that, in epilepsy, the primidone : Pb ratio should be maintained at or above 1 to avoid phenobarbital neurotoxicity (Bourgeois et al. 1982).

Valproic Acid

EVIDENCE OF INTERACTION

The steady-state levels of the primidone metabolite, phenobarbital, may increase with the addition of valproate (Adams et al. 1978, Bourgeois 1988). The addition of valproate to a regimen containing primidone caused an initial increase and then a decrease in plasma primidone levels in seven epileptic children (Windorfer et al. 1975).

MECHANISM

Valproate initially impairs phenobarbital metabolism, possibly via cytochrome P450 2C9 and 2C19; after long-term therapy (1 to 3 months), however, the metabolism may normalize.

CLINICAL IMPLICATIONS

Primidone levels should be monitored closely and dosage adjustments made as necessary during co-administration with valproate.

Section 5.8   Topiramate

Estrogens

EVIDENCE OF INTERACTION

Topiramate in doses up to 800 mg/day was studied to determine its effects on the pharmacokinetics of an oral contraceptive containing ethinyl estradiol 35 mg and norethindrone 1 mg in 12 women with epilepsy who were receiving stable doses (750 to 2500 mg/day) of valproate. Topiramate was administered during three cycles following one cycle of the oral contraceptive. The ethinyl estradiol AUC fell in a dose-related fashion by 18% to 30%, with plasma concentrations decreasing by 15% to 25%, without affecting norethindrone pharmacokinetics (Rosenfeld et al 1997).

MECHANISM
Probable induction of metabolism by topiramate.

CLINICAL IMPLICATIONS
Physicians should advise patients receiving topiramate of the potential decreased efficacy of OCs and consider OCs with an ethinyl estradiol dose at or above 35mcg.

Phenytoin and Hydantoins

EVIDENCE OF INTERACTION
Two studies monitored the effects of topiramate up to 800 mg/day on the pharmacokinetics of phenytoin in patients stabilized on phenytoin monotherapy (260 to 600 mg/day). In half of all patients, the AUC of phenytoin was approximately 25% greater during simultaneous therapy with topiramate than with phenytoin alone. However, in these patients, it was not necessary to adjust the phenytoin dose. Upon discontinuation of phenytoin, the plasma clearance of topiramate decreased 59%, compared with its clearance during the co-administration with phenytoin. This drop in clearance was accompanied by an increase in topiramate peak and average plasma concentrations, time to reach peak concentrations, and AUC (Bourgeois 1996, Gisclon 1994).

Similar results were noted in a study of 10 patients in which phenytoin increased the clearance of topiramate from 26.6 mL/min to a range of 55 to 65 mL/min; this resulted in a decrease in the AUC, C_{max}, and time to peak concentration (Sachdeo et al. 2002).

MECHANISM
Hydantoins may increase the metabolism of topiramate via induction of phase II enzymatic conjugation. Topiramate may decrease the metabolism of hydantoin via inhibition of cytochrome P450 2C19.

CLINICAL IMPLICATIONS
Physicians should carefully monitor hydantoin plasma levels and clinical response when initiating, discontinuing, or modifying the dose of either drug in patients receiving both hydantoins and topiramate.

Valproate

EVIDENCE OF INTERACTION

The effects of adding topiramate ≤800 mg/day on the pharmacokinetics of valproic acid were studied in patients stabilized on 1,000 to 4,500 mg/day valproic acid monotherapy. Following topiramate addition, the clearance of valproic acid increased about 13%, leading to an 11% decrease in the AUC of valproic acid. Upon discontinuation of the valproic acid, topiramate peak plasma concentrations and AUC increased approximately 18% (Rosenfeld 1997).

MECHANISM

Each agent may increase the metabolism of the other.

CLINICAL IMPLICATIONS

Physicians should carefully monitor valproate plasma levels and clinical response when initiating, discontinuing, or modifying the dose of either drug in patients receiving both valproate and topiramate. Adjust dosages as necessary.

Carbamazepine

EVIDENCE OF INTERACTION

The effects of up to 800 mg/day of topiramate on the pharmacokinetics of carbamazepine were studied in epilepsy patients stabilized on carbamazepine monotherapy 900 to 2,400 mg/day. Adding topiramate did not alter plasma concentrations of carbamazepine or its active epoxide metabolite. When carbamazepine was discontinued in some patients, the clearance of topiramate decreased nearly 48%, compared with those receiving both carbamazepine and topiramate. This effect was accompanied by an increase in topiramate peak plasma concentrations, time to reach the peak concentration, and AUC (Doose 1994, Sachdeo 1996).

MECHANISM

Carbamazepine inhibits the metabolism of topiramate.

CLINICAL IMPLICATIONS

Physicians should carefully monitor clinical response when initiating, discontinuing, or modifying the dose of topiramate in patients receiving both carbamazepine and topiramate. Adjust dosages as necessary.

REFERENCES

Aanderud S et al.: The influence of carbamazepine on thyroid hormones and thyroxine binding globulin in hypothyroid patients substituted with thyroxine. Clin Endocrinol (Oxf) 15: 247, 1981.

Abbott FS et al.: The effect of aspirin on valproic acid metabolism. Clin Pharmacol Ther 40: 94, 1986.

Adams DJ et al.: Sodium valproate in the treatment of intractable seizure disorders: a clinical and electroencephalographic study. Neurology 28: 152, 1978.

Aguilera L et al.: Interaction between thiopentone and sodium valproate. An in vitro and in vivo study. Br J Anaesth 58: 1380, 1986.

Ahmad S: Renal insensitivity to frusemide caused by chronic anticonvulsant therapy. Br Med J 3: 657, 1974.

Ahmad S: Diltiazem-carbamazepine interaction. Am Heart J 120: 1485, 1990.

Akula SK et al.: Valproic acid increases cerebrospinal fluid zidovudine levels in a patient with AIDS. Am J Med Sci 313: 244, 1997.

Alestig K: Studies on the intestinal excretion of doxycycline. Scand J Infect Dis 6: 265, 1974.

Anderson GD et al.: Bidirectional interaction of valproate and lamotrigine in healthy subjects. Clin Pharmacol Ther 60: 145–156, 1996.

Andreasen PB et al.: Diphenylhydantoin half-life in man and its inhibition by phenylbutazone: the role of genetic factors. Acta Med Scand 193: 561, 1973.

Arana GW, et al.: Carbamazepine-induced reduction of plasma alprazolam concentrations: a clinical case report. J Clin Psychiatry 49: 448, 1988.

Backman JT, et al.: Concentrations and effects of oral midazolam are greatly reduced in patients treated with carbamazepine or phenytoin. Epilepsia 37: 253, 1996.

Bahls FH et al.: Interactions between calcium channel blockers and the anticonvulsants carbamazepine and phenytoin. Neurology 41: 740, 1991.

Ballek RE et al.: Inhibition of diphenylhydantoin metabolism by chloramphenicol. Lancet 1: 150, 1973.

Bartle WR et al.: Dose-dependent effect of cimetidine on phenytoin kinetics. Clin Pharmacol Ther 33: 649, 1983.

Bauer LA: Interference of oral phenytoin absorption by continuous nasogastric feedings. Neurology 32: 570, 1982.

Baylis EM et al.: Influence of folic acid on blood-phenytoin levels. Lancet 1: 62, 1971.

Bearden DT et al: Telithromycin: an oral ketolide for respiratory infections. Pharmacotherapy 21: 1204–1222, 2001.

Beattie B et al.: Verapamil-induced carbamazepine neurotoxicity. A report of two cases. Eur Neurol 28: 104, 1988.

Bell J et al.: The use of serum methadone levels in patients receiving methadone maintenance. Clin Pharmacol Ther 43: 623, 1988.

Berbel Garcia A, et al.: Protease inhibitor-induced carbamazepine toxicity. Clin Neuropharmacol. 23: 216, 2000.

Bergendal L et al.: The clinical relevance of the interaction between carbamazepine and dextropropoxyphene in elderly patients in Gothenburg, Sweden. Eur J Clin Pharmacol 53: 203, 1997.

Besag FM et al.: Carbamazepine toxicity with lamotrigine: pharmacokinetic or pharmacodynamic interaction? Epilepsia 39: 183, 1998.

Besag FMC et al.: Methsuximide lowers lamotrigine blood levels: A pharma-cokinetic antiepileptic drug interaction. Epilepsia 41: 624, 2000.

Besag FM et al.: Methsuximide reduces valproic acid serum levels. Ther Drug Monit 23: 694, 2001.

Binnie CD et al.: Acute effects of lamotrigine (BW430C) in persons with epilepsy. Epilepsia 27: 248, 1986.

Binnie CD et al.: Double-blind crossover trial of lamotrigine (Lamictal) as add-on therapy in intractable epilepsy. Epilepsy Res 4: 222, 1989.

Blackshear JL et al.: Thyroxine replacement requirements in hypothyroid patients receiving phenytoin. Ann Intern Med 99: 341, 1983.

Block SH: Carbamazepine-isoniazid interaction. Pediatrics 69: 494, 1982.

Blum RA et al.: Effect of fluconazole on the disposition of phenytoin. Clin Pharmacol Ther 49: 420, 1991.

Bochner F et al.: Factors involved in an outbreak of phenytoin intoxication. J Neurol Sci 16: 481, 1972.

Bollini P et al.: Decreased phenytoin level during antineoplastic therapy: a case report. Epilepsia 24: 75, 1983.

Booker HE et al.: Concurrent administration of phenobarbital and diphenyl-hydantoin: lack of an interference effect. Neurology 21: 383, 1971.

Bourgeois BF et al.: Interactions between primidone, carbamazepine, and nicotinamide. Neurology 32: 1122, 1982.

Bourgeois BFD: Pharmacologic interactions between valproate and other drugs. Am J Med 84(Suppl 1A): 29, 1988.

Bourgeois BF: Drug interaction profile of topiramate. Epilepsia 37 (Suppl 2): S14, 1996.

Bowdle TA et al.: Effects of carbamazepine on valproic acid kinetics in normal subjects. Clin Pharmacol Ther 26: 629, 1979.

Brennan RW et al.: Diphenylhydantoin intoxication attendant to slow inacti-vation of isoniazid. Neurology 20: 687, 1970.

Brodie MJ and MacPhee GJ: Carbamazepine neurotoxicity precipitated by dil-tiazem. Br Med J (Clin Res Ed). 292: 1170, 1986.

Brooks SM et al.: Adverse effects of phenobarbital on corticosteroid metabolism in patients with bronchial asthma. N Engl J Med 286: 1125, 1972.

Browne TR et al.: Carbamazepine increases phenytoin serum concentration and reduces phenytoin clearance. Neurology 38: 1146, 1988.

Browne TR: Interaction between clonazepam and sodium valproate (reply). N Engl J Med 300: 678, 1979.

Bruni J et al.: Valproic acid and plasma levels of phenobarbital. Neurology 30: 94, 1980a.

Bruni J et al.: Interactions of valproic acid with phenytoin. Neurology 30: 1233, 1980b.

Buchanan RA and Allen RJ: Diphenylhydantoin (Dilatin) and phenobarbital blood levels in epileptic children. Neurology 21: 866, 1971.

Burroughs Wellcome.: Lamotrigine (Lamictal), 1994.

Capewell S et al.: Gross reduction in felodipine bioavailability in patients tak-ing anticonvulsants. Br J Clin Pharmacol 24: 243, 1987.

Carranco E et al.: Carbamazepine toxicity induced by concurrent erythromy-cin therapy. Arch Neurol 42: 187, 1985.

Cathro DM and Hardman RP: Sub-normal serum thyroxine levels associated with carbamazepine and valproic acid treatment. Nebr Med J 70: 235, 1985.

Cereghino JJ et al.: Preliminary observations of serum carbamazepine concentration in epileptic patients. Neurology 23: 357, 1973.

Cereghino JJ et al.: The efficacy of carbamazepine combinations in epilepsy. Clin Pharmacol Ther 18: 733, 1975.

Chalk JB et al.: Phenytoin impairs the bioavailability of dexamethasone in neurological and neurosurgical patients. J Neurol Neurosurg Psychiatry 47: 1087, 1984.

Chapron DJ et al.: Effect of calcium and antacids on phenytoin bioavailability. Arch Neurol 36: 436, 1979.

Chaudhry RP and Waters BG: Lithium and carbamazepine interaction: possible neurotoxicity. J Clin Psychiatry 44: 30, 1983.

Choi Y et al.: Effect of diphenylhydantoin on cortisol kinetics in humans. J Pharmacol Exp Ther 176: 27, 1971.

Christensen LK and Skovsted L: Inhibition of drug metabolism by chloramphenicol. Lancet 2: 1397, 1969.

Christiansen J and Dam M: Influence of phenobarbital and diphenylhydantoin on plasma carbamazepine levels in patients with epilepsy. Acta Neurol Scand 49: 543, 1973.

Clinical study of lamotrigine and valproic acid in patients with epilepsy: using a drug interaction to advantage? Morris RG, et al. Ther Drug Monit.2000; 22:656.

Cohen AF et al.: Lamotrigine, a new anticonvulsant: pharmacokinetics in normal humans. Clin Pharmacol Ther 42: 535, 1987.

Connell JM et al.: Changes in circulating thyroid hormones during short-term hepatic enzyme induction with carbamazepine. Eur J Clin Pharmacol 26: 453, 1984.

Cooney GF et al.: Effects of carbamazepine on cyclosporine metabolism in pediatric renal transplant recipients. Pharmacotherapy 15: 353, 1995.

Coulam CB and Annegers JF: Do anticonvulsants reduce the efficacy of oral contraceptives? Epilepsia 20: 519, 1979.

Crawford P et al.: Gabapentin as an antiepileptic drug in man. J Neurol Neurosurg Psychiatry 50: 682, 1987.

Crawford P et al.: The interaction of phenytoin and carbamazepine with combined oral contraceptive steroids. Br J Clin Pharmacol 30: 892, 1990.

Dalton MJ et al.: The influence of cimetidine on single-dose carbamazepine pharmacokinetics. Epilepsia 26: 127, 1985.

Dalton MJ et al.: Cimetidine and carbamazepine: a complex drug interaction. Epilepsia 27: 553, 1986.

Dam M et al.: Interaction between carbamazepine and propoxyphene in man. Acta Neurol Scand 56: 603, 1977.

Danan G et al.: Self-induction by erythromycin of its own transformation into a metabolite forming an inactive complex with reduced cytochrome P-450. J Pharmacol Exp Ther 218: 509, 1981.

Data JL et al.: Interaction of quinidine with anticonvulsant drugs. N Engl J Med 294: 699, 1976.

Depot M et al.: Kinetic effects of multiple oral doses of acetaminophen on a single oral dose of lamotrigine. Clin Pharmacol Ther 48: 346, 1990.

Dhillon S and Richens A: Valproic acid and diazepam interaction in vivo. Br J Clin Pharmacol 13: 553, 1982.

Dillard ML et al.: Ciprofloxacin-phenytoin interaction. Ann Pharmacother 26: 263, 1992.

Doose DR et al.: Effect of topiramate or carbamazepine on the pharmacokinetics of an oral contraceptive containing norethindrone and ethinyl estradiol in healthy obese and nonobese female subjects. Epilepsia 44: 540, 2003.

Doose DR et al.: Epilepsia 35(suppl 8): 54, 1994.

Dravet C et al.: Interaction between carbamazepine and triacetyloleandomycin. Lancet 1: 810, 1977.

Ebert U et al.: Effects of rifampicin and cimetidine on pharmacokinetics and pharmacodynamics of lamotrigine in healthy subjects. Eur J Clin Pharmacol 56: 299, 2000.

Edwards J et al.: Antidepressants and seizures: epidemiological and clinical aspects. In: Trimble M (ed.): *The Psychopharmacology of Epilepsy*, Chichester, John Wiley, p. 119, 1985.

Ehrnebo M and Odar-Cederlof I: Distribution of pentobarbital and diphenylhydantoin between plasma and cells in blood: effect of salicylic acid, temperature and total drug concentration. Eur J Clin Pharmacol 11: 37, 1977.

Eimer M and Carter BL: Elevated serum carbamazepine concentrations following diltiazem initiation. Drug Intell Clin Pharm. 21: 340, 1987.

Eriksson AS et al.: Pharmacokinetic interactions between lamotrigine and other antiepileptic drugs in children with intractable epilepsy. Epilepsia 37: 769, 1996.

Faigle J et al.: The biotransformation of carbamazepine. In: Birkmayer W (ed.): *Epileptic Seizures Behavior and Pain*, Baltimore, University Press, 1976.

Farringer JA, et al. Drug Intell Clin Pharm 9: 461, 1985.

Fattore C et al.: Induction of ethinyl estradiol and levonorgestrel metabolism by oxcarbazepine in healthy women. Epilepsia 40: 783, 1999.

Fincham RW et al.: The influence of diphenylhydantoin on primidone metabolism. Arch Neurol 30: 259, 1974.

Fincham RW and Schottelius DD: Decreased phenytoin levels in antineoplastic therapy. Ther Drug Monit 1: 277, 1979.

Fine A et al.: Malabsorption of frusemide caused by phenytoin. Br Med J 2: 1061, 1977.

Finelli PF: Letter: Phenytoin and methadone tolerance. N Engl J Med 294: 227, 1976.

Fleitman JS et al.: Albumin-binding interactions of sodium valproate. J Clin Pharmacol 20: 514, 1980.

Frantzen E et al.: Phenytoin (Dilantin) intoxication. Acta Neurol Scand 43: 440, 1967.

Fraser DG et al.: Displacement of phenytoin from plasma binding sites by salicylate. Clin Pharmacol Ther 27: 165, 1980.

Frattore C et al.: Induction of ethinyl estradiol and levonorgestrel metabolism by oxcarbazepine in healthy women. Epilepsia. 40: 783, 1999

Freeman DJ et al.: Evaluation of cyclosporin-phenytoin interaction with observations on cyclosporin metabolites. Br J Clin Pharmacol 18: 887, 1984.

Frey BM et al.: Phenytoin modulates the pharmacokinetics of prednisolone and the pharmacodynamics of prednisolone as assessed by the inhibition of the mixed lymphocyte reaction in humans. Eur J Clin Invest 14: 1, 1984.

Fulop M et al.: Possible diphenylhydantoin-induced arrhythmia in hypothyroidism. JAMA 196: 454, 1966.

Furlanut M et al.: Effects of folic acid on phenytoin kinetics in healthy subjects. Clin Pharmacol Ther 24: 294, 1978.

Garoner-Thorpe C et al. (eds.): *Clinical Pharmacology of Antiepileptic Drugs*, New York, Springer, 1975, p. 189.

Gadde K and Calabrese JR: Diltiazem effect on carbamazepine levels in manic depression. J Clin Psychopharmacol 10: 378, 1990.

Garnett WR: Bioavailability of phenytoin administered with antacids. Ther Drug Monit 1: 435, 1979.

Garrettson LK et al.: Methylphenidate interaction with both anticonvulsants and ethyl biscoumacetate. JAMA 207: 2053, 1969.

Gilbar PJ et al.: Phenytoin and fluorouracil interaction. Ann Pharmacother 35: 1367, 2001.

Gisclon LG et al.: Epilepsia 35(suppl 8): 54, 1994.

GlaxoSmithKline.: Lamictal package insert. Research Park Triangle, NC., GlaxoSmithKline, 1994.

Glue et al.: Pharmacokinetic interactions of felbamate: in vitro–in vivo correlation. Clin Pharmacokinet 33: 214, 1997.

Gore JM et al.: Interaction of amiodarone and diphenylhydantoin. Am J Cardiol 54: 1145, 1984.

Goulden KJ et al.: Clinical valproate toxicity induced by acetylsalicylic acid. Neurology 37: 1392, 1987.

Griffin G et al.: Primidone-phenobarbital intoxication. Drug Ther 60: 76, 1976.

Grimaldi R et al.: In vivo plasma protein binding interaction between valproic acid and naproxen. Eur J Drug Metab Pharmacokinet 9: 359, 1984.

Hall TG et al.: Effect of sucralfate on phenytoin bioavailability. Drug Intell Clin Pharm 20: 607, 1986.

Hansen JM et al.: Dicoumarol-induced diphenylhydantoin intoxication. Lancet 2: 265, 1966.

Hansen JM et al.: Sulthiame (Ospolot) as inhibitor of diphenylhydantoin metabolism. Epilepsia 9: 17, 1968.

Hansen JM et al.: Carbamazepine-induced acceleration of diphenylhydantoin and warfarin metabolism in man. Clin Pharmacol Ther 12: 539, 1971.

Hansen JM et al.: The effect of different sulfonamides on phenytoin metabolism in man. Acta Med Scand Suppl 624: 106, 1979.

Hansen BS et al.: Influence of dextropropoxyphene on steady state serum levels and protein binding of three anti-epileptic drugs in man. Acta Neurol Scand 61: 357, 1980.

Hansen J: Potentiation of warfarin by co-trimoxazole. Br Med J 1: 684, 1975.

Hansson O and Sillanpaa M: Letter: Pyridoxine and serum concentration of phenytoin and phenobarbitone. Lancet 1: 256, 1976.

Hansten P: Interactions between anticonvulsant drugs: primidone, diphenylhydantoin an phenobarbital. Northwest Med 1: 17, 1974.

Haque N et al.: Studies on dexamethasone metabolism in man: effect of diphenylhydantoin. J Clin Endocrinol Metab 34: 44, 1972.

Hatton RC: Dietary interaction with phenytoin. Clin Pharm 3: 110, 1984.

Hayden M et al.: Danazol-carbamazepine interaction. Med J Aust 155: 851, 1991.

Hedrick R et al.: Carbamazepine—erythromycin interaction leading to carbamazepine toxicity in four epileptic children. Ther Drug Monit 5: 405, 1983.

Hetzel DJ et al.: Cimetidine interaction with phenytoin. Br Med J (Clin Res Ed) 282: 1512, 1981.

Hillebrand G et al.: Valproate for epilepsy in renal transplant recipients receiving cyclosporine. Transplantation 43: 915, 1987.

Hommes OR and Obbens EA: The epileptogenic action of Na-folate in the rat. J Neurol Sci 16: 271, 1972.

Hooper WD et al.: Epilepsia. 1996 Jan;37 (1):91-7 Effect of felbamate on valproic acid disposition in healthy volunteers: inhibition of betaoxidation.

Hooper WD et al.: Preliminary observations on the clinical pharmacology of carbamazepine ('Tegretol'). Proc Aust Assoc Neurol 11: 189, 1974.

Hooper WD et al.: Effect of felbamate on valproic acid disposition in healthy volunteers: inhibition of beta-oxidation. Epilepsia 37: 91, 1996.

Houghton GW and Richens A: Phenytoin intoxication induced by sulthiame in epileptic patients. J Neurol Neurosurg Psychiatry 37: 275, 1974.

Houghton GW and Richens A: Inhibition of phenytoin metabolism by other drugs used in epilepsy. Int J Clin Pharmacol Biopharm 12: 210, 1975.

Houghton GW: Inhibition of phenytoin metabolism by sulthiame in epileptic patients. Br J Clin Pharmacol 1: 59, 1974.

Howitt KM and Oziemski MA: Phenytoin toxicity induced by fluconazole. Med J Aust 151: 603, 1989.

Hull RL: Possible phenytoin-ciprofloxacin interaction. Ann Pharmacother 27: 1283, 1993.

Hunninghake DB: Drug interactions. Postgrad Med 47: 71, 1970.

Hussein G et al.: Gabapentin interaction with felbamate. Neurology 47: 1106, 1996.

Ishizaki T et al.: The effects of neuroleptics (haloperidol and chlorpromazine) on the pharmacokinetics of valproic acid in schizophrenic patients. J Clin Psychopharmacol 4: 254, 1984.

Iteogu MO et al.: Effect of cimetidine on single-dose phenytoin kinetics. Clin Pharm 2: 302, 1983.

Jaillon P and Kates RE: Phenytoin-induced changes in quinidine and 3-hydroxyquinidine pharmacokinetics in conscious dogs. J Pharmacol Exp Ther 213: 33, 1980.

Jann MW et al.: Increased valproate serum concentrations upon carbamazepine cessation. Epilepsia 29: 578, 1988.

Janz D and Schmidt D: Letter: Anti-epileptic drugs and failure of oral contraceptives. Lancet 1: 1113, 1974.

Janz D: The teratogenic risk of antiepileptic drugs. Epilepsia 16: 159, 1975.

Jawad S et al.: Lamotrigine: single-dose pharmacokinetics and initial 1 week experience in refractory epilepsy. Epilepsy Res 1: 194, 1987.

Jensen ON and Olesen OV: Subnormal serum folate due to anticonvulsive therapy. A double-blind study of the effect of folic acid treatment in patients with drug-induced subnormal serum folates. Arch Neurol 22: 181, 1970.

Johannessen S et al.: The influence of phenobarbital and phenytoin on carbamazepine serum level. In: Schneider H JD, Garoner-Thorpe C et al. (eds.): *Clinical Pharmacology of Anti-Epileptic Drugs*, New York, Springer, p. 201, 1975.

Jubiz W et al.: Effect of diphenylhydantoin on the metabolism of dexamethasone. N Engl J Med 283: 11, 1970.

Karlin JM and Kutt H: Acute diphenylhydantoin intoxication following halothane anesthesia. J Pediatr 76: 941, 1970.

Karlsson E et al.: Plasma levels of lidocaine during combined treatment with phenytoin and procainamide. Eur J Clin Pharmacol 7: 455, 1974.

Kater RM et al.: Increased rate of clearance of drugs from the circulation of alcoholics. Am J Med Sci 258: 35, 1969.

Kato Y et al.: Potential interaction between ritonavir and carbamazepine. Pharmacotherapy 20: 851, 2000.

Keilholz U, et al.: Adverse effect of phenytoin on mineralocorticoid replacement with fludrocortisone in adrenal insufficiency. Am J Med Sci 291: 280, 1986.

Kendall AG and Boivin M: Warfarin-carbamazepine interaction. Ann Intern Med 94: 280, 1981.

Kenyon IE: Unplanned pregnancy in an epileptic. Br Med J 1: 686, 1972.

Ketter TA et al.: Principles of clinically important drug interactions with carbamazepine. Part II. J Clin Psychopharmacol 11: 306, 1991.

Ketter TA et al.: Principles of clinically important drug interactions with carbamazepine. Part I. J Clin Psychopharmacol 11: 198, 1991.

Ketter TA et al.: Synergy of carbamazepine and valproic acid in affective illness: case report and review of the literature. J Clin Psychopharmacol 12: 276, 1992.

Ketter TA, Pazzaglia PJ, Post RM Synergy of carbamazepine and valproic acid in affective illness: case report and review of the literature. J Clin Psychopharmacol. 1992 Aug;12(4):276-81.

Kiorboe E: Phenytoin intoxication during treatment with Antabuse (disulfiram). Epilepsia 7: 246, 1966.

Klosterskov Jensen P, et al.: Oxcarbazepine does not affect the anticoagulant activity of warfarin. Epilepsia 33: 1145, 1992.

Knopp RH et al.: Diphenylhydantoin and an insulin-secreting islet adenoma. Arch Intern Med 130: 904, 1972.

Kramer G et al.: Carbamazepine-danazol drug interaction: its mechanism examined by a stable isotope technique. Ther Drug Monit 8: 387, 1986.

Kulshrestha VK et al.: Interaction between phenytoin and antacids. Br J Clin Pharmacol 6: 177, 1978.

Kumar D et al.: Diagnostic use of glucagon-induced insulin response. Studies in patients with insulinoma or other hypoglycemic conditions. Ann Intern Med 80: 697, 1974.

Kupferberg HJ et al.: Effect of methylphenidate on plasma anticonvulsant levels. Clin Pharmacol Ther 13: 201, 1972.

Kutt H et al.: Depression of parahydroxylation of diphenylhydantoin by antituberculosis chemotherapy. Neurology 16: 594, 1966.

Kutt H et al.: The effect of phenobarbital on plasma diphenylhydantoin level and metabolism in man and in rat liver microsomes. Neurology 19: 611, 1969.

Kutt H et al.: Diphenylhydantoin intoxication. A complication of isoniazid therapy. Am Rev Respir Dis 101: 377, 1970.

Kutt H: Interactions of antiepileptic drugs. Epilepsia 16: 393, 1975.

Laengner H and Detering K: Letter: Anti-epileptic drugs and failure of oral contraceptives. Lancet 2: 600, 1974.

Lai ML et al.: Effect of single- and multiple-dose carbamazepine on the pharmacokinetics of diphenylhydantoin. Eur J Clin Pharmacol 43: 201, 1992.

Lamictal [package insert]. Research Park Triangle, NC: GlaxoSmithKline; December 1994.

Lander CM et al.: Interactions between anticonvulsants. Proc Aust Assoc Neurol 12: 111, 1975.

Lang M: Depression of drug metabolism in liver microsomes after treating rats with unsaturated fatty acids. Gen Pharmacol 7: 415, 1976.

Lazarus A: Tardive dyskinesia-like syndrome associated with lithium and carbamazepine. J Clin Psychopharmacol 14: 146, 1994.

Lele P et al.: Cyclosporine and Tegretol—another drug interaction. Kidney Int 27: 344, 1985.

Leonard RF et al.: Phenytoin-salicylate interaction. Clin Pharmacol Ther 29: 56, 1981.

Lertora JJ et al.: Pharmacokinetic interaction between zidovudine and valproic acid in patients infected with human immunodeficiency virus. Clin Pharmacol Ther 56: 272, 1994.

Levine M et al.: Differential effect of cimetidine on serum concentrations of carbamazepine and phenytoin. Neurology 35: 562, 1985.

Levy RH et al.: Carbamazepine/valproic acid interaction in man and rhesus monkey. Epilepsia 25: 338, 1984.

Linnoila M et al.: Effects of sodium valproate on tardive dyskinesia. Br J Psychiatry 137: 240, 1980.

Luder PJ et al.: Treatment of hydatid disease with high oral doses of mebendazole. Long-term follow-up of plasma mebendazole levels and drug interactions. Eur J Clin Pharmacol 31: 443, 1986.

Lumholtz B et al.: Sulfamethizole-induced inhibition of diphenylhydantoin, tolbutamide, and warfarin metabolism. Clin Pharmacol Ther 17: 731, 1975.

Lunde PK et al.: Plasma protein binding of diphenylhydantoin in man. Interaction with other drugs and the effect of temperature and plasma dilution. Clin Pharmacol Ther 11: 846, 1970.

Macphee GJ et al.: Effects of cimetidine on carbamazepine auto- and heteroinduction in man. Br J Clin Pharmacol 18: 411, 1984.

Macphee GJ et al.: Verapamil potentiates carbamazepine neurotoxicity: a clinically important inhibitory interaction. Lancet 1: 700, 1986.

Mallette LE: Letter: Anticonvulsants, acetazolamide and osteomalacia. N Engl J Med 293: 668, 1975.

Mallette LE: Acetazolamide-accelerated anticonvulsant osteomalacia. Arch Intern Med 137: 1013, 1977.

Mamiya K et al.: Synergistic effect of valproate co-administration and hypoalbuminemia on the serum-free phenytoin concentration in patients with severe motor and intellectual disabilities. Clin Neuropharmacol 25: 230, 2002.

Maoz E et al.: Carbamazepine neurotoxic reaction after administration of diltiazem. Arch Intern Med 152: 2503, 1992.

Marcoux A. Carbamazepine neurotoxic reaction after administration of diltiazem. Arch Intern Med. 152: 2503, 1992.

Marsden JR: Effect of isotretinoin on carbamazepine pharmacokinetics. Br J Dermatol. 119: 403, 1988.

Massey EW: Effect of carbamazepine on Coumadin metabolism. Ann Neurol 13: 691, 1983.

Mateu-de Antonio J et al.: Ritonavir-induced carbamazepine toxicity. Ann Pharmacother 35: 125, 2001.

Mattson RH et al.: Folate therapy in epilepsy. A controlled study. Arch Neurol 29: 78, 1973.

Mattson RH et al.: Valproic acid in epilepsy: clinical and pharmacological effects. Ann Neurol 3: 20, 1978.

Mattson GF et al.: Interaction between valproic acid and carbamazepine: an in vitro study of protein binding. Ther Drug Monit 4: 181, 1982.

Maxwell JD et al.: Folate deficiency after anticonvulsant drugs: an effect of hepatic enzyme induction? Br Med J 1: 297, 1972.

May CA et al.: Effects of three antacids on the bioavailability of valproic acid. Clin Pharm 1: 244, 1982.

May TW et al.: Influence of oxcarbazepine and methsuximide on lamotrigine concentrations in epileptic patients with and without valproic acid co-medication: results of a retrospective study. Ther Drug Monit 21: 175, 1999.

McGovern B et al.: Possible interaction between amiodarone and phenytoin. Ann Intern Med 101: 650, 1984.

McKauge L et al.: Factors influencing simultaneous concentrations of carbamazepine and its epoxide in plasma. Ther Drug Monit 3: 63, 1981.

McLelland J and Jack W: Phenytoin/dexamethasone interaction: A clinical problem. Lancet 1: 1096, 1978.

McLeod R: Comment: unexpectedly low phenytoin concentration in a patient receiving ciprofloxacin. Ann Pharmacother 32: 1110, 1998.

Meikle AW et al.: Effect of diphenylhydantoin on the metabolism of metyrapone and release of ACTH in man. J Clin Endocrinol Metab 29: 1553, 1969.

Meikle AW et al.: Kinetics and interconversion of prednisolone and prednisone studied with new radioimmunoassays. J Clin Endocrinol Metab 41: 717, 1975.

Mendez JS et al.: Diphenylhydantoin. Blocking of levodopa effects. Arch Neurol 32: 44, 1975.

Mesdjian E et al.: Carbamazepine intoxication due to triacetyloleandomycin administration in epileptic patients. Epilepsia 21: 489, 1980.

Metz DC et al.: Helicobacter pylori gastritis therapy with omeprazole and clarithromycin increases serum carbamazepine levels. Dig Dis Sci 40: 912, 1995.

Miles MV et al.: Erythromycin effects on multiple-dose carbamazepine kinetics. Ther Drug Monit 11: 47, 1989.

Minton NA et al.: Fatal paracetamol poisoning in an epileptic. Hum Toxicol 7: 33, 1988.

Mirkin BL and Wright F: Drug interactions: effect of methylphenidate on the disposition of diphenylhydantoin in man. Neurology 21: 1123, 1971.

Mitsch RA: Carbamazepine toxicity precipitated by intravenous erythromycin. DICP 23: 878, 1989.

Monks A and Richens A: Effect of single doses of sodium valproate on serum phenytoin levels and protein binding in epileptic patients. Clin Pharmacol Ther 27: 89, 1980.

Morris RG et al.: Clinical study of lamotrigine and valproic acid in patients with epilepsy: using a drug interaction to advantage? Ther Drug Monit 22: 656, 2000.

Morris RG et al.: Clinical study of lamotrigine and valproic acid in patients with epilepsy: using a drug interaction to advantage? Ther Drug Monit 22: 656, 2000.

Morselli PL et al.: Interaction between phenobarbital and diphenylhydantoin in animals and in epileptic patients. Ann NY Acad Sci 179: 88, 1971.

Müller T et al.: Neuroleptic malignant syndrome after clozapine plus carbamazepine. Lancet 2: 1500, 1988.

Murray FJ: Outbreak of unexpected reactions among epileptics taking isoniazid. Am Rev Respir Dis 86: 729, 1962.

Nair DR et al.: Potential fluconazole-induced carbamazepine toxicity. Ann Pharmacother 33: 790, 1999.

Nappi JM: Warfarin and phenytoin interaction. Ann Intern Med 90: 852, 1979.

Neuvonen PJ and Penttila O: Interaction between doxycycline and barbiturates. Br Med J 1: 535, 1974.

Neuvonen PJ et al.: Effect of antiepileptic drugs on the elimination of various tetracycline derivatives. Eur J Clin Pharmacol 9: 147, 1975.

Neuvonen PJ et al.: Antipyretic analgesics in patients on antiepileptic drug therapy. Eur J Clin Pharmacol 15: 263, 1979.

Neuvonen PJ et al.: Cimetidine-phenytoin interaction: effect on serum phenytoin concentration and antipyrine test in man. Naunyn Schmiedebergs Arch Exp Pathol Pharmakol 313(suppl): R60, 1980.

Norris JW: A controlled study of folic acid in epilepsy. A controlled study of folic acid in epilepsy. Neurology 21: 659, 1971.

O'Brien LS et al.: Failure of antacids to alter the pharmacokinetics of phenytoin. Br J Clin Pharmacol 6: 176, 1978.

Oettinger L: Interaction of methylphenidate and diphenylhydantoin. Drug Ther 5: 107, 1976.

Oles KS et al.: Catastrophic neurologic signs due to drug interaction: Tegretol and Darvon. Surg Neurol 32: 144, 1989.

Olesen OV: The influence of disulfiram and calcium carbimide on the serum diphenylhydantoin. Excretion of HPPH in the urine. Arch Neurol 16: 642, 1967.

Olesen OV et al.: Drug—interaction between sulthiame (Ospolot (R)) and phenytoin in the treatment of epilepsy. Dan Med Bull 16: 154, 1969.

Olivesi A: Modified elimination of prednisolone in epileptic patients on carbamazepine monotherapy, and in women using low-dose oral contraceptives. Biomed Pharmacother 40: 301, 1986.

Organon: NuvaRing package insert, 2001.

Orr JM et al.: Interaction between valproic acid and aspirin in epileptic children: serum protein binding and metabolic effects. Clin Pharmacol Ther 31: 642, 1982.

ORTHO-McNeil: Ortho Evra package insert, 2003.

Otero MJ et al.: Interaction between phenytoin and ciprofloxacin. Ann Pharmacother 33: 251, 1999.

Package insert. Voriconazole (Vfend). Pfizer Labz. May 2002

Palomeras E et al.: Dystonia in a patient treated with propranolol and gabapentin. Arch Neurol 57: 570, 2000.

Panesar SK et al.: The effect of carbamazepine on valproic acid disposition in adult volunteers. Br J Clin Pharmacol 27: 323, 1989.

Patel IH et al.: Phenobarbital–valproic acid interaction. Clin Pharmacol Ther 27: 515, 1980.

Patsalos PN et al.: Effect of sodium valproate on plasma protein binding of diphenylhydantoin. J Neurol Neurosurg Psychiatry 40: 570, 1977.

Paxton JW: Effects of aspirin on salivary and serum phenytoin kinetics in healthy subjects. Clin Pharmacol Ther 27: 170, 1980.

Peck AW: Clinical pharmacology of lamotrigine. Epilepsia 32 (suppl 2): S9, 1991.

Penttila O et al.: Interaction between doxycycline and some antiepileptic drugs. Br Med J 2: 470, 1974.

Perel JM and Black N: In vitro metabolism studies with methylphenidate. Fed Proc 29: 315, 1970.

Perucca E et al.: Paracetamol disposition in normal subjects and in patients treated with antiepileptic drugs. Br J Pharmacol 7: 201, 1971.

Petereit LB et al.: Effectiveness of prednisolone during phenytoin therapy. Clin Pharmacol Ther 22: 912, 1977.

Petro DJ et al.: Letter: Diazoxide-diphenylhydantoin interaction. J Pediatr 89: 331, 1976.

Pinder RM et al.: Sodium valproate: a review of its pharmacological properties and therapeutic efficacy in epilepsy. Drugs 13: 81, 1977.

Pisani F et al.: Valproic acid-ethosuximide interaction: a pharmacokinetic study. Epilepsia 25: 229, 1984.

Pisani F et al.: Carbamazepine-viloxazine interaction in patients with epilepsy. J Neurol Neurosurg Psychiatry 49: 1142, 1986.

Pisani F et al.: Interaction of lamotrigine with sodium valproate. Lancet 341: 1224, 1993.

Pollack PT et al.: Ann Pharmacother. 31:61, 1997.

Porro MG et al.: Phenytoin: an inhibitor and inducer of primidone metabolism in an epileptic patient. Br J Clin Pharmacol 14: 294, 1982.

Price WA et al.: Verapamil-carbamazepine neurotoxicity. J Clin Psychiatry 49: 80, 1988.

Privitera MR et al.: Interference by carbamazepine with the dexamethasone suppression test. Biol Psychiatry 17: 611, 1982.

Product Information. Lamotrigine (Lamictal). Burroughs Wellcome. December, 1994.

Pugh RN et al.: Interaction of phenytoin with chlorpheniramine. Br J Clin Pharmacol 2: 173, 1975.

Raitasuo V et al.: Carbamazepine and plasma levels of clozapine. Am J Psychiatry 150: 169, 1993.

Rajaonarison JF et al.: 3'-azido-3'-deoxythymidine drug interactions. Screening for inhibitors in human liver microsomes. Drug Metab Dispos 20: 578, 1992.

Ramsay RE et al.: Carbamazepine metabolism in humans: effect of concurrent anticonvulsant therapy. Ther Drug Monit 12: 235, 1990.

Rane A et al.: Kinetics of carbamazepine and its 10,11-epoxide metabolite in children. Clin Pharmacol Ther 19: 276, 1976.

Rapport DJ et al.: Interactions between carbamazepine and birth control pills. Psychosomatics 30: 462, 1989.

Renton KW: Inhibition of hepatic microsomal drug metabolism by the calcium channel blockers diltiazem and verapamil. Biochem Pharmacol 34: 2549, 1985.

Reunanen M et al.: Low serum valproic acid concentrations in epileptic patients on combination therapy. Curr Ther Res Clin Exp 28: 456, 1980.

Reutens DC et al.: Disabling tremor after lamotrigine with sodium valproate. Lancet 342: 185, 1993.

Reynolds EH: Effects of folic acid on the mental state and fit-frequency of drug-treated epileptic patients. Lancet 1: 1086, 1967.

Reynolds ES et al.: Massive hepatic necrosis after fluroxene anesthesia—a case of drug interaction? N Engl J Med 286: 530, 1972.

Reynolds EH: Anticonvulsants, folic acid, and epilepsy. Lancet 1: 1376, 1973.

Richens A et al.: Phenytoin intoxication caused by sulthiame. Lancet 2: 1442, 1973.

Roe TF et al.: Drug interaction: diazoxide and diphenylhydantoin. J Pediatr 87: 480, 1975.

Rösche J et al.: Possible oxcarbazepine interaction with cyclosporine serum levels: a single case study. Clin Neuropharmacol 24: 113, 2001.

Rose JQ et al.: Intoxication caused by interaction of chloramphenicol and phenytoin. JAMA 237: 2630, 1977.

Rose JQ et al.: Prednisolone pharmacokinetics in relation to dose. J Pediatr 94: 1014, 1979.

Rosemergy I et al.: Phenytoin toxicity as a result of 5-fluorouracil administration. NZ Med J 115: U124, 2002.

Rosenberry KR et al.: Reduced theophylline half-life induced by carbamazepine therapy. J Pediatr 102: 472, 1983.

Rosenfeld WE et al.: Effect of topiramate on the pharmacokinetics of an oral contraceptive containing norethindrone and ethinyl estradiol in patients with epilepsy. Epilepsia 38: 317, 1997.

Rosenfeld WE et al.: Comparison of the steady-state pharmacokinetics of topiramate and valproate in patients with epilepsy during monotherapy and concomitant therapy. Epilepsia 38: 324, 1997.

Rothermich N: Diphenylhydantoin intoxication. Lancet 2: 640, 1966.

Rotne H et al.: Pharmacokinetics of 2-propylaleric acid (Depakene) in epileptic children. In: Johannessen S (ed.): *Antiepileptic Therapy: Advances in Drug Monitoring*, New York, Raven, p. 57, 1980.

Roy-Byrne PP et al.: Carbamazepine and thyroid function in affectively ill patients. Clinical and theoretical implications. Arch Gen Psychiatry 41: 1150, 1984.

Sabers A et al.: Lamotrigine plasma levels reduced by oral contraceptives. Epilepsy Res 47: 151, 2001.

Sabers A et al.: Oral contraceptives reduce lamotrigine plasma levels. Neurology 61: 570, 2003.

Sachdeo RC et al.: Steady-state pharmacokinetics of topiramate and carbamazepine in patients with epilepsy during monotherapy and concomitant therapy. Epilepsia 37: 774, 1996.

Sachdeo RC et al.: Topiramate and phenytoin pharmacokinetics during repetitive monotherapy and combination therapy to epileptic patients. Epilepsia 43: 691, 2002.

Salem RB et al.: Effect of cimetidine on phenytoin serum levels. Epilepsia 24: 284, 1983.

Sälke-Kellermann RA et al.: Influence of ethosuximide on valproic acid serum concentrations. Epilepsy Res 26: 345, 1997.

Samara EE et al.: Effect of valproate on the pharmacokinetics and pharmacodynamics of lorazepam. J Clin Pharmacol 37: 442, 1997.

Schmidt D: Effects of ethanol intake on phenytoin metabolism in volunteers. Experientia 31: 1313, 1980.

Schneider H: Carbamazepine: the influence of other antiepileptic drugs on its serum level. In: Schneider H, Clinical Pharmacology of Antiepileptic Drugs, New York, Springer, p.189, 1975.

Schobben F et al.: Pharmacokinetics, metabolism and distribution of 2-propylpentanoate (sodium valproate) and the influence of salicylate comedication. In: Meinardi HaR, AJ (ed.): Advances in Epileptology, Amsterdam, Swet and Zeiftinger, p. 271, 1978.

Schofield OM et al.: Cyclosporin A in psoriasis: interaction with carbamazepine. Br J Dermatol 122: 425, 1990.

Seirbaek-Neilsen K et al.: Sulphamethizole-induced inhibition of diphenylhydantoin and tolbutamide metabolism in man. Clin Pharmacol Ther 14: 148, 1973.

Shoeman DW et al.: Diphenylhydantoin potency and plasma protein binding. J Pharmacol Exp Ther 195: 84, 1975.

Shukla S et al.: Lithium-carbamazepine neurotoxicity and risk factors. Am J Psychiatry 141: 1604, 1984.

Sisodiya SM et al.: Carbamazepine toxicity during combination therapy with levetiracetam: a pharmacodynamic interaction. Epilepsy Res 48: 217, 2002.

Skovsted L et al.: The effect of different oral anticoagulants on diphenylhydantoin (DPH) and tolbutamide metabolism. Acta Med Scand 199: 513, 1976.

Smart HL et al.: The effects of sucralfate upon phenytoin absorption in man. Br J Clin Pharmacol 20: 238, 1985.

Solomon HM et al.: Interactions between digitoxin and other drugs in vitro and in vivo. Ann N Y Acad Sci 179: 362, 1971.

Solomon GE et al.: Coagulation defects caused by diphenylhydantoin. Neurology 22: 1165, 1972.

Sonne J et al.: Lack of interaction between cimetidine and carbamazepine. Acta Neurol Scand 68: 253, 1983.

Sotaniemi E et al.: The clinical significance of microsomal enzyme induction in the therapy of epileptic patients. Ann Clin Res 2: 223, 1970.

Soto Alvarez J et al.: Effect of carbamazepine on cyclosporin blood level. Nephron 58: 235, 1991.

Speidel BD et al.: Epilepsy, anticonvulsants and congenital malformations. Drugs 8: 354, 1974.

Spina E et al.: Effect of phenobarbital on the pharmacokinetics of carbamazepine-10,11-epoxide, an active metabolite of carbamazepine. Ther Drug Monit 13: 109, 1991.

Spina E et al.: Clinically significant pharmacokinetic drug interactions with carbamazepine. An update. Clin Pharmacokinet 31: 198, 1996.

Spina E et al.: Elevation of plasma carbamazepine concentrations by ketoconazole in patients with epilepsy. Ther Drug Monit 19: 535, 1997.

Stafstrom CE et al.: Erythromycin-induced carbamazepine toxicity: a continuing problem. Arch Pediatr Adolesc Med 149: 99, 1995.

Stjernholm MR et al.: Effects of diphenylhydantoin, phenobarbital, and diazepam on the metabolism of methylprednisolone and its sodium succinate. J Clin Endocrinol Metab 41: 887, 1975.

Strauss RG et al.: Folic acid and Dilantin antagonism in pregnancy. Obstet Gynecol 44: 345, 1974.

Sutton G et al.: Isoniazid as an inhibitor of primidone metabolism. Neurology 25: 1179, 1975.

Sylvester RK et al.: Impaired phenytoin bioavailability secondary to cisplatinum, vinblastine, and bleomycin. Ther Drug Monit 6: 302, 1984.

Syversen GB et al.: Acetazolamide-induced interference with primidone absorption. Case reports and metabolic studies. Arch Neurol 34: 80, 1977.

Taylor J et al.: The interaction of phenytoin and theophylline. Drug Intell Clin Pharm 14: 638, 1980.

Tong TG et al.: Phenytoin-induced methadone withdrawal. Ann Intern Med 94: 349, 1981.

Tyndel F: Interaction of gabapentin with other antiepileptics. Lancet 343: 1363, 1994.

Tyrer JH et al.: Outbreak of anticonvulsant intoxication in an Australian city. Br Med J 4: 271, 1970.

Valsalan VC et al.: Carbamazepine intoxication caused by interaction with isoniazid. Br Med J (Clin Res Ed) 285: 261, 1982.

Vapaatalo H et al.: Variations of serum diphenylhydantoin concentrations in epileptic out-patients. Eur Neurol 5: 303, 1971.

Vauzelle-Kervroedan F et al.: Influence of concurrent antiepileptic medication on the pharmacokinetics of lamotrigine as add-on therapy in epileptic children. Br J Clin Pharmacol 1996; 41: 325.

Wagner ML et al.: Effect of felbamate on carbamazepine and its major metabolites. Clin Pharmacol Ther 53: 536, 1993.

Wagner ML et al.: The effect of felbamate on valproic acid disposition. Clin Pharmacol Ther 56: 494, 1994.

Warner T et al.: Lamotrigine-induced carbamazepine toxicity: an interaction with carbamazepine-10,11-epoxide. Epilepsy Res 11: 147, 1992.

Wassner SJ et al.: The adverse effect of anticonvulsant therapy on renal allograft survival. A preliminary report. J Pediatr 88: 134, 1976.

Watkins JS et al.: Drug interactions of macrolides: emphasis on dirithromycin. Ann Pharmacother 31: 349, 1997.

Watson WA: Interaction between clonazepam and sodium valproate. N Engl J Med 300: 678, 1979.

Watts RW et al.: Lack of interaction between ranitidine and phenytoin. Br J Clin Pharmacol 15: 499, 1983.

Webster LK et al.: Effect of cimetidine and ranitidine on carbamazepine and sodium valproate pharmacokinetics. Eur J Clin Pharmacol 27: 341, 1984.

Wells DG: Folic acid and neuropathy in epilepsy. Lancet 1: 146, 1968.

Werk EE, Jr. et al.: Failure of metyrapone to inhibit 11-hydroxylation of 11-deoxycortisol during drug therapy. J Clin Endocrinol Metab 27: 1358, 1967.

Werk EE, Jr. et al.: Interference in the effect of dexamethasone by diphenylhydantoin. N Engl J Med 281: 32, 1969.

Wilder BJ et al.: Valproic acid: interaction with other anticonvulsant drugs. Neurology 28: 892, 1978.

Windorfer A, Jr. et al.: Elevation of diphenylhydantoin and primidone serum concentration by addition of dipropylacetate, a new anticonvulsant drug. Acta Paediatr Scand 64: 771, 1975.

Windorfer A, Jr. et al.: Drug interactions during anticonvulsant therapy in childhood: diphenylhydantoin, primidone, phenobarbitone, clonazepam, nitrazepam, carbamazepine and dipropylacetate. Neuropadiatrie 8: 29, 1977.

Witassek F et al.: Chemotherapy of larval echinococcosis with mebendazole: microsomal liver function and cholestasis as determinants of plasma drug level. Eur J Clin Pharmacol 25: 85, 1983.

Wong YY et al.: Effect of erythromycin on carbamazepine kinetics. Clin Pharmacol Ther 33: 460, 1983.

Wood RA: Sinoatrial arrest: an interaction between phenytoin and lignocaine. Br Med J 1: 645, 1971.

Wright JM et al.: Isoniazid-induced carbamazepine toxicity and vice versa: a double drug interaction. N Engl J Med 307: 1325, 1982.

Yee GC et al.: Pharmacokinetic drug interactions with cyclosporin (Part I). Clin Pharmacokinet 19: 319, 1990.

Yokochi K et al.: Phenytoin–allopurinol interaction: Michaelis–Menten kinetic parameters of phenytoin with and without allopurinol in a child with Lesch–Nyhan syndrome. Ther Drug Monit 4: 353, 1982.

Yu YL et al.: Interaction between carbamazepine and dextropropoxyphene. Postgrad. Med J 62: 231, 1986.

Yuen AW et al.: Sodium valproate acutely inhibits lamotrigine metabolism. Br J Clin Pharmacol 33: 511, 1992.

Zaccara G et al.: Influence of single and repeated doses of oxcarbazepine on the pharmacokinetic profile of felodipine. Ther Drug Monit 15: 39, 1993.

Zielenski J et al.: Carbamazepine-phenytoin interactions: elevation of plasma phenytoin concentrations due to carbamazepine interaction. Ther Drug Monit 7: 51, 1983.

Zielinski JJ et al.: Clinically significant danazol-carbamazepine interaction. Ther Drug Monit 9: 24, 1987.

Zitelli BJ et al.: Erythromycin-induced drug interactions. An illustrative case and review of the literature. Clin Pediatr 26: 117, 1987.

Electroconvulsive Therapy

WAYNE L. CREELMAN
DONNA JEAN ECKLESDAFER
CHARLES A. WELCH

Anesthetics: Anticholinergics

EVIDENCE OF INTERACTION

The effects of atropine have been carefully studied in electroconvulsive therapy (ECT) (Altschule 1950, Anton et al. 1977, Bouckoms et al. 1989, Miller et al. 1987, Perrin 1961). Atropine increases the heart rate, reduces the number of dropped beats, and reduces the number of premature atrial beats. It virtually eliminates poststimulus asystole and bradyarrhythmias. It reduces oral secretions. Glycopyrrolate has similar effects (Swartz and Saheba 1989), although it may not cross the blood–brain barrier to the extent that atropine does. Atropine blocks the vagal effect more consistently than glycopyrrolate (APA 2001).

MECHANISM

Vagal blockade causes the cardiovascular effects of anticholinergic agents. Identical effects are seen after sectioning the vagus in experimental animals.

CLINICAL IMPLICATIONS

Anticholinergics should not be administered routinely during ECT, but should be reserved for patients who demonstrate bradyarrhythmias or prolonged poststimulus asystole. Anticholinergic medications also should be used to prevent asystole and bradycardia during stimulus dose titration (Mayur et al. 1998, Kellner et al. 1997, APA 2001). Elderly patients with coronary artery disease are at risk

The chapter on Electroconvulsive Therapy for the 2nd edition was written by Charles A. Welch. Wayne L. Creelman and Donna Jean Ecklesdafer revised and updated this chapter for the 3rd edition.

for cardiac ischemia due to the increase in cardiac rate caused by anticholinergics.

Anesthetics: Barbiturates and Nonbarbiturate Anesthetics

EVIDENCE OF INTERACTION

Methohexital, thiopental, etomidate, propofol, and ketamine are the most commonly used anesthetics for narcosis during ECT. Most short-acting anesthetics have an anticonvulsant effect and raise the seizure threshold (Standtland et al. 2002). Methohexital and thiopental both shorten the seizure duration by 40% to 50% (Lunn et al. 1981, Mokriski et al. 1992), with methohexital having a slightly less pronounced effect on seizure duration. Thiopental is associated with cardiovascular depression (Kellner et al. 1997). Seizure length is longer with etomidate than with thiopental (Saffer et al. 1998). A greater increase in postictal arrhythmias occurs with thiopental than with methohexital (APA 2001). One study showed adding remifentanil, a short-acting opioid, to methohexital increased seizure duration compared to either medication alone (Andersen et al. 2001). Etomidate is associated with adrenal suppression and less anticonvulsant properties. Less cardiovascular depression occurs with etomidate, and it may be the anesthetic of choice in patients with heart failure due to its less negative impact on the heart's contractibility (Kellner et al. 1997). Propofol is a hypnotic, nonbarbiturate anesthetic that also has anticonvulsant properties. It is metabolized rapidly and gives greater hemodynamic stability than the barbiturates. It has an antinausea and antiemetic effect. Although a decrease in seizure duration occurs with propofol, there may not be a reduced efficacy of ECT (Martin et al. 1998) or in the quality of the seizure (mean integrated amplitude, postictal suppression index) (Geretsegger et al. 1998). Propofol markedly reduces the duration and intensity of seizures (Boey and Lai 1990), although in one study, ECT with propofol has been found as effective as ECT with methohexital (Malsch et al. 1992). Propofol has a smoother emergence syndrome than other brief anesthetics. Methohexital and thiopental both induce cardiac arrhythmias, although methohexital is significantly less likely to do so (Mokriski et al. 1992). With methohexital, a postictal increase of pulse and blood pressure occurs, which is not evident with propofol (Geretsegger et al. 1998). Ketamine is a proconvulsant (Kellner et al. 1997). It is associated with high blood pressure, tachycardia, hallucinations, and psychotic symptoms. Midazolam given immediately after ECT helps relieve postictal agitation (Krystal et al. 2003).

MECHANISM

The central depressant effects of anesthetics are responsible for their effect on seizure duration (Standtland et al. 2002). The mechanism of their hypotensive effect is unknown.

CLINICAL IMPLICATIONS

Methohexital continues to be the choice for routine use in ECT (Kellner et al. 1997). Although propofol is associated with a more benign emergence syndrome, its inhibitory effect on the ictal process is impressive. Although the quality of the seizure is good with propofol (Geretsegger et al. 1998), individual patients may present in whom this reduces the effectiveness of the treatment. Alternatively, ketamine offers an interesting alternative for narcosis, because it actually increases the intensity and duration of the ECT seizure (Staton et al. 1986). However, recovery from treatment takes approximately an hour, making this strategy impractical. Then injection of etomidate does not have the pain associated with it as does methohexital and propofol (Standtland et al. 2002).

Anesthetics: Succinylcholine

EVIDENCE OF INTERACTION

Succinylcholine, a depolarizing paralytic agent, provides almost complete paralysis of skeletal muscle at doses averaging 0.75 mg/kg, although doses vary considerably from patient to patient. Typically, the effects of succinylcholine last 5 to 10 minutes, although individuals with pseudocholinesterase deficiency may take 6 to 12 hours to regain ventilatory competency. Although cholinesterase deficiency is usually hereditary, it also is associated with cardiac failure, uremia, malnutrition, hypothyroidism, and hepatic failure. It also may result from exposure to insecticides or neuroleptics (Marco and Randels 1979). Extended apnea with succinylcholine also may be associated with quinidine, kanamycin, gentamicin, or streptomycin. Succinylcholine causes an increase in serum potassium, which may put the patient with hyperkalemia or widespread third-degree burns at more of a risk for cardiotoxic effects. Caution must also be used for patients with a personal or family history of malignant hyperthermia, and individuals with hypercalcemia, severe neuromuscular disease or injury, or severe muscular rigidity (APA 2001).

MECHANISM

Succinylcholine normally induces a slight and transient increase in serum potassium due to its effect of triggering a single firing of skeletal muscle prior to paralysis. In denervated muscle, this effect is more pronounced.

CLINICAL IMPLICATIONS

Succinylcholine is the muscle relaxant of choice for ECT. Fasciculations from depolarizing muscle relaxants can cause muscle aches that can be pretreated with aspirin, acetaminophen, nonsteroidal antiinflammatory drugs (NSAIDs), or even a nondepolarizing muscle relaxant. Patients who are at a higher risk when using succinylcholine can be switched to a nondepolarizing muscle relaxer, such as atracurium, mivacurium, curare, rocuronium, or rapacuronium (APA 2001). These nondepolarizing muscle relaxers require a reversal agent, such as neostigmine, edrophonium, or physostigmine (APA 2001). Patients with cholinesterase deficiency, thermal injury, or recent stroke may be treated safely using mivacurium 0.25 mg/kg, with reversal by edrophonium 0.5 mg/kg and atropine 0.005 mg/kg (McCain et al. 1992).

Anticholinesterase Inhibitors

EVIDENCE OF INTERACTION

An 81-year-old woman who was treated with the acetylcholinesterase inhibitor rivastigmine received eight unilateral ECTs. The dose of rivastigmine was decreased during ECT to adjust for ECT-induced alterations in the permeability of the blood–brain barrier. No deterioration in cognitive function occurred, nor was there prolonged paralysis or apnea with the use of succinylcholine and rivastigmine (Zink et al. 2002).

MECHANISM

The exact mechanism of action is unknown, however, rivastigmine is thought to enhance cholinergic function (PDR 2003).

CLINICAL IMPLICATIONS

ECT appears safe for patients with mild memory impairment who are being treated with rivastigmine. Whether the use of rivastigmine during ECT protects against cognitive and memory disturbances is an intriguing but inadequately studied question (Zink et al. 2002).

Anticoagulants

EVIDENCE OF INTERACTION

A total of six cases have been reported of patients receiving ECT during anticoagulant therapy (Loo et al. 1985, Tancer and Evans 1989):

three patients were heparinized, and three were receiving warfarin. No complications were associated with anticoagulant therapy.

MECHANISM

In the early use of ECT, some deaths were attributed to cerebral hemorrhage (Madow 1956), and postmortem study of ECT patients has demonstrated petechial hemorrhages (Impastato 1957). Theoretically, the use of anticoagulants could predispose patients to these complications.

CLINICAL IMPLICATIONS

The theoretical concern regarding intracranial hemorrhage in anticoagulated ECT patients appears not to be borne out in clinical practice. Consequently, anticoagulated patients should be treated according to standard contemporary techniques. However, meticulous attention should be given to blood pressure, and, if significant hypertensive responses occur, they should be attenuated with short-acting intravenous β-blockade (i.e., esmolol 100 to 300 mg intravenously 2 minutes prior to stimulus).

Anticonvulsants

EVIDENCE OF INTERACTION

Anticonvulsants raise the seizure threshold and decrease the quality of the seizure (APA 2001). The principal in vivo effect of all anticonvulsants is to antagonize the initiation, proliferation, and duration of ictal events. Carbamazepine has been reported to interfere with the induction of seizure activity during ECT (Roberts and Attah 1988).

MECHANISM

Varies with specific agents.

CLINICAL IMPLICATIONS

Patients who are taking anticonvulsants for clinical indications, such as epilepsy, usually should remain on these drugs throughout ECT, because discontinuation often results in an exacerbation of the underlying illness. In these patients, an abrupt withdrawal of these medications increases the risk for status epilepticus (Abrams 1997). Because ECT has anticonvulsant properties, some physicians reduce or stop the doses of anticonvulsant medications during an index course/acute series. It is important to maintain serum levels of anticonvulsants in the low therapeutic range. It is generally recommended that, with maintenance ECT treatment, one or two doses should be withheld prior to each session

(APA 2001). It is possible to override the anticonvulsant effect with a modest increase in the intensity of the ECT stimulus and induce seizures that are of adequate duration, generalization, and effectiveness.

Antidepressants: Monoamine Oxidase Inhibitors (MAOIs)

EVIDENCE OF INTERACTION

Some psychiatrists and anesthesiologists discontinue monoamine oxidase inhibitors (MAOIs) 7 to 14 days before ECT treatments. However, considerable documentation exists of the use of ECT while the patient is taking these medications, with few cases of adverse effects (APA 2001). The concurrent use of ECT and MAOIs appears to be safe. In a controlled prospective study of patients undergoing ECT or elective surgery, no differences in cardiovascular function were noted between patients with or without MAOIs (El-Ganzouri et al. 1985). One flawed study (Monaco and DelaPlaine 1964) found no augmentation of efficacy with MAOIs, but this question remains to be adequately researched.

MECHANISM

Theoretically, the concurrent use of MAOIs would predispose patients either to hypotensive episodes through their antihypertensive effect, or to hypertension and arrhythmias through their interference with the degradation of circulating catecholamines.

CLINICAL IMPLICATIONS

At this time, no evidence suggests that patients on MAOIs must be taken off these drugs for a course of ECT (Freese 1985, Remick et al. 1987). MAOIs may enhance the efficacy of ECT, and the empirical use of this combination in treatment-resistant patients is reasonable. The extensive clinical experience with MAOIs and ECT indicate that combining the therapies does not increase the risks of ECT (Dunlop 1960, Imlah et al. 1965, Muller 1961). Certain precautions should be allowed when treating hypotension during ECT (phenylphrine [Neo-Synephrine] should be used instead of ephedrine). Meperidine is contraindicated with the use of MAOIs.

Antidepressants: Tricyclics

EVIDENCE OF INTERACTION

Tricyclic antidepressant medications have been shown to be safe and effective when used with ECT, although caution must be used with patients who take more than one antidepressant and with those patients who have a preexisting cardiovascular disease (APA 2001). In one study, patients who were treated with combined ECT and tricyclic antidepressants had better outcomes and in some cases, fewer treatments were required. In an index series, the combination of imipramine and ECT was more effective than paroxetine and ECT (Kellner et al. 1998). When administered concurrently with a course of ECT, tricyclics have been found to increase neither the incidence of cardiac ectopy (Janowsky et al. 1981), nor the seizure duration (Markowitz and Brown 1987). One case report, however, documents increased cardiac irritability following an acute discontinuation of tricyclics prior to ECT (Raskin 1984). The efficacy of ECT appears not to be affected negatively or positively by concurrent tricyclic therapy (Seager and Bird 1962). However, one retrospective study has reported better outcomes in patients receiving combination ECT–TCA than ECT alone (Nelson and Benjamin 1989).

MECHANISM

Patients on chronic tricyclic therapy appear to derive some cardiac antiarrhythmic effect, which is protective during a course of ECT (Glassman et al. 1987).

CLINICAL IMPLICATIONS

Patients on chronic tricyclic therapy should not be abruptly withdrawn immediately prior to a course of ECT. At the clinician's discretion, they should be withdrawn either well prior to the initiation of treatment, gradually withdrawn during a course of treatment, or maintained on a tricyclic throughout their course, with the intention to continue it after ECT is completed.

The augmentation of ECT with tricyclics is a reasonable and safe strategy in treatment-resistant patients, although the evidence for its effectiveness is equivocal.

Antidepressants: Selective Serotonin Reuptake Inhibitors and Others

EVIDENCE OF INTERACTION

Several cases suggest combining selective serotonin reuptake inhibitors (SSRIs) with ECT is safe, with little increased risk for prolonged seizures (APA 2001). Patients treated with fluoxetine and ECT were compared with patients receiving ECT alone (Gutierrez-Esteinou and Pope 1989). No differences were observed in seizure duration, although a trend appeared for shorter seizures to occur as fluoxetine dosage increased. No evidence suggests that fluoxetine or other SSRIs alter the cardiovascular response to ECT, although this is based on fewer than 20 case reports in the literature. As yet, no evidence suggests that fluoxetine augments the effectiveness of ECT. Evidence suggests that the combination of paroxetine and ECT is effective in sustaining remission (Kellner et al. 1998) and does not increase the incidence of adverse effects. Citalopram does not alter seizure length during ECT (Papakostas et al. 2000). A small study demonstrated the safety of venlafaxine and ECT, with no alterations in seizure duration or cardiovascular function (Bernardo et al. 2000). Another study combining venlafaxine (<300 mg/day) and ECT showed this to be a safe and effective combination (Gonzalez-Pinto et al. 2002). The safe use of mirtazapine or trazodone also has been reported with ECT (Farah 1997). On the other hand, seizure length may increase when ECT is administered during bupropion treatment (APA 2001). Some clinicians recommend bupropion discontinuation or dose reduction prior to ECT.

MECHANISM

The mechanism by which SSRIs might decrease seizure length is unknown.

CLINICAL IMPLICATIONS

No adverse effect appears to occur when continuing SSRIs throughout a course of ECT. SSRIs may be continued through a course of ECT when their use is clinically indicated. If SSRIs are discontinued, clinicians should be aware that withdrawal may cause symptoms similar to the side effects of ECT, such as headache, myalgia, nausea, and fatigue. Patients may report these symptoms as side effects of ECT when they may be symptoms of SSRI withdrawal (Markowitz 1998).

Antihypertensives: β-Blockers

EVIDENCE OF INTERACTION

The use of short-acting injectable β-blockers to attenuate the sympathetic discharge during ECT has been studied extensively (Castelli et al. 1995, Foster and Ries 1988, Howie et al. 1990, 1992, Kovac et al, 1990, 1991, McCall et al. 1991, Stoudemire et al. 1990, Weigner et al. 1991a). These studies have all reported a reduction in heart rate and in systolic and diastolic blood pressure relative to placebo in ECT patients. Both esmolol and labetalol have been associated with shortening of seizure duration in some studies (Howie et al. 1990, Weigner et al. 1991a), but in one study, no such effect was noted (Kovac et al. 1990). Although esmolol may reduce seizure length, it does not appear to decrease ECT efficacy, and it decreases tachycardia and hypertension in high-risk patients (van den Broek et al 1999). Labetalol and nicardipine also blunt the hyperdynamic response to ECT (Avramov et al. 1998). Hydralazine decreases blood pressure within 10 to 80 minutes after administration, but it is associated with hypotension and tachycardia (Kellner et al. 1997).

MECHANISM

β-Blockers blunt the sympathetic discharge at the postsynaptic receptor during ECT-induced seizures. Esmolol is selective for the β-1-receptor, whereas labetalol is not (Gilman et al. 1985). In addition, labetalol has some α-1-blocking activity (McCarthy and Bloomfield 1983). Because of the widespread distribution of these receptors, effects are seen on peripheral vascular resistance, cardiac rate, and cardiac contractility. Pretreatment with esmolol reduces the surge in circulating catecholamines (epinephrine and norepinephrine) during ECT, but labetalol does not (Weigner et al. 1991b).

CLINICAL IMPLICATIONS

Blunting the cardiovascular response to ECT has not been shown to reduce the overall incidence of adverse effects (Kellner 1991). On the other hand, it is clear that specific patients can be more safely treated with the use of these agents. Criteria for use of β-blockers are not yet established, but their use is widespread in patients with preexisting hypertension, coronary artery disease, and ventricular ectopy. These drugs have not been associated with a significant incidence of hypotension or bradycardia during ECT, and they are probably the ideal strategy for protecting the vulnerable cardiac patient from the sympathetic outflow which occurs during ECT.

Antihypertensives: Nitroprusside

EVIDENCE OF INTERACTION

Nitroprusside is a potent antihypertensive given by direct intravenous infusion. It has a rapid onset and short duration of action, and blood pressure is controlled by infusion rate.

MECHANISM

Nitroprusside is a peripheral vasodilator.

CLINICAL IMPLICATIONS

Although a potent antihypertensive, nitroprusside has the disadvantage of producing reflex tachycardia, which, in addition to the sympathetic outflow during a seizure, may induce extremely high cardiac rates. In addition, it may decrease cardiac perfusion. Consequently, its use is not recommended during ECT.

Antihypertensives: Nifedipine

EVIDENCE OF INTERACTION

Nifedipine lowers blood pressure more than β-blockers do and has an antibradycardiac effect (Beyer et al. 1998). Nifedipine has been shown to blunt the hypertensive response to ECT (Kalayam and Alexopoulos 1989, Wells et al. 1989). When administered at a dose of 10 mg sublingually 5 to 10 minutes, or orally 20 to 30 minutes before treatment (Kellner et al. 1997, Abrams 1997).

MECHANISM

Nifedipine selectively inhibits calcium ion influx across the cell membrane of cardiac muscle and vascular smooth muscle. The clinical effects of this mechanism include coronary artery dilation, increased coronary perfusion, and peripheral vasodilation.

CLINICAL IMPLICATIONS

In patients whose pressure is inadequately controlled by injectable β-blockers during ECT, nifedipine is an effective and safe means of augmenting the antihypertensive regimen. In one study, no significant changes occurred in the heart rate or complications; however, the potential for tachycardia exists (Abrams 1997).

Antipsychotics

EVIDENCE OF INTERACTION

The extensive literature on ECT and antipsychotic drugs has been reviewed (Klapheke 1993). Both retrospective and prospective studies indicate that, for some chronic schizophrenic or acutely psychotic patients, the combination of ECT and antipsychotics results in a faster or more pronounced response to treatment, earlier discharge, and lower subsequent relapse rate, relative to treatment with either agent alone. It is important to note that the improved efficacy is not universal, and some individual patients show a dramatic response, whereas others show none, from combined therapy. The presence of affective symptoms is not a prerequisite for good response to combined therapy (Brandon et al. 1985, Dodwell and Goldberg 1989, Taylor and Fleminger 1980). Reports of antipsychotics (older and atypical) and ECT suggest that the combination is safe and effective (APA 2001). Many trials have used clozapine and ECT in schizophrenia, treatment-resistant schizophrenia, and clozapine-resistant schizophrenia. All show clinical improvements in patients (Tang et al. 2002, Chanpattana 2000, Fink 1998, Bhatia et al. 1998, Kupchik et al. 2000, Kales et al. 1999, APA 2001). Seizure durations must be monitored, because seizure threshold is lowered by clozapine (Bhatia et al. 1998). Concerns have surfaced that clozapine and ECT may cause prolonged or spontaneous seizures, but this is rare (APA 2001). During the sympathetic discharge a surge in blood pressure occurs, possibly changing the patency of the blood–brain barrier. This might cause more clozapine to pass into the brain (Fink 1998). Other studies have shown that risperidone is safe and effective, especially when used with psychotic or aggressive patients (Hirose et al. 2001, Kellner et al. 1997). No evidence suggests that neuroleptics improve the effectiveness of ECT in the treatment of major depression (Thase 1992).

In a review of the literature, Friedel (1986) reported no evidence of any harmful interactions with ECT and high-potency neuroleptics. Although rarely prescribed as an antipsychotic, reserpine use during ECT has been associated with death and should be avoided (APA 2001).

MECHANISM

The therapeutic mechanism of the combined use of ECT and neuroleptics is unknown.

CLINICAL IMPLICATIONS

Based on the available literature, the combined use of ECT and neuroleptics is indicated in schizophrenic patients who have not responded optimally to neuroleptic treatment alone (Klapheke 1993). Target symptoms are both positive and negative signs of schizophrenia, and patients without depressive symptomatology may derive dramatic benefit from combined therapy. Patients may respond to less than 12 ECTs, although larger numbers of treatments are commonplace. Both unilateral and bilateral ECT have been reported effective in schizophrenia (Gujavarty et al. 1987, Small 1985).

Benzodiazepines

EVIDENCE OF INTERACTION

Benzodiazepines have anticonvulsant properties, which can shorten seizure length and may interfere with seizure quality, making ECT less effective (APA 2001). Higher doses of benzodiazepines (e.g., lorazepam) are related to shorter EEG seizure length (Boylan et al. 2000). Benzodiazepines should be withheld for at least 8 hours before ECT treatments.

If they cannot be discontinued or withheld pre-ECT, flumazenil may be given to reverse the action of benzodiazepines (APA 2001). Flumazenil is a benzodiazepine-competitive antagonist. It is safe and effective with ECT. No difference is observed in seizure duration or efficacy of the treatment (Krystal et al. 1998). The use of flumazenil may cause benzodiazepine withdrawal symptoms, which can be treated with midazolam postictal. Chloral hydrate and other sedative hypnotics have anticonvulsant effects similar to benzodiazepines (APA 2001).

MECHANISM

A fully generalized tonic-clonic (grand mal) seizure is the essential therapeutic component of ECT. Benzodiazepines reduce the effectiveness of ECT, probably through inhibition of the ictal process, by binding to the γ-aminobutyric acid (GABA)-benzodiazepine receptor complex (Enna and Mohler 1987). Intravenous benzodiazepines are highly effective in terminating excessively long seizure activity during ECT. It is important to keep in mind that midazolam has potent, but brief, respiratory depressant activity.

CLINICAL IMPLICATIONS

Benzodiazepines decrease the efficacy of ECT by shortening the seizure length and interfering with seizure quality. They should be discontinued or at least withheld for 8 hours before ECT. If this is not possible, flumazenil may be given to reverse benzodiazepine action (APA 2001). One case report documents severe post ECT agitation when droperidol was added to midazolam. This allowed for lower doses of each medication to control a severely agitated postictal patient (Hines et al. 1997).

Digitalis

EVIDENCE OF INTERACTION

No systematic study has reported the interaction between digitalis and ECT. On the other hand, a strong theoretical basis supports concern regarding postictal bradycardia or even cardiac arrest in digitalized patients. Because the effect of digitalis is dose related, heightened concern is warranted with digitalis levels above the therapeutic range. Digitalis may slightly prolong succinylcholine's metabolism (Beyer et al. 1998) but should be continued throughout the ECT treatments (Kellner et al. 1997).

MECHANISM

Digitalis glycosides have a vagomimetic action, resulting in slowed conduction at the sinoatrial and atrioventricular nodes. By this mechanism, digitalis glycosides exert a dose-related negative chronotropic effect.

CLINICAL IMPLICATIONS

Any digitalized patient should have blood levels checked prior to ECT. Although routine pretreatment with atropine is probably unwarranted, atropine should be available in the event of postictal bradycardia. Patients with digitalis levels above the therapeutic range must not receive ECT until blood levels are reduced.

Lithium

EVIDENCE OF INTERACTION

Lithium in combination with ECT may put patients at higher risk for prolonged seizures and delirium or neurotoxicity (APA 2001). An index course of ECT in combination with lithium is not deemed safe due to neurotoxicity and the potential for prolonged seizures. Lithium should be discontinued 2 to 7 days before treatments begin and withheld 2 to 7 days after treatments stop (Gupta et al. 1998). Although many patients have had ECT treatments with lithium in combination without adverse effects, it is best to discontinue the use of lithium during ECT. If lithium cannot be stopped, then a case-by-case decision must be made. It is advisable to decrease the dose of lithium to a low to moderate therapeutic range (APA 2001).

Continuation/maintenance ECT combined with lithium may be an effective and safe treatment in specific cases (Stewart 2000). In the past two decades, numerous case reports have documented severe delirium associated with the concurrent use of ECT and lithium (Mukherjee 1993). Only one retrospective study (Small et al. 1980) compared 25 patients receiving ECT and lithium in combination versus 25 patients receiving ECT alone. Patients receiving the combined treatment demonstrated more severe memory loss, a lower therapeutic response, and lower scores on neuropsychological testing during and after treatment.

Two prospective studies report no evidence of ECT-lithium interaction. Coppen et al. (1981) found no evidence of increased encephalopathy in patients who were started on lithium during a course of ECT. Martin and Kramer (1982) likewise reported no increased morbidity associated with concurrent lithium during a course of ECT.

MECHANISM

The mechanism of interaction between ECT and lithium is hypothetical and unknown.

CLINICAL IMPLICATIONS

About 10% to 30% of bipolar patients switch from depression to mania during a course of ECT (Angst et al. 1992). Consequently, some clinical basis supports the continuation of lithium during a course of ECT. On the other hand, the case reports in the literature cannot be ignored. Although evidence for an ECT-lithium interaction is weak, and may indeed be attributed to other issues such as lithium toxicity, certain individual patients may indeed be sensitive to the combined regimen. If clear indications exist for the continuation of lithium, it may be reasonable and even therapeutically advantageous. On the other hand, the emergence of delirium or encephalopathy during a course of ECT should be grounds for the immediate discontinuation of lithium. All patients receiving the combined regimen should be informed of the potential interaction prior to the initiation of treatment.

Sympathomimetics (Methylxanthines)

EVIDENCE OF INTERACTION

Theophylline is more likely to cause prolonged seizures and even status epilepticus when combined with ECT, even at therapeutic levels (APA 2001). For patients who must take theophylline during ECT, serum levels should be in the range of 10 to 20 μg/mL. Seizures should be carefully monitored (Fink et al. 1998). Theophylline at a dose of 200 to 400 mg orally the night before treatment is associated with a lengthening of seizure duration (Swartz and Lewis 1991), but theophylline may cause prolonged seizures (Devanand 1988, Peters et al. 1984). One study showed that aminophylline increased seizure length with no adverse effects (Stern et al. 1999). Caffeine augmentation of ECT has been extensively studied (Calev et al. 1993, Coffey et al. 1987, 1990). The use of caffeine sodium benzoate in doses of 500 to 2,000 mg intravenously prior to ECT is associated with an increase in seizure duration, a reduction in number of treatments (Calev 1993), and a decrease in seizure threshold (Coffey et al. 1990). Caffeine increases seizure length but does not seem to lower the seizure threshold. Rare cases occur of cardiovascular complications and possibly other adverse effects in the combination of caffeine and ECT. It is questionable whether any real benefit accrues to the use of caffeine and ECT, compared to the potential adverse effects (APA 2001).

MECHANISM

Methylxanthines may act as proconvulsants by acting as a competitive inhibitor of adenosine, an endogenous anticonvulsant, at the adenosine receptor (Snyder and Sklar 1984).

CLINICAL IMPLICATIONS

The use of methylxanthines may be indicated for patients in whom it is difficult to initiate seizure activity, or in patients who have brief seizures (<20 seconds). On the other hand, these augmentation strategies occasionally have resulted in protracted seizures (Coffey et al. 1987) or an increase in cardiac ectopy. Consequently, if a patient is showing a reasonable clinical response to ECT, adding methylxanthines to the treatment format is probably unwarranted.

Thyroid Hormone

EVIDENCE OF INTERACTION

The combined use of thyroid hormone and ECT was evaluated by Stern et al. (1993). Patients receiving 50 μmg/day of triiodothyronine were compared with patients receiving placebo. The patients receiving thyroid hormone had significantly longer seizures than the placebo group and required significantly fewer treatments. In addition, patients receiving thyroid hormone performed better on cognitive testing post-ECT and reported a higher degree of subjective improvement. No increase was observed in cardiovascular complications in the treatment group.

MECHANISM

The mechanism of interaction between thyroid hormone and ECT is unknown. One possible mechanism is the suppression of thyrotropin-releasing hormone, which is known to have anticonvulsant activity.

CLINICAL IMPLICATIONS

The concurrent use of thyroid hormone and ECT is not associated with cardiovascular or central nervous system toxicity, and indeed the combined regimen may be more effective in the treatment of depression than ECT alone. The evidence for potentiation is not strong enough to warrant the routine administration of thyroid hormone to patients receiving ECT, but in treatment-resistant patients, an empirical trial of thyroid augmentation is a reasonable strategy.

Tryptophan

EVIDENCE OF INTERACTION

The administration of tryptophan does not augment the effectiveness of ECT (Kirkegaard et al. 1978), but it does increase seizure duration (Raotma 1978).

MECHANISM

The mechanism of tryptophan's anticonvulsant action is unknown.

CLINICAL IMPLICATIONS

Tryptophan is contraindicated during ECT.

REFERENCES

Abrams R: *Electroconvulsive Therapy*, New York Oxford, Oxford University Press, pgs. 87, 94, 202, 1997.

Altschule MD: Further observations on vagal influences on the heart during electroshock therapy for mental disease. Am Heart J 39: 88, 1950.

Andersen FA et al.: Effects of combined methohexitone-remifentanil anaesthesia in electroconvulsive therapy. Acta Anaesthesiol Scand 45(7): 830–833, 2001.

Angst J et al.: ECT-induced and drug-induced hypomania. Convulsive Ther 8: 179, 1992.

Anton AH et al.: Autonomic blockade and the cardiovascular and catecholamine response to electroshock. Anesth Analg 56: 46, 1977.

APA Task Force Report: *The Practice of Electroconvulsive Therapy, Recommendations for Treatment, Training, and Privileging*, 2nd ed., 2001, pgs. 18–19, 33–35, 37–45, 61–64, 69, 82–88, 91–92, 118–119, 131–136.

Avramov MN et al.: Effects of nicardipine and labetalol on the acute hemodynamic response to electroconvulsive therapy. J Clin Anesth 10(5): 394–400, 1998.

Bernardo M et al.: Seizure activity and safety in combined treatment with venlafaxine and ECT: a pilot study. J ECT 16(1): 38–42, 2000.

Beyer J L et al.: *Electroconvulsive Therapy—A Programmed Text*, 2nd ed., Washington, DC, London, American Psychiatric Press, Inc., 1998, pgs. 41, 44.

Bhatia SC et al.: Concurrent administration of clozapine and ECT: a successful therapeutic strategy for a patient with treatment resistant schizophrenia. J ECT: 14(4) 280–283, 1998.

Boey WK, Lai FO: Comparison of propofol and thiopentone as anaesthetic agents for electroconvulsive therapy. Anaesthesia 45: 623, 1990.

Bouckoms AJ et al.: Atropine in electroconvulsive the rapy. 5: 48, 1989.

Boylan Laura S et al.: Determinants of seizure threshold in ECT: benzodiazepine use, anesthetic dosage, and other factors. J ECT 16(1): 3–18, 2000.

Bracha S, Hes J: Death occurring during combined reserpine-electroshock treatment. Am J Psychiatry 113: 257, 1956.

Brandon S et al.: Leicester ECT trial: results in schizophrenia. Br J Psychiatry 146: 177, 1985.

Calev A et al.: Caffeine pretreatment enhances clinical efficacy and reduces cognitive effects of electroconvulsive therapy. Convulsive Ther 9: 95, 1993.

Castelli I et al.: Comparative effects of esmolol and labetalol to attenuate hyperdynamic states after electroconvulsive therapy. Anesth Analg 80: 11, 1995.

Chanpattana W: Combined ECT and clozapine in treatment-resistant mania. J ECT: 16(2) 204–207, 2000.

Coffey CE et al.: Augmentation of ECT seizures with caffeine. Biol Psychiatry 22: 637, 1987.

Coffey CE et al.: Caffeine augmentation of ECT. Am J Psychiatry 147: 579, 1990.

Conway CR, Nelson LA: The combined use of bupropion, lithium, and venlafaxine during ECT: a case of prolonged seizure activity. J ECT 17(3): 216–218, 2001.

Coppen A, et al.: Lithium continuation therapy following electroconvulsive therapy. Br J Psychiatry 139: 284, 1981.

Dannon PN et al.: Labetalol does not lengthen asystole during electroconvulsive therapy. J ECT: 14(4) 245–250, 1998.

Devanand DP et al.: Status epilepticus during ECT in a patient receiving theophylline. J Clin Psychopharmacol 8: 153, 1988.

Dodwell D, Goldberg D: A study of factors associated with response to electroconvulsive therapy in patients with schizophrenic symptoms. Br J Psychiatry 154: 635, 1989.

Dunlop E: Electroshock and monoamine oxidase inhibitors in the treatment of depressed reactions. Dis Nerv Syst 21: 130, 1960.

Dwersteg JF, Avery DH: Atracurium as a muscle relaxant for electroconvulsive therapy in a burned patient. Convulsive Ther 3: 49, 1987.

El-Ganzouri A et al.: Monoamine oxidase inhibitors: Should they be discontinued preoperatively? Anesth Analg 64: 592, 1985.

Enna SJ, Mohler H: Gamma-aminobutyric acid (GABA) receptors and their association with benzodiazepine recognition sites. In Meltzer HY (ed.), *Psychopharmacology: The Third Generation of Progress*, New York, Raven Press, 1987, p. 265.

Farah A: Mirtazapine and ECT combination therapy. Convulsive Ther 13(2): 116–117, 1997.

Fink, M: *Electroshock—Restoring the Mind*, New York, Oxford, Oxford University Press, 1999.

Fink M: ECT and clozapine in schizophrenia. J ECT 14(4): 223–226, 1998.

Fink M, Sackiem HA: Theophylline and ECT. J ECT 14(4): 286–290, 1998.

Foster S, Ries R: Delayed hypertension with electroconvulsive therapy. J Nerv Ment Dis 176: 374, 1988.

Freese KJ: Can patients safely undergo electroconvulsive therapy while receiving monoamine oxidase inhibitors? Convulsive Ther 1: 190, 1985.

Friedel RO: The combined use of neuroleptics and ECT in drug resistant schizophrenic patients. Psychopharmacol Bull 22: 928, 1986.

Geretsegger C et al.: Propofol and methohexital as anesthetic agents for electroconvulsive therapy (ECT): a comparison of seizure-quality measures and vital signs. J ECT 14(1): 28–35, 1998.

Gilman A et al.: *Pharmacological Basis of Therapeutics*, 7th ed., New York, Macmillan, 1985, p. 693.

Glassman AH et al.: Cardiovascular effects of tricyclic antidepressants. In Meltzer HY (ed.), *Psychopharmacology: The Third Generation of Progress*, New York, Raven Press, 1987, p. 1437.

Gonzalez-Pinto A et al.: Efficacy and safety of venlafaxine-ECT combination in treatment-resistant depression. J Neuropsychiatry Clin Neurosci 14(2): 206–209, 2002.

Gujavarty K et al.: Electroconvulsive therapy and neuroleptic medication in therapy-resistant positive-symptom psychosis. Convulsive Ther 3: 185, 1987.

Gupta S et al.: Lithium and maintenance electroconvulsive therapy. J ECT 14(4): 241–244, 1998.

Gutierrez-Esteinou R, Pope HG: Does fluoxetine prolong electrically induced seizures? Convulsive Ther 5: 344, 1989.

Hines AH, Labbate LA: Combination midazolam and droperidol for severe post-ECT agitation. Convulsive Ther 13(2): 113–117, 1997.

Hirose S et al.: Effectiveness of ECT combined with risperidone against aggression in schizophrenia. J ECT 17(1): 22–26, 2001.

Howie et al.: Esmolol reduces the autonomic hypersensitivity and length of seizures induced by electroconvulsive therapy. Anesth Analg 71: 384, 1990.

Howie et al.: Defining the dose range for esmolol used in electroconvulsive therapy hemodynamic attenuation. Anesth Analg 75: 805, 1992.

Imlah NW et al.: The influence of antidepressant drugs on the response to electroconvulsive therapy and on subsequent relapse rates. Neuropsychopharmacology 4: 438, 1965.

Impastato D: Prevention of fatalities in electroshock therapy. Dis Nerv Syst 18(suppl): 34, 1957.

Janowsky EC et al.: Psychotropic agents. In Smith NT, Miller RD, Corbascio AN (eds.), *Drug Interactions and Anesthesia*, Philadelphia, Lea & Febiger, 1981, p. 177.

Kalayam B, Alexopoulos GS: Nifedipine in the treatment of blood pressure rise after ECT. Convulsive Ther 5: 110, 1989.

Kales HC et al.: Combined electroconvulsive therapy and clozapine in treatment-resistant schizophrenia. Prog Neuropsychopharmacol Biol Psychiatry 23(3): 547–556, 1999.

Kellner CH et al.: *Handbook of ECT*, Washington, DC, London, American Psychiatric Press, pgs. 24, 27, 31, 61–63, 68–70, 1997.

Kellner CH, Bourgon LN: Combining ECT and antidepressants: time to reassess. J ECT 14(2): 65–67, 1998.

Kellner CH: Labetalol and ECT (letter). J Clin Psychiatry 52: 386, 1991.

Kellner CH et al.: ECT-drug interactions: a review. Psychopharmacol Bull 27: 595, 1991.

Kirkegaard C et al.: Addition of L-tryptophan to electroconvulsive treatment in endogenous depression: a double-blind study. Acta Psychiatr Scand 58: 457, 1978.

Klapheke MM: Combining ECT and antipsychotic agents: benefits and risks. Convulsive Ther 9: 241, 1993.

Kovac et al.: Esmolol bolus and infusion attenuates increases in blood pressure and heart rate during electroconvulsive therapy. Can J Anaesth 37: 58, 1990.

Kovac et al.: Comparison of two esmolol bolus doses on the haemodynamic response and seizure duration during electroconvulsive therapy. Can J Anaesth 38: 204, 1991.

Krahn LE et al.: Electroconvulsive therapy and cardiovascular complications in patients taking trazodone for insomnia. J Clin Psychiatry 62(2): 108–110, 2001.

Krystal AD et al.: The use of flumazenil in the anxious and benzodiazepine-dependent ECT patient. J ECT 14(1): 5–14, 1998.

Krystal AD et al.: Comparison of seizure duration, ictal EEG, and cognitive effects of ketamine and methohexital anesthesia with ECT. J Neuropsychiatry Clin Neurosci 15:1, 27–34, 2003.

Kupchik M et al.: Combined electroconvulsive-clozapine therapy. Clin Neuropharmacol 23(1): 14–16, 2000.

Loo H et al.: Electroconvulsive therapy during anticoagulant therapy. Convulsive Ther 1: 258, 1985.

Lunn RJ et al.: Anesthetics and electroconvulsive therapy seizure duration: implications for therapy from a rat model. Biol Psychiatry 16: 1163, 1981.

Madow L: Brain changes in electroshock therapy. Am J Psychiatry 113: 337, 1956.

Malsch E et al.: Efficacy of electroconvulsive therapy after propofol or methohexital anesthesia. Anesth Analg 72: S192, 1992.

Marco LA, Randels PM: Succinylcholine drug interactions during electroconvulsive therapy. Biol Psychiatry 14: 433, 1979.

Markowitz JC, Brown RP: Seizures with neuroleptics and antidepressants. Gen Hosp Psychiatry 9: 135, 1987.

Markowitz John S: Selective serotonin reuptake inhibitor discontinuation with ECT and withdrawal symptoms. J ECT 14(1): 55, 1998.

Martin BA, et al.: Propofol anesthesia, seizure duration, and ECT: a case report and literature review. J ECT 14(2): 99–108, 1998.

Martin BA, Kramer PM: Clinical significance of the interaction between lithium and a neuromuscular blocker. Am J Psychiatry 139: 1326, 1982.

Mayur PM et al.: Atropine premedication and the cardiovascular response to electroconvulsive therapy. Br J Anaesth 81(3): 466–467, 1998.

McCain J et al.: Is mivacurium chloride, a new short-acting non-depolarizing muscle relaxant, useful in ECT procedures? A report of four cases (abstract). Presented at the Gulf Atlantic Residents Meeting, New Orleans, September 5, 1992.

McCall WV et al.: Effects of labetalol on hemodynamics and seizure duration during ECT. Convulsive Ther 7: 5, 1991.

McCall WV et al.: Effect of esmolol pretreatment on EEG seizure morphology in RUL ECT. Convulsive Ther 13(3): 175–180, 1997.

McCarthy EP, Bloomfield SS: Labetalol: a review of its pharmacology, pharmacokinetics, clinical uses and adverse effects. Pharmacology 3: 193, 1983.

McCleane GJ, Howe JP: Electroconvulsive therapy and serum potassium. Ulster Med J 58: 172, 1989.

Miller ME et al.: Atropine sulfate premedication and cardiac arrhythmia in electroconvulsive therapy (ECT). Convulsive Ther 3: 10, 1987.

Mokriski BK et al.: Electroconvulsive therapy-induced cardiac arrhythmias during anesthesia with methohexital, thiamylal, or thiopental sodium. J Clin Anesthes 4: 208, 1992.

Monaco JT, DelaPlaine RP: Tranylcypromine with ECT. Am J Psychiatry 120: 1, 1964.

Mukherjee S: Combined ECT and lithium therapy. Convulsive Ther 9: 274, 1993.

Muller D: Nardil (phenelzine) as a potentiator of electroconvulsive therapy. J Ment Sci 107: 994, 1961.

Nelson JP, Benjamin L: Efficacy and safety of combined ECT and tricyclic antidepressant drugs in the treatment of depressed geriatric patients. Convulsive Ther 5: 321, 1989.

Nettelbladt P: Factors influencing number of treatments and seizure duration in ECT: drug treatment, social class. Convulsive Ther 4: 160, 1988.

Olesen AC et al.: Effect of a single nighttime dose of oxazepam on seizure duration in electroconvulsive therapy. Convulsive Ther 5: 3, 1989.

Papakostas Y, et al.: Administration of citalopram before ECT: seizure duration and hormone responses. J ECT 16(4): 356–360, 2000.

Physician's Desk Reference (PDR), 2003, 57th Edition, Thomson PDR, 2003, pgs. 2260–2263.

Perrin GM: Cardiovascular aspects of electric shock therapy. Acta Psychiatr Scand 36: 7, 1961.

Peters SG et al.: Status epilepticus as a complication of concurrent electroconvulsive and theophylline therapy. Mayo Clin Proc 59: 568, 1984.

Pettinati HM et al.: Evidence for less improvement in depression in patients taking benzodiazepines during unilateral ECT. Am J Psychiatry 147: 1029, 1990.

Raotma H: Has tryptophan any anticonvulsive effect? Acta Psychiatr Scand 57: 253, 1978.

Raskin DA: Cardiac irritability, tricyclic antidepressants, and electroconvulsive therapy. J Clin Psychopharmacol 4: 237, 1984.

Remick RA et al.: Monoamine oxidase inhibitors in general anesthesia: a reevaluation. Convulsive Ther 3: 196, 1987.

Roberts MA, Attah JR: Carbamazepine and ECT. Br J Psychiatry 153: 418, 1988.

Saffer S, Berk M: Anesthetic induction for ECT with etomidate is associated with longer seizure duration than thiopentone. J ECT 14(2): 89–93, 1998.

Seager CP, Bird RL: Imipramine with electrical treatment in depression—a controlled trial. J Ment Sci 108: 704, 1962.

Small JG et al.: Complications with electroconvulsive treatment combined with lithium. Biol Psychiatry 15: 103, 1980.

Small JG: Efficacy of electroconvulsive therapy in schizophrenia, mania, and other disorders, I: schizophrenia. Convulsive Ther 1: 263, 1985.

Snyder SH, Sklar P: Behavioral and molecular actions of caffeine: focus on adenosine. J Psychiatr Res 18: 91, 1984.

Standish-Barry HMAS et al.: The relationship of concurrent benzodiazepine administration to seizure duration in ECT. Acta Psychiatr Scand 71: 269, 1985.

Standtland C et al.: A switch from propofol to etomidate during an ECT course increases EEG and motor seizure duration. J ECT 18(1): 22–25, 2002.

Staton RD et al.: The electroencephalographic pattern during electroconvulsive therapy, IV: spectral energy distributions with methohexital, Innovar and ketamine anesthesias. Clin Electroencephal 17: 203, 1986.

Stern L et al.: Aminophylline increases seizure length during electroconvulsive therapy. J ECT 15(4): 252–257, 1999.

Stern RA et al.: Combined use of thyroid hormone and ECT. Convulsive Ther 9: 285, 1993.

Stewart JT: Lithium and maintenance ECT. J ECT 16(3): 300–301, 2000.

Stoudemire A et al.: Labetalol in the control of cardiovascular responses to electroconvulsive therapy in high-risk depressed medical patients. J Clin Psychiatry 51: 508, 1990.

Swartz CM: Anesthesia for ECT. Convulsive Ther 9: 301, 1993.

Swartz CM, Lewis RK: Theophylline reversal of electroconvulsive therapy (ECT) seizure inhibition. Psychosomatics 32: 47, 1991.

Swartz CM, Saheba NC: Comparison of atropine with glycopyrrolate for use in ECT. Convulsive Ther 5: 56, 1989.

Tancer ME, Evans DL: Electroconvulsive therapy in geriatric patients undergoing anticoagulation therapy. Convulsive Ther 5: 102, 1989.

Tang WK et al.: Effect of piracetam on ECT-induced cognitive disturbances: a randomized, placebo-controlled, double-blind study.

Tang WK, Ungvari Gabor S: Efficacy of electroconvulsive therapy combined with antipsychotic medication in treatment-resistant schizophrenia: a prospective, open trial. J ECT 18(2): 90–94, 2002.

Taylor P, Fleminger JJ: ECT for schizophrenia. Lancet 1: 1380, 1980.

Thase ME: Long-term treatments of recurrent depressive disorders. J Clin Psychiatry 53: 32, 1992.

van den Broek WW et al.: Low-dose esmolol bolus reduces seizure duration during electroconvulsive therapy: a double-blind, placebo-controlled study: Br J Anaesth 83(2): 271–274, 1999.

Weigner MB et al.: Prevention of the cardiovascular and neuroendocrine response to electroconvulsive therapy: I. Effectiveness of pretreatment regimens on hemodynamics. Anesth Analg 73: 556, 1991a.

Weigner MB et al.: Prevention of the cardiovascular and neuroendocrine response to electroconvulsive therapy, II: effects of pretreatment regimens on catecholamines, ACTH, vasopressin, and cortisol. Anesth Analg 73: 563, 1991b.

Weiss DM: Changes in blood pressure with electroshock therapy in a patient receiving chlorpromazine hydrochloride (Thorazine). Am J Psychiatry 111: 617, 1955.

Wells DG et al.: Attenuation of electroconvulsive therapy induced hypertension with sublingual nifedipine. Anaesth Intensive Care 17: 31, 1989.

Zink M et al.: Electroconvulsive therapy in a patient receiving rivastigmine. J ECT 18(3): 162–164, 2002.

Drug Interactions of Importance in Substance Abuse

CLIFFORD M. KNAPP

TABLE A1.1. BUPRENORPHINE DRUG INTERACTIONS

Anticonvulsants (carbamazepine, phenytoin, phenobarbital)	These anticonvulsant agents may increase the activity of the CYP3A4 enzyme, potentially leading to an increase in the metabolism of buprenorphine.
Antiretrovirals (indinavir, ritonavir, saquinavir)	These retroviral agents may reduce buprenorphine metabolism by inhibiting the activity of the CYP3A4 enzyme.
Azole antifungal agents (fluconazole, itraconazole, ketoconazole, voriconazole)	Ketoconazole and other azole antifungal agents that inhibit CYP3A4 activity may decrease buprenorphine metabolism.
Barbiturate anesthetics (methohexital, thiopental)	Additive CNS and respiratory depressant effects may occur when barbiturates are co-administered with buprenorphine.
Benzodiazepines	Additive CNS and respiratory depressant effects leading to coma and death may occur when benzodiazepines are administered in combination with buprenorphine. The risk of these effects occurring is greatly increased when these agents are intravenously injected.
CNS depressants (alcohol, antihistamine, phenothiazine)	Buprenorphine may enhance sedation and related effects produced by other CNS depressant agents.
Macrolide antibiotics (erythromycin)	Macrolide antibiotics, such as erythromycin, that inhibit the activity of the CYP3A4 enzyme may reduce the metabolism of buprenorphine.

(continued)

TABLE A1.1. BUPRENORPHINE DRUG INTERACTIONS (CONTINUED)

Monoamine oxidase inhibitors	MAO inhibitors may potentiate the CNS depressant effects of buprenorphine.
Opioid antagonists (nalmefene, naloxone, naltrexone)	Opioid antagonists may block the actions of buprenorphine.
Rifamycins (rifampin, rifabutin, rifapentine)	Rifamycins may reduce buprenorphine plasma concentrations by increasing the rate of its metabolism. Buprenorphine patients should be monitored for signs of withdrawal when started on a rifamycin.

TABLE A1.2. METHADONE DRUG INTERACTIONS

Anticonvulsants (carbamazepine, fosphenytoin, mephenytoin phenobarbital, phenytoin, primidone)	These agents may enhance the metabolism of methadone, leading to a reduction in levels of this opioid. Methadone patients started on these anticonvulsant agents should be monitored for signs of opioid withdrawal, and their methadone dose may need to be increased.
Antiretrovirals (amprenavir, delavirdine efavirenz, nelfinavir, nevirapine, ritonavir)	These agents may reduce methadone plasma concentrations by increasing the rate of methadone metabolism. Methadone patients should be monitored for signs of opioid withdrawal when started on these antiretrovirals.
Azole antifungal agents (fluconazole, itraconazole, ketoconazole, voriconazole)	Azole antifungal agents that inhibit the CYP3A4 enzyme activity may produce increases in methadone plasma concentrations. This may lead to respiratory depression.
Barbiturates (butalbital, methohexital, mephobarbital, pentobarbital, phenobarbital, thiamylal, thiopental)	Additive CNS and respiratory depressant effects when barbiturate anesthetic agents are co-administered with methadone. Chronic administration of barbiturates, on the other hand, may lead to an increase in the metabolism of methadone.
Cimetidine	Cimetidine may decrease methadone metabolism. This interaction has resulted in respiratory depression and fatalities in some cases.
Opioid antagonists (nalmefene, naloxone, naltrexone)	The administration of opioid antagonists may block the actions of methadone. This may result in severe withdrawal in opioid-dependent individuals.

(continued)

TABLE A1.2.   METHADONE DRUG INTERACTIONS (CONTINUED)

Desipramine	Concurrent administration of methadone and desipramine may lead to an increase in desipramine plasma concentrations.
Quinolones (ciprofloxacin, enoxacin, norfloxacin)	The administration of ciprofloxacin and other quinolones may increase methadone plasma levels by inhibiting its metabolism. This may occur through inhibition of the CYP3A4 and CYP1A2 enzymes.
Rifamycins (rifampin, rifabutin, rifapentine)	Methadone patients may exhibit signs of withdrawal when treated with rifamycins. This may result from the induction of methadone metabolism by this class of medications.
Somatostatin	Somatostatin may decrease the analgesic effects of methadone.
SSRIs (fluvoxamine, fluoxetine, paroxetine)	Plasma concentrations of methadone may be increased by the administration of these agents.
St. John's wort	Withdrawal symptoms may occur in methadone patients treated with St. John's wort as a result of induction of CYP3A4 activity or altered P-glycoprotein transport.
Urinary acidifiers (ammonium chloride, potassium acid phosphate)	Agents that decrease the urine pH level below 6 may promote the renal excretion of methadone.
Zidovudine	Methadone may increase the plasma concentrations of zidovudine by delaying its excretion.

TABLE A1.3.   NALTREXONE DRUG INTERACTIONS

Opioid agonists	Naltrexone will block the actions of opioid agonists.
Acamprosate	Acamprosate levels are increased when administered with naltrexone. The clinical implications are not known.
Thioridazine	Concurrent use of naltrexone and thioridazine may produce lethargy and somnolence.

TABLE A1.4. ETHANOL DRUG INTERACTIONS

Acetaminophen	Chronic excessive alcohol consumption increases susceptibility to acetaminophen-induced hepatotoxicity. Acute intoxication theoretically protects against acetaminophen toxicity because less hepatotoxic metabolite is generated.
Anticoagulants (oral)	Chronic ethanol consumption induces hepatic metabolism of warfarin, decreasing hypoprothrombinemic effect. Very large acute ethanol doses (more than 3 drinks/day) may impair the metabolism of warfarin and increase hypothrombinemic effect. Vitamin K–dependent clotting factors may be reduced in alcoholics with liver disease, also affecting coagulation.
Antidepressants (See Chapter 2)	Enhanced sedative effects of alcohol and psychomotor impairment are possible. Acute ethanol impairs metabolism. Fluoxetine, paroxetine, fluvoxamine, and probably other SSRIs do not interfere with psychomotor or subjective effects of ethanol.
Antipyrine	Chronic ethanol consumption (>1 ml/kg/day) enhances antipyrine metabolism.
Ascorbic acid	Ascorbic acid increases ethanol clearance and serum triglyceride levels and improves motor coordination and color discrimination after ethanol consumption.
Barbiturates	Phenobarbital decreases blood ethanol concentration; acute intoxication inhibits pentobarbital metabolism; chronic intoxication enhances hepatic pentobarbital metabolism. Combined central nervous system depression.
Benzodiazepines	Psychomotor impairment increased with the combination.
Bromocriptine	Ethanol increases gastrointestinal side effects of bromocriptine.
Caffeine	Caffeine has no effect on ethanol-induced psychomotor impairment.
Calcium channel blockers	Verapamil (Calan) inhibits ethanol metabolism and increases intoxication.
Cephalosporin antibiotics	Ethanol produces flushing, nausea, headaches, tachycardia, and hypotension. Cephalosporin antibiotics that have a methyltetrazolethiol side chain produce this disulfiramlike reaction (e.g.,

(continued)

TABLE A1.4.   ETHANOL DRUG INTERACTIONS (CONTINUED)

	cefoperazone [Cefobid], cefamandole [Mandol], cefotetan [Cefotan], and moxalactam).
Chloral hydrate	Elevation of plasma trichloroethanol (a chloral hydrate metabolite) and blood ethanol. Combined central nervous system depression. Vasodilation, tachycardia, headache.
Chloroform	Ethanol increases chloroform hepatotoxicity.
Doxycycline	Chronic consumption of ethanol induces hepatic metabolism of doxycycline and may lower serum concentration of the antibiotic.
Erythromycin	Ethanol may interfere with absorption of the ethylsuccinate salt. Effects on other formulations are unknown.
Furazolidone (Furoxone)	When ethanol is ingested, nausea, flushing, lightheadedness, and dyspnea may occur (i.e., a disulfiramlike reaction).
Glutethimide	Blood ethanol concentration increases while plasma glutethimide concentration decreases.
H^2–Antagonists	Cimetidine (Tagamet) potentiates ethanol effects. Increases peak plasma ethanol concentrations and area under the plasma ethanol concentration time curve. Central nervous system toxicity from increased cimetidine serum concentration. Nizatidine (Axid), and ranitidine (Zantac) may also increase blood alcohol levels slightly by inhibiting gastric alcohol dehydrogenase. Famotidine (Pepcid) does not affect blood alcohol levels.
Isoniazid (INH)	Consumption of ethanol with INH increases risk of hepatotoxicity. Tyramine containing alcoholic beverages may cause hypertensive reaction.
Ketoconazole (Nizoral) and metronidazole (Flagyl)	When ethanol is ingested, nausea, flushing, lightheadedness, and dyspnea may occur (i.e., a disulfiramlike reaction may occur with metronidazole). A sunburnlike rash has been reported with ethanol consumption and ketoconazole. A similar reaction may occur with itraconazole (Sporanox), although no reports exist.
Meprobamate	Synergistic central nervous system depression.
Metoclopramide (Reglan)	Enhances sedative effects of ethanol.

(continued)

**TABLE A1.4. ETHANOL DRUG
INTERACTIONS (CONTINUED)**

Milk	Reduces ethanol absorption by delaying gastric emptying.
Monoamine oxidase inhibitors	Tyramine-containing alcoholic beverages may cause a hypertensive crisis. Pargyline may inhibit aldehyde dehydrogenase and cause a disulfiramlike interaction with ethanol.
Narcotic analgesics	Volume of distribution of intravenous meperidine increases with increasing ethanol consumption. Clinical significance unknown. Potential for enhanced CNS depression.
Oral hypoglycemic agents	Chlorpropamide (Diabinese) tolbutamide and tolazamide may cause flushing, lightheadedness, nausea, and dyspnea if alcohol is ingested (i.e., a disulfiramlike reaction).
Paraldehyde	Possible metabolic acidosis.
Phenothiazines	Potentiates psychomotor effects of ethanol.
Phenytoin	Chronic ethanol ingestion induces phenytoin metabolism.
Quinacrine	Possibly inhibits acetaldehyde oxidation.
Salicylates	Increases gastric bleeding associated with aspirin; may increase chance of gastrointestinal hemorrhage.
Tetrachloroethylene	Combined central nervous system depression.
Trichloroethylene	Flushing, lacrimation, blurred vision, tachypnea may occur when patients exposed to trichloroethylene drink alcohol.

B

Interactions of Psychotropics with Herbals*

ANN MARIE CIRAULO
DOMENIC A. CIRAULO

Herbals & Supplements	Herbal Use	Interacting Drugs	Clinical Implications
Belladonna	Irritable bowel, premenstrual symptoms	Anticholinergics	Potentiation of anticholinergic effects.
Betel palm	Mild stimulant	Anticholinergic anti-Parkinson agents: Cogentin, Artane, and Akineton	Arecoline is an active component of betel palm. Its cholinergic actions may reverse the effect of anticholinergic antiparkinson agents. Onset of extrapyramidal symptoms has been reported.
Black cohosh	PMS, menopausal symptoms		May contain estrogen and have interactions similar to that hormone. Also lowers blood pressure and could interact with psychotropics that affect blood pressure.
Brewer's yeast	Irritable bowel, diarrhea, gastritis	MAOIs	Concomitant use may result in severe hypertension.

(continued)

Herbals & Supplements	Herbal Use	Interacting Drugs	Clinical Implications
Broom	Smoked to induce relaxation and euphoria, orally as diuretic, antiarrhythmic, emetic	TCAs	Broom contains sparteine, which is a type 1A antiarrhythmic and may have additive conduction effects with TCAs.
Bupleurum	Fever, hepatitis	Benzodiazepines and other sedative hypnotics	Additive CNS depression with benzodiazepines and other sedative hypnotics.
Butcher's broom	Arthritis, edema, varicose veins, peripheral vascular disease	MAOIs	Hypertensive crisis possible with MAOIs.
Caffeine	Stimulant	Clozapine	Clozapine plasma levels may increase in the presence of caffeine. Alterations in clinical and adverse effects have been reported. Caffeine doses of 400–1000 mg/qd were reported to interact. Inhibition of 1A2 by caffeine is suspected.
		Lithium	Caffeine may promote renal excretion of lithium, and increased plasma lithium levels have been reported in patients who abruptly discontinue caffeine intake.
Cat's claw	Joint pain, inflammation, viral infections, diarrhea	Agents metabolized by 3A4	Cat's claw inhibits 3A4.
Chamomile	Insomnia, anxiety	CNS depressants	Additive sedation.
Chaparral	Bronchitis, fever, diabetes, cancer	Drugs with hepatic toxicity	Chaparral is associated with

(continued)

Herbals & Supplements	Herbal Use	Interacting Drugs	Clinical Implications
			hepatic and renal toxicity. Its use should be avoided in patients taking medications that are associated with hepatotoxicity.
Chaste tree	Premenstrual symptoms	Drugs that act on dopamine	Chaste tree enhances dopamine activity and has the potential to interact with antipsychotics and antiparkinson drugs.
Chromium	Diabetes, elevated cholesterol, depression	Antidepressants	Chromium may potentiate antidepressant response.
Clary	Anxiety, depression	ETOH and other CNS depressants	Clary has an additive sedative effect with alcohol and sedative-hypnotics.
Coenzyme Q10	Heart failure, angina, high blood pressure, Alzheimer disease	Antidepressants	Antidepressants lower coenzyme Q10 levels. Clinical importance not known.
Corkwood	Stimulant, antispasmodic, nausea	TCAs and other anticholinergics	Contains scopolamine.
Cowslip	Anxiety, restlessness	Sedatives	Additive sedation.
Dandelion	Laxative, diuretic	Lithium	Lithium toxicity possible.
Devil's claw	Appetite enhancement, antiinflammatory	Drugs metabolized by 2C8/9/19 and 3A4	Moderate inhibition of 2C8/9/19 and 3A4; low inhibition of IA2 and 2D6.
DHEA	Depression, memory disorders	Androgen/ estrogen hormones	May complicate hormone therapy.
Echinacea	Immune stimulant, prophylaxis against cold, flu	Drugs metabolized by 3A4	May increase hepatic 3A4 activity. However may inhibit intestinal 3A4 metabolism; effects may offset each other.

(continued)

Herbals & Supplements	Herbal Use	Interacting Drugs	Clinical Implications
Ephedra	Stimulant	MAOIs, TCAs	Hypertensive crisis.
		Phenothiazines (Thorazine, Stelazine, etc.)	Tachycardia.
Eucalyptus oil	Decongestant, antimicrobial	Sedatives	Additive sedative effect. 3A4 inhibition.
Feverfew	Migraine prevention	Drugs metabolized by 1A2 and 2C9	Inhibits 1A2 and 2C9. Moderate inhibition of 2C8/19/3A4. Low inhibition of 2D6.
Galanthamine	Alzheimer disease	MAOIs, depolarizing muscle relaxants	Acetylcholinesterase inhibitor.
Ginkgo	Memory, depression, impotence caused by SSRIs	Alprazolam	Slight decrease in alprazolam AUC; no effect on $t_{1/2}$.
		Trazodone	A single case report of increased risk of sedation with the continuation.
		Haloperidol	Increased antipsychotic effectiveness and decreased EPS, although improvement on combination was slight and of limited clinical importance.
Ginseng	Stimulant	MAOIs	CNS effects may be increased (e.g., maniclike symptoms, headache, insomnia, tremulousness), (Phenelzine) incident of manic episode.
Grapefruit juice		Clomipramine	Possible improvement of OCD symptoms when co-administered. A reduction of desmethyl-clomipramine

(continued)

Herbals & Supplements	Herbal Use	Interacting Drugs	Clinical Implications
			concentrations occurs and an increase in clomipramine levels. Grapefruit juice may inhibit intestinal CYP3A3/4 and subsequently the demethylation of clomipramine.
		Fluvoxamine	The pharmacologic and adverse effects of the drug may be elevated due to increased fluvoxamine plasma concentrations. The mechanism may be either the inhibition of fluvoxamine metabolism or the alteration of P-glycoprotein–mediated transport by the grapefruit juice.
		Methadone	Inhibition of gut 3A4 may increase methadone plasma levels.
		Buspirone	Elevates plasma levels, increasing pharmacologic effects and adverse effects.
		Carbamazepine	Increases plasma levels and bioavailability.
		Midazolam	Delayed onset and increase in pharmacologic effects.
		Triazolam	Delayed onset and increase in pharmacologic action.
Herbal diuretics (goldenrod,		Lithium	Potential for reduced excretion of lithium,

(continued)

Herbals & Supplements	Herbal Use	Interacting Drugs	Clinical Implications
Equisetum hyemale, *Uva ursi*, *Ovate buchu*, corn silk, juniper bromelain)			but data are limited. Lithium case report with Eskalith, increased risk of lithium toxicity.
High fiber diet		TCAs	Several case reports indicate that TCA-treated patients experienced diminished therapeutic effect when they added high amounts of fiber to their diet.
Hops	Hypnotic, sedative depression	ETOH, sedative hypnotics, antidepressants, carbamazepine	Additive sedation, cytochrome induction.
Horehound	Digestive aid, expectorant	SSRIs	Serotonergic effects enhanced.
Jamaican dogwood	Asthma, insomnia	Sedatives	Enhanced effect of sedatives.
		Opioids	Enhanced effect of opioids.
Jimsonweed (illegal in the United States)	Hallucinogen	L-Dopa	Interaction may decrease gastric absorption
		Phenothiazines TCAs	Anticholinergic properties potentiated.
Kava	Anxiety, depression, psychosis	Benzodiazepines	CNS effects may be increased. Broad inhibition of cytochromes IA2, 2C9/19, 2C8, 2D6, 3A4.
Khat	Depression, fatigue	MAOIs	Hypertension; additive psychostimulant effects.
Lavender	Insomnia, restlessness, nervousness	Benzodiazepines	Enhanced effect.
		Opioids	Enhanced effect.

(continued)

Herbals & Supplements	Herbal Use	Interacting Drugs	Clinical Implications
Melatonin	Sleep aid	Fluvoxamine	Elevated melatonin plasma levels, possibly through the inhibition of melatonin metabolism by fluvoxamine. Increased effects of melatonin, such as drowsiness, may occur.
Mistletoe	Depression, anxiety	MAOIs	Elevated blood pressure.
New Zealand prickly spinach		MAOIs	Elevated blood pressure, possibly due to a tyraminelike reaction.
Nutmeg	Anxiety, depression	Antipsychotics	Potential for CNS toxicity, increase in psychotic symptoms.
Parsley	Asthma, cough, hypertension	Antidepressants, Opioids	Serotonin syndrome is possible.
		Lithium	Lithium toxicity is possible.
Passionflower	Sedative	Sedative hypnotics, seizure medications	Additive sedation.
		Opioids	May decrease opioid withdrawal symptoms.
		Seizure medications	
		MAOIs	Potentiation of MAO inhibitors.
Peppermint oil	Antispasmodic, irritable bowel syndrome		Moderate inhibition of most cytochromes, but not 3A4.
Plantain	As a bulk forming laxative, mucilloid	Lithium	Decreased absorption of lithium from GI tract with decreased plasma concentration, decreased efficacy of lithium.

(continued)

Herbals & Supplements	Herbal Use	Interacting Drugs	Clinical Implications
Primrose (evening)	Anxiety, pain, PMS	Phenothiazines	Evening primrose oil lowers seizure threshold when used with some antipsychotics.
Rauwolfia	Hypertension, anxiety, insomnia	TCAs	Alterations in blood pressure.
		L-Dopa	L-Dopa effects antagonized.
		MAOIs	Excitement, hypertension.
Red clover	Menopause, elevated cholesterol, diabetes		Moderate inhibition of many cytochromes.
St. John's wort	Anxiety, depression mild to moderate, insomnia	Drugs metabolized by 1A2, 2C9, 3A4	St. John's wort induces 1A2, 2C9, 3A4. Also induces P-glycoprotein transporter.
		SSRIs	Serotonin syndrome may occur. Symptoms are CNS irritability, shivering, myoclonus, altered consciousness.
		TCAs	TCA plasma concentrations and metabolites may be reduced.
		Alprazolam	Induction of CYP3A4 decreases the AUC of alprazolam twofold and increases clearance twofold.
		Methadone	The actions of methadone may be decreased, causing withdrawal symptoms for those patients in methadone maintenance or receiving chronic methadone

(continued)

Herbals & Supplements	Herbal Use	Interacting Drugs	Clinical Implications
			treatment. The documentation is from noncontrolled trials.
		Midazolam	Reduction in plasma levels of midazolam, decreasing pharmacologic effects via induction of enzymes (CYP3A4).
		Nefazodone	Serotonin syndrome, CNS irritability, shivering, myoclonus, altered conscious may occur. Additive serotonin reuptake inhibition is suspected. 3A4 metabolism of nefazodone is increased.
Valerian	Anxiety	Sedative hypnotics	Excessive sedation.
		MAOIs	Reversal of antidepressant activity.
		Phenytoin	Antagonism of anticonvulsant activity.

*The reader is cautioned that drug–herbal interactions are not adequately studied. Some of the listed interactions are based on clinical reports or assumptions of mechanisms of action. The term "herbal use" does not indicate established efficacy.

Suggested Readings and Internet Resources

Abebe W: Herbal medication: potential for adverse interactions with analgesic drugs. J Clin Pharm Thera 27: 391–401, 2002.

Basch E et al.: *Natural Standard Herb & Supplement Handbook: The Clinical Bottom Line*. St. Louis, Missouri, Elsevier Mosby, 2005.

Comfort A: Hypertensive reaction to New Zealand prickly spinach in woman taking phenelzine. Lancet 2: 472, 1981.

Cupp MJ: Herbal remedies: adverse effects and drug interactions. Am Fam Phys 59(5): 1239–1245, 1999.

Davidson JR et al.: Effectiveness of chromium in atypical depression: a placebo-controlled trial. Biol Psychiatry 53: 261–264, 2003.

Deahl M: Betel nut-induced extrapyramidal syndrome: an unusual drug interaction. Mov Disord 4: 330–332, 1989.

Desai AK et al.: Herbals and botanicals in geriatric psychiatry. Am J Geriatr Psychiatry 11(5): 498–506, 2003.

Dresser GK et al.: St. John's Wort induces intestinal and hepatic CYP3A4 and P-glycoprotein in healthy volunteers. Clin Pharmacol Ther 69: 23, 2001.

Drug Interactions Facts: Herbal Supplements and Food. St. Louis, Missouri, Wolters Kluwer Health, Inc, 2004.

Drugfacts.com. www.factsandcomparisons.com.

Eich-Hochi D et al.: Methadone maintenance treatment and St. John's wort—a case report. Pharmacopsychiatry 36: 35–37, 2003.

Ernst E: The risk-benefit profile of commonly used herbal therapies: gingko, St. John's wort, ginseng, echinacea, saw palmetto, and kava. Ann Intern Med 136: 42–53, 2002.

Facciolá G et al.: Cytochrome P450 isoforms involved in melatonin metabolism in human liver microsomes. Eur J Clin Pharmacol 56: 881–888, 2001.

FDA Center for Food Safety and Applied Nutrition. www.cfsan.fda.gov.

Gordon JB: SSRIs and St. John's wort: possible toxicity? Am Fam Physician 57(5): 950–953, 1998.

Greenblatt DJ: Interaction of warfarin with drugs, natural substances, and foods. J Clin Pharmacol 45(2):127–132, 2005.

Härtter S et al.: Differential effects of fluvoxamine and other antidepressants on the biotransformation of melatonin. J Clin Psychopharmacol 21: 167–174, 2001.

Härtter S et al.: Increased bioavailability of oral melatonin after fluvoxamine coadministration. Clin Pharmacol Ther 67: 1–6, 2000.

HerbMed: www.herbmed.org.

Hori H et al.: Grapefruit juice-fluvoxamine interaction—is it risky or not? J Clin Psychopharmacol 23: 422–424, 2003.

Johne A et al.: Decreased plasma levels of amitriptyline and its metabolites on comedication with an extract from St. John's wort (*Hypericum perforatum*). J Clin Psychopharmacol 22(1): 46–54, 2002.

Jones BD et al.: Interaction of ginseng with phenelzine. J Clin Psychopharmacol 7: 201–202, 1987.

Lantz MS et al.: St. John's wort and antidepressant drug interactions in the elderly. J Geriatr Psychiatry Neurol 12(1): 7–10, 1999.

Laplaud PM et al.: Antioxidant action of *Vaccinum myrtillus* extract on human low density lipoproteins in vitro: Initial observations. Fund Clin Pharmacol 11: 35–40, 1997.

McLeod MN et al.: Chromium potentiation of antidepressant pharmacotherapy for dysthymic disorder in 5 patients. J Clin Psychiatry 60(4): 237–240, 1999.

Miller LG: Herbal medicinals: selected clinical considerations focusing on known or potential drug-herb interactions. Arch Intern Med 158: 2200–2211, 1998.

Miyazawa M et al.: Roles of human CYP2A6 and 2B6 and rat CYP2C11 and 2B1 in the 10-hydroxylation of (-)-verbenone by liver microsomes. Drug Metabol Dispos 31: 1049–1053, 2003.

Morazzoni P et al.: Effects of *V. myrtillis* anthocynosides on prostacyclin-like activity in rat arterial tissue. Fitoterapia 57: 11–14, 1986.

National Center for Complementary and Alternative Medicine: www.nccam.nih.gov.

Oesterheld J et al.: Grapefruit juice and clomipramine: shifting metabolic ratios. J Clin Psychopharmacol 17: 62–63, 1997.

Office of Dietary Supplements. www.ods.od.nih.gov.

Perloff MD et al.: Rapid assessment of P-glycoprotein inhibition and induction in vitro. Pharm Res 20(8): 1177–1183, 2003.

Perloff MD et al.: St. John's wort: an in vitro analysis of P-glycoprotein induction due to extended exposure. Br J Pharmacol 134(8): 1601–1608, 2001.

Physician's Desk Reference for Herbal Medicines, 3rd ed. Montvale, NJ, Thomson PDR, 2004.

Shader RI et al.: More on oral contraceptives, drug interactions, herbal medicines, and hormone replacement therapy. J Clin Psychopharmacol 20(4): 397–398, 2000.

Shader RI et al.: Phenelzine and the dream machine—ramblings and reflections. J Clin Psychopharmacol 5: 65, 1985.

Skidmore-Roth L: *Mosby's Handbook of Herbs and Natural Supplements*. St. Louis, Missouri, Mosby, Inc. 2004.

Stewart DE: High-fiber diet and serum tricyclic antidepressant levels. J Clin Psychopharmacol 12(6): 438–440, 1992.

Unger M et al.: Simultaneous determination of the inhibitory potency of herbal extracts on the activity of six major cytochrome P450 enzymes using liquid chromatography/mass spectrometry and automated online extraction. Rapid Comm Mass Spectrom 18: 2273–2281, 2004.

Wang Z et al.: The effects of St. John's wort (Hypericum perforatum) on human cytochrome P450 activity. Clin Pharmacol Ther 70: 317–326, 2001.

C

Drugs (Including Metabolites) That Are Substrates of Cytochrome P450

DOMENIC A. CIRAULO
DAVID J. GREENBLATT
RICHARD I. SHADER

TABLE A3.1.

Drugs Metabolized by 3A4

Antianxiety (non-benzodiazepine)
  Buspirone

Antiarrhythmic Agents
  Amiodarone (Cordarone®)
  Lidocaine (also 2C19 and 2D6)
  Quinidine
  Propafenone (Rythmol®) (see 2D6)
  Disopyramide (Norpace®)

Antidepressants
  Nefazodone
  Trazodone
  Amitriptyline
  Imipramine
  Clomipramine
  Trimipramine
  Doxepin
  Mirtazapine

Antihistamines
  Terfenadine (Seldane®) (no longer marketed in the U.S.)
  Astemizole (Hismanal®) (no longer marketed in the U.S.)
  Loratadine (Claritin®)
  Chlorpheniramine

(continued)

TABLE A3.1. (CONTINUED)

Antimicrobial Agents
Erythromycin
Clarithromycin (Biaxin®)
Troleandomycin (Tao®)
Dapsone

Antineoplastic
Paclitaxel (Taxol®)

Antipsychotics
Aripiprazole
Haloperidol

Antiulcer (proton pump inhibiting) Agents
Omeprazole (Prilosec®) (also possibly 2C)

Benzodiazepines
Alprazolam (Xanax®)
Triazolam
Midazolam
Diazepam

Calcium Channel Blockers
Diltiazem (Cardizem®)
Verapamil (Calan ®) (also 1A2)
Nifedipine (Procardia®)
And others

HIV Agents
Ritonavir
Indinavir
Saquinavir
Nelfinavir

Hormones/Steroids
Tamoxifen (Nolvadex®)
Testosterone
Cortisol
Progesterone
Ethinyl Estradiol

Hypnotics
Zolpidem (and others)
Zaleplon

Immunosuppressant Agents
Cyclosporine (Sandimmune®)
Tacrolimus (Prograf®)

Opioid Analgesics
Alfentanil (Alfenta®)
Codeine (mainly 2D6)
Dextromethorphan (also 2D6)

(continued)

TABLE A3.1. (CONTINUED)

Statins
Atorvastatin
Lovastatin
Cerivastatin (Rosuvastatin, Simvastatin, and Pravastatin not 3A4)

Drugs Metabolized by the CYP 2C
S-Mephenytoin (Mesantoin®) (2C19)
Phenytoin (Dilantin®) (2C9)
Tolbutamide (2C9)
S-Warfarin (Coumadin®) (2C9)
Ibuprofen (2C9)
Diclofenac (Voltaren®)
Naproxen (2C9)

Antidepressants
Amitriptyline
Imipramine
Clomipramine
Trimipramine
Doxepin

Antipsychotics
Clozapine
Olanzapine

Drugs Metabolized by CYP 1A2
Caffeine (also 2E1 and 3A4)
Theophylline
Aminophylline

Antidepressants
Amitriptyline
Imipramine
Trimipramine
Doxepin
Mirtazapine
Maprotiline

Antipsychotics
Risperidone
Haloperidol
Perphenazine
Thioridazine
Aripiprazole
Chlorpromazine

Drugs Metabolized by CYP 2D6
Propranolol (Inderal®) (and possibly 2C19)
Metoprolol
Timolol

(continued)

TABLE A3.1.   (CONTINUED)

Mexiletine (Mexitil®)
Propafenone (Rythmol®) (also CYP and CYP 1A2)
Codeine (also CYP 3A4)
Dextromethorphan (also CYP 3A4)

Antidepressants
  Amitriptyline
  Imipramine
  Clomipramine
  Trimipramine
  Nortriptyline
  Desipramine
  Protriptyline
  Mirtazapine
  Bupropion (mainly 2B6)
  Venlafaxine

TABLE A3.2.   COMMON ENZYME INHIBITORS

ANTIDEPRESSANTS: Fluvoxamine (1A2, 2C9/19, 3A4, 2D6); Fluoxetine (2C9/19, 2D6), Tranylcypromine (2C19), Nefazodone (3A3/4, 2D6), Paroxetine (2D6, 3A4), Sertraline (3A4), Venlafaxine (2D6), Bupropion (2D6), Duloxetine (2D6)

ANTIBIOTICS: Erythromycin (3A4, 1A2,), Clarithromycin (3A4), Ciprofloxacin (3A4, 1A2), Norfloxacin (3A4, 1A2), Troleandomycin (3A4), Sulfonamides (2C9), Doxorubicin (2D6)

PROTEASE INHIBITORS: Ritonavir (2D6, 3A4), Indinavir (3A4), Lopinavir (3A4), Nelfinavir (2D6, 3A4), Amprenavir (3A4), Saquinavir (3A4)

NON-NUCLEOSIDE REVERSE TRANSCRIPTASE INHIBITORS: Delavirdine (3A4), Efavirenz (3A4, 2C9/19)

ANTIFUNGALS: Ketoconazole (2A6, 2C9/19), Itraconazole (3A4), Fluconazole (3A4), Metronidazole (2C9)

CALCIUM CHANNEL BLOCKERS: Diltiazem (3A4), Verapamil (3A4)

BETA BLOCKERS: Propranolol (2D6), Labetalol (2D6), Pindolol (2D6)

ANTICONVULSANTS: Felbamate (2C19)

H2 ANTAGONISTS: Cimetidine (1A2, 2C8-10, 2C18, 2D6, 3A3/4), Ranitidine (2D6, 3A4, clinical effects weak)

PROTON PUMP INHIBITORS: Omeprazole (2C8, 2C19)

TABLE A3.3.   COMMON ENZYME INDUCERS

ANTIDEPRESSANTS: St. John's Wort (3A4, 1A2, 2C9)

STIMULANTS: Modafinil (1A2, 3A4)

PROTEASE INHIBITORS: Efavirenz (3A4), Nevirapine (3A4)

ANTICONVULSANTS: Phenobarbital (1A2, 2B6, 2C8, 3A4), Primidone (1A2, 2B6, 2C8, 3A4), Phenytoin (2B6, 2C9, 3A4), Carbamazepine (2C9,3A4)

PROTON PUMP INHIBITORS: Omeprazole (1A2)

ANTITUBERCULARS: Rifampin (1A2, 2C9/19, 3A4)

GLUCOCORTICOIDS: Dexamethasone (3A4, 2D6), Prednisone (3A4)

Index

Page numbers followed by *f* denote figures; those
followed by *t* denote tables.